RELIABLE DESIGN OF
MEDICAL DEVICES

SECOND EDITION

RELIABLE DESIGN OF MEDICAL DEVICES

SECOND EDITION

RICHARD FRIES

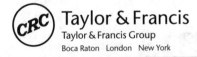

Taylor & Francis
Taylor & Francis Group
Boca Raton   London   New York

A CRC title, part of the Taylor & Francis imprint, a member of the
Taylor & Francis Group, the academic division of T&F Informa plc.

Published in 2006 by
CRC Press
Taylor & Francis Group
6000 Broken Sound Parkway NW, Suite 300
Boca Raton, FL 33487-2742

International Standard Book Number-10: 0-8247-2375-9 (Hardcover)
International Standard Book Number-13: 978-0-8247-2375-0 (Hardcover)
Library of Congress Card Number 2005043942

Library of Congress Cataloging-in-Publication Data

Fries, Richard C.
    Reliable design of medical devices / Richard C. Fries.--2nd ed.
        p. cm.
    Includes bibliographical references and index.
    ISBN 0-8247-2375-9
    1. Medical instruments and apparatus--Reliability. 2. Medical instruments and apparatus--Design and construction. 3. Medical instruments and apparatus--Quality control. 4. Medical instruments and apparatus--Standards. I. Title.

R856.6.F749 2005
681'.761--dc22

                                                2005043942

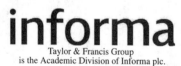

Preface

The design and functional complexity of medical devices have increased during the past 50 years, evolving from the use of a metronome circuit for the initial cardiac pacemaker to functions that include medical book-keeping, electro-cardiogram analysis, delivery of anesthesia, laser surgery, magnetic resonance imaging, and intravenous delivery systems that adjust dosages based on patient feedback. As device functionality becomes more intricate, concerns arise regarding efficacy, safety, and reliability. Both the user and the patient want the device to operate as specified, perform in a safe manner, and continue to perform over a long period of time without failure. To be successful, the designer and manufacturer of medical devices must ensure that all devices meet these requirements.

In almost every major medical system developed or acquired by commercial or governmental organizations, software or firmware plays a major part and has become an increasing management concern. In many cases it takes too long to develop, causing the entire system to slip its schedule, and commensurately raising development costs. When delivered, it may not perform as expected. Requirements that were to be implemented in software have had to be scaled down to achieve a reasonable delivery schedule, or the software is shipped with known bugs. As a result, major management attention has been focused on the productivity of software development, the costs associated with its development, and the resultant quality of the delivered product.

Software productivity, or the rate at which software can be delivered, is limited by current development practice. Software scientists generally believe that software productivity will not dramatically improve without major technological breakthroughs creating more automated programming techniques. Many scientists believe, however, that the rigorous employment of modern disciplined software engineering practice can achieve significant software quality improvement over current practice without a corresponding increase in cost. By concentrating on engineering practices to achieve software quality and reliability, concomitant improvements in the overall reliability of the device will also be obtained.

Medical device development is therefore a complex process that requires the careful integration of diverse disciplines, technical activities, standards, regulatory requirements, and administrative project controls. The need for systematic approaches to product development and maintenance is necessary to ensure a safe and effective device for the user and patient, an economical and competitive success for the manufacturer, and a reliable, cost-effective investment for the user.

Reliability engineering provides the theoretical and practical tools by which the probability and capability of systems and their components to perform required functions can be specified, predicted, designed-in, tested, and demonstrated. It is an integral part of the product development process and of problem solving activities related to manufacturing and field failures. Reliability, however, is more than a science. It is also a philosophy – a way of structuring professional activities so details are planned before action is taken and problems are anticipated so they may be eliminated prior to occurring in the field.

The primary goal of this text is to acquaint the developer of medical devices, as well as the purchaser of medical equipment, with the basic concepts and major issues of medical device reliability, to describe current product development processes and techniques, and to provide a basis for evaluating new technologies. Developers may use this information to improve their own design, validation, and manufacturing processes. Purchasers may use this information to ask more pertinent questions and make a more educated assessment of their suppliers. This text may also be used by non-medical developers and purchasers because the reliability process is relevant to all product development.

The text provides a practical approach to the formation and operation of a reliability assurance program. The emphasis of the book is on the practical, hands-on approach to product development. The mathematics included in the text is that which is necessary to conduct everyday tasks. Equations, where needed, are merely given, not derived. It is assumed the reader has a basic knowledge of statistics. For those wishing to delve deeper into the mathematics of the subject, references are given at the end of each chapter.

The layout of the text follows the typical product development process. Section 1 introduces the reader to the basics of reliability engineering and failures. Failures and reliability are discussed from the hardware, software, and systems levels.

Section 2 deals with myriad device standards and regulations, both domestic and international. Particular emphasis is placed on FDA regulations, the medical device directives, and the quality system regulation.

Section 3 deals with the specification of a medical device. The section covers the definition of a medical device, defining the device and establishing product requirements, safety and risk analysis, liability, and intellectual property.

Section 4 deals with the design of a medical device. The discussion begins with a review of Six Sigma methodology and some of the tools involved, including axiomatic and robust design. The section then addresses both hardware and software design, software coding, the use of metrics, and human factors.

Section 5 discusses verification and validation. The section begins with a review of various types of testing, then discusses in detail hardware and software testing. The section concludes with the analysis of test data that has been accumulated and the calculation of reliability parameters.

Section 6 deals with manufacturing as a continuation of the product development process. A device may be designed reliably, but if it is not manufactured reliably, it will not be a success. Configuration management and its many implications are reviewed. Finally, techniques for the analysis of field data are discussed in relation to building an efficient database for all product development personnel.

Reliability engineering is essential to the success of any medical device company. It helps develop a more profitable product, contributes to a more satisfied customer base, reduces the risk of liability, and builds confidence in meeting requirements of standards and regulatory agencies. Knowledge of reliability engineering is also an asset in evaluating potential vendors of medical devices and addressing device problems. It is hoped this text will assist in establishing and operating a viable reliability engineering program. In addition it is hoped this text will assist the purchaser of medical devices in developing an effective program of vendor evaluation.

I am deeply indebted to many people for their encouragement, help, and constructive criticism in the preparation of this book. I particularly want to thank my wife, June, who constantly encouraged me and who sacrificed much quality time together during the writing of this text.

Richard C. Fries, PE, CRE

Editor

Richard C. Fries holds degrees in biology from Loyola University in Chicago and in electrical/biomedical engineering from Marquette University in Milwaukee. He has nearly 30 years' experience in the health care field, holding positions in reliability engineering, software design, programming, quality assurance, platelet studies, and pharmaceutical research. He is currently the corporate manager of reliability engineering for Baxter Healthcare, in Round Lake, Illinois.

Mr. Fries is a licensed professional engineer in the state of Wisconsin and is certified as a reliability engineer by the American Society for Quality. He is also certified as an ISO 9001 TickIT lead auditor. He is co-inventor of United States Patent 5,682,876.

He is currently a member of the Industrial Advisory Board for the Biomedical Engineering Department and a member of the Advisory Board for the Reliability Engineering Curriculum at Vanderbilt University. He is a project advisor and lecturer for a senior biomedical engineering design course at Vanderbilt. He is a member of the Industrial Advisory Board and a guest lecturer for the Biomedical Engineering Department at Marquette University.

He is past co-chair of the AAMI Medical Device Software Task Force and past chair of the HIMA Software Task Force. He was a member of Working Group 1 to ISO TC210, and is currently a member of the IEEE Software Engineering Standards Subcommittee.

Mr. Fries is the author of several books and numerous articles in professional journals on reliability engineering, medical device design, software quality, standards and regulations.

Table of Contents

Preface v

Section 1
Basics of reliability................................. 1

Chapter 1   Reliability 3

1.1   History of reliability.. 3
1.2   The definition of reliability 4
1.3   Quality versus reliability..................................... 5
1.4   Reliability versus unreliability............................... 6
1.5   Types of reliability 7
      1.5.1   Electronic reliability 7
            1.5.1.1   Infant mortality........................... 7
            1.5.1.2   Useful life 8
            1.5.1.3   Wearout 8
      1.5.2   Mechanical reliability 8
      1.5.3   Software reliability................................... 9
      1.5.4   Device reliability.................................... 10
1.6   Optimizing reliability 12
1.7   Reliability assurance... 12
1.8   Reliability's effect on medical devices 12
      References 13

Chapter 2   The concept of failure................................. 15

2.1   Failure 15
2.2   Causes of failure 16
2.3   The practical aspects of failures............................. 17
2.4   Failure rate 18
2.5   Hardware failures 18
      2.5.1   Early failures 19
      2.5.2   Chance failures 19
      2.5.3   Wearout failures..................................... 19
2.6   Software failures 20
2.7   Failures due to human error................................... 21
2.8   Failures from the customer's point of view.................... 21
      References 22

Section 2
Regulations and standards 23

Chapter 3   The Food and Drug Administration........................ 25

3.1   History of device regulation 26
3.2   Device classification.. 28
    3.2.1   Class I devices... 28
    3.2.2   Class II devices.. 28
    3.2.3   Class III devices 29
3.3   Registration and listing... 30
3.4   The 510(k) process 31
    3.4.1   Determining substantial equivalency 31
    3.4.2   The regular 510(k)...................................... 31
        3.4.2.1   Types of 510(k)s................................. 31
        3.4.2.2   The 510(k) format 33
    3.4.3   The Special 510(k)...................................... 35
        3.4.3.1   Special 510(k) content 38
    3.4.4   The Abbreviated 510(k)................................. 38
        3.4.4.1   Abbreviated 510(k) content 39
3.5   Declaration of conformance to a recognized standard.............. 40
3.6   The PMA application 40
    3.6.1   The PMA process 41
    3.6.2   Contents of a PMAA................................... 41
3.7   Investigational Device Exemptions (IDEs) 42
    3.7.1   Institutional Review Boards (IRBs) 42
    3.7.2   IDE format 43
3.8   Good laboratory practices (GLPs)................................. 44
3.9   Good manufacturing practices (GMPs) 44
3.10 Human factors 44
3.11 Design control 45
3.12 The FDA and software.. 46
3.13 Software classification 47
3.14 The FDA inspection.. 48
3.15 Advice on dealing with the FDA 48
    References 49

Chapter 4   The Medical Devices Directives 53

4.1   Definition of a medical device 54
4.2   The Medical Devices Directives process.......................... 55
4.3   Choosing the appropriate directive................................ 56
    4.3.1   Active Implantable Medical Devices Directive (AIMDD).... 56
    4.3.2   Medical Devices Directive (MDD) 56
    4.3.3   *In Vitro* Diagnostic Medical Devices
        Directive (IVDMDD)................................... 56

4.4   Identifying the applicable essential requirements 56
4.5   Identification of corresponding harmonized standards.............. 58
4.6   Assurance that the device meets the essential requirements and
      harmonized standards and documentation of the evidence......... 59
      4.6.1   Essential requirement 1 59
              4.6.1.1   Hazard analysis.................................. 60
              4.6.1.2   Safety review 61
      4.6.2   Essential requirement 2 62
              4.6.2.1   Peer review 62
              4.6.2.2   Safety review 62
      4.6.3   Essential requirement 3 62
              4.6.3.1   Specification reviews............................ 62
              4.6.3.2   Validation testing............................... 62
      4.6.4   Essential requirement 4 63
              4.6.4.1   Environmental testing............................ 63
              4.6.4.2   Environmental stress screening................... 63
              4.6.4.3   Use/misuse evaluation 64
4.7   Classification of the device 64
4.8   Decision on the appropriate conformity assessment procedure...... 66
      4.8.1   Medical Devices Directive 66
              4.8.1.1   Annex II 66
              4.8.1.2   Annex III 66
              4.8.1.3   Annex IV... 66
              4.8.1.4   Annex V 66
              4.8.1.5   Annex VI... 67
              4.8.1.6   Annex VII.. 67
              4.8.1.7   Class I 67
              4.8.1.8   Class IIa 67
              4.8.1.9   Class IIb 67
              4.8.1.10 Class III.. 67
      4.8.2   Active Implantable Medical Devices Directive.............. 68
              4.8.2.1   Alternative 1.................................... 68
              4.8.2.2   Alternative 2.................................... 68
      4.8.3   *In Vitro* Diagnostic Medical Devices Directive 68
4.9   Type testing.. 68
4.10 Identification and choice of a Notified Body...................... 69
4.11 Establishing a declaration of conformity 72
4.12 Application of the CE mark 73
4.13 Conclusion... 74
      References 74

Chapter 5 Quality system regulation 77

5.1   History of the quality system regulations......................... 78
5.2   Scope 79
5.3   General provisions 79

5.4   Quality system 81
5.5   Design controls 81
5.6   Document controls 83
5.7   Purchasing controls 84
5.8   Identification and traceability 85
5.9   Production and process controls 85
5.10 Acceptance activities 88
5.11 Non-conforming product 89
5.12 Corrective and preventive action 89
5.13 Labeling and packaging controls 90
5.14 Handling, storage, distribution, and installation 91
5.15 Records 92
5.16 Servicing requirements 93
      References 94

Chapter 6   Domestic standards 95

6.1   Domestic standards organizations 95
      6.1.1   AAMI 95
      6.1.2   ANSI 96
      6.1.3   ASQC 96
      6.1.4   ASTM 96
      6.1.5   IEEE 96
      6.1.6   IES 96
      6.1.7   IPC 97
      6.1.8   NEMA 97
      6.1.9   NFPA 97
      6.1.10 OSHA 97
      6.1.11 UL 97
6.2   Software standards and regulations 98
      References 99

Chapter 7   International standards 101

7.1   The international notion of standards 102
7.2   The international regulatory scene 103
      7.2.1   BSI 103
      7.2.2   CEN 103
      7.2.3   CENELAC 103
      7.2.4   CISPR 104
      7.2.5   CSA 104
      7.2.6   DIN 104
      7.2.7   DoH 104
      7.2.8   IEC 105
      7.2.9   IEE 105
      7.2.10 ISO 105
      7.2.11 JSA 105

      7.2.12   Other Japanese standards organizations................... 105
7.3   The TickIT program... 106
7.4   The Software Quality System Registration program 106
7.5   The ISO guidance documents for ISO 9001 and 9002 107
7.6   Proposed regulatory requirements for Canada..................... 108
7.7   ISO 14000 series.. 108
7.8   Medical informatics 110
      References 111

Section 3
Specifying the product............................ 113

Chapter 8   The medical device as an entity 115

8.1   What is a medical device?.. 115
      8.1.1   Food and Drug Administration........................... 116
      8.1.2   The Medical Device Directives........................... 116
8.2   A brief history of medical devices............................... 117
8.3   Current medical devices 117
      References 119

Chapter 9   Defining the device 121

9.1   The product definition process................................... 122
      9.1.1   Surveying the customer 123
      9.1.2   Defining the company's needs............................ 123
      9.1.3   What are the company's competencies?.................... 123
      9.1.4   What are the outside competencies? 124
      9.1.5   Completing the product definition 124
9.2   Overview of quality function deployment 124
9.3   The QFD process 125
      9.3.1   The voice of the customer 125
      9.3.2   The technical portion of the matrix 126
      9.3.3   Overview of the QFD process............................ 127
9.4   Summary of QFD 131
9.5   The business proposal 133
      9.5.1   Project overview, objectives, major milestones,
            and schedule.. 134
      9.5.2   Market need and market potential 134
      9.5.3   Product proposal 135
      9.5.4   Strategic fit... 135
      9.5.5   Risk analysis and research plan 135
      9.5.6   Economic analysis 137
      9.5.7   Core project team 137
      References 138

Chapter 10   Requirements engineering 139

10.1   Requirements, design, verification, and validation 140
        10.1.1   Refinement of requirements 141
        10.1.2   Assimilation of requirements 141
        10.1.3   Requirements versus design 143
10.2   The product specification 144
10.3   The reliability goal 145
10.4   Specification review 147
10.5   The design specification 147
10.6   The software quality assurance plan (SQAP) 148
        10.6.1   Purpose 149
        10.6.2   Reference documents 149
        10.6.3   Management 149
        10.6.4   Documentation 149
        10.6.5   Standards, practices, conventions, and metrics 149
        10.6.6   Review and audits 150
        10.6.7   Test 150
        10.6.8   Problem reporting and corrective action 150
        10.6.9   Tools, techniques, and methodologies 150
        10.6.10 Code control 150
        10.6.11 Media control 150
        10.6.12 Supplier control 150
        10.6.13 Records collection, maintenance, and retention 151
        10.6.14 Training 151
        10.6.15 Risk management 151
        10.6.16 Additional sections as required 151
10.7   Software requirements specification (SRS) 151
        10.7.1   Purpose 151
        10.7.2   Scope 152
        10.7.3   Definitions, acronyms, and abbreviations 152
        10.7.4   References 152
        10.7.5   Overview 152
        10.7.6   Product perspective 152
        10.7.7   Product functions 152
        10.7.8   User characteristics 152
        10.7.9   General constraints 153
        10.7.10 Assumptions and dependencies 153
        10.7.11 Specific requirements 153
10.8   The software design description (SDD) 153
        10.8.1   Decomposition description 154
        10.8.2   Dependency description 154
        10.8.3   Interface description 155
        10.8.4   Detailed design description 155
        References 155

Chapter 11 Safety and risk management 157

11.1   Risk 158
11.2   Deciding on acceptable risk................................... 160
11.3   Factors important to medical device risk assessment 160
        11.3.1 Device design and manufacture 160
        11.3.2 Materials.. 161
        11.3.3 Device users... 161
        11.3.4 Human factors 162
        11.3.5 Medical device systems 162
11.4   Risk management 162
11.5   The risk management process................................... 162
        11.5.1 Identifying the risk factors........................... 164
        11.5.2 Assessing risk probabilities and effects on
                the project 164
        11.5.3 Developing strategies to mitigate identified risks 165
        11.5.4 Monitoring risk factors............................... 165
        11.5.5 Invoking a contingency plan........................... 166
        11.5.6 Managing the crisis................................... 166
        11.5.7 Recovering from the crisis 166
11.6   Tools for risk estimation 166
        11.6.1 Hazard/risk analysis.................................. 166
        11.6.2 Failure mode and effects analysis 169
                11.6.2.1   The FMEA process........................... 169
        11.6.3 Fault tree analysis.................................... 172
                11.6.3.1   The fault tree process........................ 172
                11.6.3.2   Example of a fault tree analysis............... 173
        References 176

Chapter 12 Liability 177

12.1   Negligence 178
12.2   Strict liability 179
12.3   Breach of warranty.. 179
        12.3.1 Implied warranties 179
        12.3.2 Exclusion of warranties............................... 180
12.4   Defects... 180
12.5   Failure to warn of dangers 182
12.6   Plaintiff's conduct 182
12.7   Defendant's conduct 183
12.8   Defendant-related issues....................................... 183
12.9   Manufacturer's and physician's responsibilities.................. 183
12.10   Conclusion... 184
        References 185

Chapter 13 Intellectual property 187

13.1 Patents... 188
      13.1.1 What qualifies as a patent 188
              13.1.1.1 Patentable subject matter 189
              13.1.1.2 Usefulness.................................... 189
              13.1.1.3 Novelty 189
              13.1.1.4 Non-obviousness 189
              13.1.1.5 Improvement of an existing invention.......... 190
              13.1.1.6 A design 190
      13.1.2 The patent process 191
      13.1.3 Patent claims... 192
      13.1.4 Protecting your rights as an inventor 192
      13.1.5 Patent infringement..................................... 193
13.2 Copyrights 194
      13.2.1 What can be copyrighted? 195
      13.2.2 The copyright process 196
              13.2.2.1 Copyright notice 196
              13.2.2.2 Copyright registration 197
      13.2.3 Copyright duration...................................... 197
      13.2.4 Protecting your copyright rights 198
      13.2.5 Infringement 198
13.3 Trademarks 198
      13.3.1 Selecting a trademark 199
              13.3.1.1 What is a distinctive trademark?.............. 200
      13.3.2 The trademark process 201
      13.3.3 Intent to use registration 201
      13.3.4 Protecting your trademark rights 202
13.4 Trade secrets 202
      13.4.1 What qualifies for trade secrecy........................ 203
      13.4.2 Trade secrecy authorship 203
      13.4.3 How trade secrets are lost 203
      13.4.4 Duration of trade secrets 204
      13.4.5 Protecting your trade secret rights 204
      13.4.6 A trade secrecy program................................. 204
      13.4.7 Use of trade secrecy with copyrights and patents........ 205
              13.4.7.1 Trade secrets and patents.................... 205
              13.4.7.2 Trade secrets and copyrights................. 205
      References 205

Section 4
Designing the product 207

Chapter 14 Six Sigma and product design........................... 209

14.1 Design for Six Sigma 210
14.2 Methodologies 210

14.3   Structure...212
14.4   Design for Six Sigma tools 213
        14.4.1 Robust design..213
                14.4.1.1 Why use the robust design methodology? 213
                14.4.1.2 Typical problems addressed by
                          robust design...................................214
                14.4.1.3 Robustness strategy 214
                          14.4.1.3.1 P-diagram 216
                14.4.1.4 Quality measurement 216
                14.4.1.5 Signal to noise (S/N) ratios 216
                          14.4.1.5.1 Static vs. dynamic
                                      S/N ratios 217
                          14.4.1.5.2 Steps in robust parameter
                                      design 217
        14.4.2 Quality function deployment..............................218
        14.4.3 Robust design failure mode and effects analysis..........218
                14.4.3.1 Benefits of a robust DFMEA...................219
                14.4.3.2 The parameter diagram.......................219
                14.4.3.3 Performing a robust DFMEA 221
                14.4.3.4 Conclusion 225
        14.4.4 Axiomatic design..226
                14.4.4.1 What is axiomatic design? 226
                14.4.4.2 Mapping of axiomatic design 227
        References 229

Chapter 15   Hardware design..231

15.1   Block diagram 232
15.2   Redundancy 232
        15.2.1 Active redundancy 233
        15.2.2 Standby redundancy.......................................234
15.3   Component selection 235
        15.3.1 Component fitness for use................................236
        15.3.2 Component reliability 236
        15.3.3 Component history...237
        15.3.4 Component safety..238
15.4   Component derating 238
15.5   Safety margin 239
15.6   Load protection..240
15.7   Environmental protection 240
15.8   Product misuse...240
15.9   Initial reliability prediction 241
        15.9.1 Parts count prediction....................................242
        15.9.2 Parts count prediction example 244
        15.9.3 Summary of reliability prediction 248
15.10   Design for variation...248

15.11   Design of experiments... 249
        15.11.1   The Taguchi method 249
15.12   Design changes... 249
15.13   Design reviews 250
        References 252

Chapter 16   Software design... 255

16.1   Software design levels 256
        16.1.1   Top-level design... 256
        16.1.2   Detailed design... 256
16.2   Design alternatives and tradeoffs 256
16.3   Software architecture.. 257
16.4   Choosing a methodology.. 259
16.5   Structured analysis 260
16.6   Object-oriented design... 260
16.7   Choosing a language 261
16.8   Software risk analysis 263
16.9   The requirements traceability matrix............................. 265
16.10   Software review 266
16.11   Design techniques 269
16.12   Performance predictability and design simulation 269
16.13   Module specifications 270
16.14   Coding... 270
16.15   Design support tools 270
16.16   Design as the basis for verification and validation activity 271
16.17   Conclusion... 272
        References 272

Chapter 17   Software coding 275

17.1   Structured coding techniques 276
17.2   Single-entry, single-exit constructs 276
17.3   Good coding practices.. 277
        17.3.1   Review every line of code.............................. 277
        17.3.2   Require coding sign-offs............................... 278
        17.3.3   Route good code examples for review.................... 278
        17.3.4   Emphasize that code listings are public assets 278
        17.3.5   Reward good code 278
        17.3.6   One easy standard...................................... 279
17.4   The coding process 279
        17.4.1   Start with a PDL....................................... 279
        17.4.2   Writing the routine declaration 279
        17.4.3   Turning the PDL into high level comments 279
        17.4.4   Fill in the code below each comment 281
        17.4.5   Check the code informally.............................. 281

17.4.6   Clean up the leftovers 281
17.4.7   Check the code formally 282
17.5   Implementation checklist 282
References 282

Chapter 18   Establishing and using metrics 285

18.1   Software metrics 286
18.2   Software complexity metrics 288
18.3   Objective and algorithmic measurements 288
18.4   Process and product metrics 289
18.5   Meta-metrics 289
18.6   Size metrics 290
        18.6.1   Lines of code 290
        18.6.2   Token count 290
        18.6.3   Function count 291
18.7   McCabe's complexity 292
18.8   Halstead measures 293
        18.8.1   Vocabulary of the software 293
        18.8.2   Length of the program 294
        18.8.3   Volume of the software 294
        18.8.4   The potential volume 294
        18.8.5   The program level 294
        18.8.6   Effort 294
18.9   Other metrics 295
18.10 Computer-aided metrics 295
18.11 Software metrics methodology 295
        18.11.1   Establish software quality requirements 295
        18.11.2   Identify software quality metrics 296
        18.11.3   Implement the software quality metrics 296
        18.11.4   Analyze the software quality metrics results 296
        18.11.5   Validate the software quality metrics 296
18.12 Establish software quality requirements 296
18.13 Identify a list of possible quality requirements 297
References 297

Chapter 19   Human factors 299

19.1   What are human factors? 300
19.2   The human element in human factors engineering 301
19.3   The hardware element in human factors 302
19.4   The software element in human factors 304
19.5   The human factors process 307
19.6   Planning 307
19.7   Analysis 307

19.8   Conduct user studies 308
      19.8.1   Observations 308
      19.8.2   Interviews 308
      19.8.3   Focus groups 309
      19.8.4   Task analysis 309
      19.8.5   Benchmark usability test 310
      19.8.6   Write user profile 310
      19.8.7   Set up an advisory panel 310
19.9   Set usability goals 310
19.10   Design user interface concepts 311
      19.10.1   Develop conceptual model 311
      19.10.2   Develop user interface structure 311
      19.10.3   Define interaction style 312
      19.10.4   Develop screen templates 312
      19.10.5   Develop hardware layout 312
      19.10.6   Develop a screenplay 312
      19.10.7   Develop a refined design 312
      19.10.8   Develop a final design 312
19.11   Model the user interface 313
19.12   Test the user interface 313
19.13   Specify the user interface 314
      19.13.1   Style guide 314
      19.13.2   Screen hierarchy map 314
      19.13.3   Screenplay 314
      19.13.4   Specification prototype 314
      19.13.5   Hardware layouts 315
19.14   Additional human factors design considerations 315
      19.14.1   Consistency and simplicity 315
      19.14.2   Safety 315
      19.14.3   Environmental/organizational considerations 316
      19.14.4   Documentation 316
      19.14.5   Anthropometry 317
      19.14.6   Functional dimensions 317
      19.14.7   Psychological elements 319
      19.14.8   Workstation design considerations 320
      19.14.9   Alarms and signals 320
      19.14.10   Labeling 323
      19.14.11   Software 324
      19.14.12   Data entry 325
      19.14.13   Displays 325
      19.14.14   Interactive control 327
      19.14.15   Feedback 328
      19.14.16   Prompts 328
      19.14.17   Defaults 329
      19.14.18   Error management/data protection 329
      References 329

Section 5
Testing and data analysis............331

Chapter 20 The basis and types of testing............333

20.1 Testing defined............334
20.2 Parsing test requirements............335
20.3 Test protocol............337
20.4 Test methodology............337
    20.4.1 Time testing............337
    20.4.2 Event testing............337
    20.4.3 Stress testing............337
    20.4.4 Environmental testing............338
    20.4.5 Time related............338
    20.4.6 Failure related............339
20.5 Purpose of the test............339
20.6 Failure definition............339
20.7 Determining sample size and test length............339
    20.7.1 Example 20-1............340
    20.7.2 Example 20-2............341
20.8 Types of testing............342
    20.8.1 Verification............342
    20.8.2 Validation............342
    20.8.3 Black box............342
    20.8.4 White box............343
    20.8.5 Hardware testing............343
    20.8.6 Software testing............343
    20.8.7 Functional testing............344
    20.8.8 Robustness testing............345
    20.8.9 Stress testing............345
    20.8.10 Safety testing............346
    20.8.11 Regression testing............347
    References............348

Chapter 21 Hardware verification and validation............349

21.1 Standard tests............350
    21.1.1 Cycle testing............350
    21.1.2 Typical use testing............350
    21.1.3 10×10 testing............350
21.2 Environmental testing............351
    21.2.1 Operating temperature testing............352
    21.2.2 Storage temperature testing............352
    21.2.3 Thermal shock testing............352
    21.2.4 Humidity testing............353
    21.2.5 Mechanical shock testing............353

        21.2.6   Mechanical vibration testing 354
        21.2.7   Impact testing 354
        21.2.8   Electrostatic discharge 355
        21.2.9   Electromagnetic compatibility 355
21.3   Accelerated testing 356
        21.3.1   Increasing sample size 356
        21.3.2   Increasing test severity 356
        21.3.3   Example 21-1 357
        21.3.4   Example 21-2 358
21.4   Sudden death testing 359
        21.4.1   Weibull testing and plotting 359
                 21.4.1.1   Example 21-3 359
                 21.4.1.2   Confidence limits 360
                 21.4.1.3   The shape of Weibull plots 361
21.5   The sudden death test 362
        21.5.1   Sudden death example 365
        References 369

Chapter 22   Software verification and validation 371

22.1   Allocation of software testing 373
22.2   Verification and validation test method commonality 373
22.3   Validation and test overview 375
        22.3.1   Techniques, methodologies, and test approach 375
        22.3.2   Software testing requirements 377
        22.3.3   Verification and validation reporting 378
22.4   The essentials of software testing 378
        22.4.1   The quality of the test process determines the success
                 of the test effort 379
        22.4.2   Prevent defect migration by using early life-cycle
                 testing techniques 379
        22.4.3   The time for software testing tools is now 379
        22.4.4   A real person must take responsibility for improving
                 the testing process 380
        22.4.5   Testing is a professional discipline requiring trained
                 and skilled people 380
        22.4.6   Cultivate a positive team attitude of creative
                 destruction 380
        References 381

Chapter 23   Analysis of test results 383

23.1   Failure rate 384
        23.1.1   Example 23-1 384
        23.1.2   Example 23-2 384
23.2   Mean time between failures (MTBF) 385
        23.2.1   Time-terminated, failed parts replaced 385

	23.2.1.1	Example 23-3	385
23.2.2	Time-terminated, no replacement		386
23.2.3	Failure-terminated, failed parts replaced		387
	23.2.3.1	Example 23-4	387
23.2.4	Failure-terminated, no replacement		387
23.2.5	No failures observed		388
	23.2.5.1	Example 23-5	388
23.3	Reliability		388
23.3.1	Example 23-6		389
23.3.2	Example 23-7		389
23.4	Confidence level		390
23.4.1	Example 23-8		390
23.5	Confidence limits		390
23.5.1	Time-terminated confidence limits		390
	23.5.1.1	Example 23-9	391
23.5.2	Failure-terminated confidence limits		391
23.6	Minimum life		392
23.7	Graphical analysis		392
23.7.1	Pareto analysis		392
23.7.2	Graphical plotting		393
	23.7.2.1	Example 23-10	393
23.7.3	Weibull plotting		394
	References		394

Section 6
The manufacturing and maintenance processes ... 395

Chapter 24	GMPs and manufacturing		397
24.1	A history of GMPs		398
24.2	The GMP regulation		400
24.2.1	Design controls		400
24.2.2	Purchasing controls		400
24.2.3	Servicing controls		401
24.2.4	Changes in critical device requirements		401
24.2.5	Harmonization		401
24.3	Design for manufacturability		402
24.3.1	The DFM process		402
24.4	Design for assembly		403
24.4.1	Overall design concept		403
24.4.2	Component mounting		403
24.4.3	Test points		403
24.4.4	Stress levels and tolerances		404
24.4.5	PCBs		404
24.4.6	Miscellaneous		404

24.4.7   Design for assembly process 404
24.5   The manufacturing process 405
24.5.1   Pre-production activity 405
24.5.2   The pilot run build 406
24.5.3   The production run 407
24.5.4   Customer delivery 407
References 407

Chapter 25   Configuration management 409

25.1   Configuration identification 410
25.1.1   Functional baseline.................................... 410
25.1.2   Allocated baseline 411
25.1.3   Developmental configuration 412
25.1.4   Product baseline....................................... 412
25.2   Configuration audits 412
25.2.1   Functional configuration audits........................ 413
25.2.2   Physical configuration audits 413
25.2.3   In-process audits 414
25.3   Configuration management metrics 414
25.4   The FDA's view of configuration management................... 414
25.5   Status accounting 415
References 416

Chapter 26   Analysis of field data 417

26.1   Analysis of field service reports................................ 418
26.1.1   The database.. 418
26.1.2   Data analysis.. 419
26.2   Failure analysis of field units 421
26.3   Warranty analysis 422
References 422

Appendices.. 423

Appendix 1   Chi square table...................................... 425
Appendix 2   Percent rank tables 427
Appendix 3   Common failure modes................................ 437
Appendix 4   Glossary 447

Index 461

Dedication

To
Avery Grace Fries
whose humor, smile, and zest for life
make being your grandfather a most enjoyable occupation

Section 1

Basics of reliability

1 Reliability

CONTENTS

1.1 History of reliability... 3
1.2 The definition of reliability 4
1.3 Quality versus reliability 5
1.4 Reliability versus unreliability..................................... 6
1.5 Types of reliability 7
    1.5.1 Electronic reliability 7
        1.5.1.1 Infant mortality..................................... 7
        1.5.1.2 Useful life 8
        1.5.1.3 Wearout 8
    1.5.2 Mechanical reliability 8
    1.5.3 Software reliability.. 9
    1.5.4 Device reliability.. 10
1.6 Optimizing reliability 12
1.7 Reliability assurance.. 12
1.8 Reliability's effect on medical devices 12
References... 13

The term reliability is a term that has been used extensively, but is often misunderstood. Reliability has been described by some as a group of statisticians spewing endless streams of data. Others have described it as testing a device ad nauseam. Reliability is neither of these.

Reliability is a characteristic that describes how good a device really is. It is a measure of the dependability of the device. It is a characteristic that must be planned for, designed, and manufactured into a device. The inclusion of reliability in manufacturing is important because, no matter how reliably a device is designed, it will not be a success unless it is manufactured and serviced reliably. Thus, reliability is the state of mind that all personnel associated with a product must be in. It is a philosophy that dictates how good a device will be.

1.1 HISTORY OF RELIABILITY

Reliability originated during World War II, when the Germans first introduced the concept to improve the operation of their V-1 and V-2 rockets. Prior to this time, most equipment was mechanical in nature and failures could usually be isolated to a simple part. Products were expected to be reliable and safety margins in stress-strength, wear or fatigue conditions were employed to assure it. Then, as electronics began to grow, so did reliability.

From 1945 to 1950, various military studies were conducted in the U.S. on equipment repair, maintenance costs and failure of electronic equipment. As a result of these studies, the Department of Defense established an ad hoc committee on reliability in 1950. This committee became a permanent group in 1952, known as the Advisory Group on the Reliability of Electronic Equipment (AGREE). In 1957, this group published a report that led directly to a specification on the reliability of military electronic equipment.

In the early 1960s, the field of reliability experienced growth and widespread application in the aerospace industry, especially following the failure of Vanguard TV3 and several satellites. During this time engineers also began to realize that, to really improve reliability, one must eliminate the source of failures. This led to the first Physics of Failure Symposium in 1962. This was followed by a period of growth in other highly technical areas, such as computers.

Today many industries and government agencies employ specialists in the area of reliability. Reliability is moving in the direction of more realistic recognition of causes and effects of failures, from the system to the component level. These companies have come to realize that poor reliability is costly, leads to poor customer reputation and the subsequent loss of market share. Industries that are regulated must also comply with reliability requirements established by the regulating agencies.

1.2   THE DEFINITION OF RELIABILITY

This idea of quality over a period of time is reflected in the more formal definition of reliability:

> The probability, at a desired confidence level, that a device will perform a required function, without failure, under stated conditions, for a specified period of time.

This definition contains four key requirements:

- *To perform a required function*, the function must have been established through such activities as customer and/or market surveys. Thus, reliability requires the device to be fully specified prior to design
- *To perform without failure*, the normal operation of the device must be defined, in order to establish what a failure is. This activity also includes anticipating the misuse to which the device could be subjected and designing around it

- *To perform under stated conditions*, the environment in which the device will operate must be specified. This includes typical temperature and humidity ranges, methods of shipping, shock and vibration experienced in normal usage and interference from associated equipment or to other equipment
- *To operate for a specified period of time*, the life expectancy of the device must be defined as well as the typical daily usage

In summary, reliability assumes that preliminary thought processes have been completed and that the device and its environment have been thoroughly defined. These conditions make the task of the designer easier and less costly in time and effort. It assumes that failure-free or failure-tolerant design principles are used. It assumes manufacturing processes are designed so that they will not reduce the reliability of the device.

The user of a medical device does not need such a formal definition. From the customer point of view, a reliable product is:

One that does what the customer wants to do, when the customer wants to do it.

Anything else is unreliable and totally unacceptable.

Reliability, like any science, depends upon other technical areas as a base for its functionality. These include:

- Basic mathematics and statistics
- Current regulatory standards
- Design principles
- Software quality assurance
- System interface principles
- Human factors
- Cost/benefit analysis
- Common sense

1.3   QUALITY VERSUS RELIABILITY

The terms "quality" and "reliability" are sometimes used interchangeably, although they are quite different. The difference grew out of the need for a time-based concept of quality. This distinction of time marks the difference between the traditional quality control concept and the modern approach to reliability.

The traditional concept of quality does not include the notion of a time base. The term *"quality"* is defined in ISO 8402 as:

The totality of features or characteristics of a product or
service that bear on its ability to satisfy stated or implied needs.

The definition refers to this totality at a particular instant of time. Thus, we may speak of the quality of a component at incoming, the quality of a subassembly in a manufacturing test, or the quality of a device at set-up.

In terms of this definition, a medical device is assessed against a specification or set of attributes. Having passed the assessment, the device is delivered to a customer, accompanied by a warranty, so that the customer is relieved of the cost implications of early failures. The customer, upon accepting the device, realizes that it might fail at some future time, hopefully far into the future. This approach provides no measure of the quality of the device outside the warranty period. It assumes this is the customer's responsibility and not the company's.

Reliability, on the other hand, is quality over a specific time period, such as the 5-year expected life of a device or an 8-hour operation. It has been described as the science of estimating, controlling and managing the probability of failure over time.

If the medical device is assessed against a specification or set of attributes, but was additionally designed for a mean time between failures of 5 years prior to being sent to the customer, reliability is being designed into the product (a mean time between failure of 5 years means 63% of the units in the field would have failed once within the 5-year period). A company must realize that, if they want to be successful and build a satisfied customer base, the responsibility for the quality of the device outside the warranty period belongs to them.

1.4   RELIABILITY VERSUS UNRELIABILITY

If reliability is a measure of how good a device is, unreliability is a measure of the potential for the failure of a device. It is the result of the lack of planning for design and manufacturing activities. It is a philosophy that states the manufacturer does not care how good their device will be. The consequences of such a philosophy include:

- High cost
- Wasted time
- Customer inconvenience
- Poor customer reputation

Because reliability is preferable to unreliability, processes should be instituted to avoid the causes of unreliability, including:

- Improper design
- Improper materials
- Manufacturing errors
- Assembly and inspection errors

- Improper testing
- Improper packaging and shipping
- User abuse
- Misapplication

1.5 TYPES OF RELIABILITY

Reliability is composed of three primary subdivisions, each with their own particular attributes:

- Electronic reliability
- Mechanical reliability
- Software reliability

1.5.1 ELECTRONIC RELIABILITY

Electronic reliability (Figure 1-1) is a function of the age of a component or assembly. The failure rate is defined in terms of the number of malfunctions occurring during a period of time. As is evident from the figure, the graph is divided into three distinct time periods:

- Infant mortality
- Useful life
- Wearout

1.5.1.1 Infant mortality

Infant mortality is the beginning of the life of an electronic component or assembly. This period is characterized by an initial high failure rate, which decreases rapidly and then stabilizes. These failures are caused by gross, built-in flaws, due to faulty workmanship, bad processes, manufacturing deviations

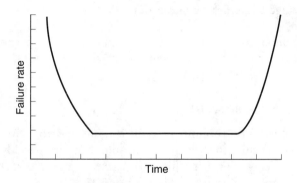

FIGURE 1-1 Electronic reliability curve

from the design intent or transportation damage. Examples of early failures include:

- Poor welds or seals
- Poor solder joints
- Contamination on surfaces or in materials
- Voids, cracks, or thin spots on insulation or protective coatings

Many of these failures can be prevented by improving the control over the manufacturing process or by screening components. Improvements in design or materials are necessary for these manufacturing deviations.

1.5.1.2   Useful life

The useful life period of a component or assembly is the largest segment of the life cycle and is characterized by a constant failure rate. During this period, the failure rate reaches its lowest level and remains relatively constant. Failures occurring during this period are either stress related or occur by chance. These are the most difficult to repeat or analyze.

1.5.1.3   Wearout

The final period in the life cycle occurs when the failure rate begins to increase rapidly. Wearout failures are due primarily to deterioration of the design strength of the components or assemblies, as a consequence of operation and/or exposure to environmental fluctuations. Such deterioration may result from:

- Corrosion or oxidation
- Insulation breakdown or leakage
- Ionic migration of metals on surfaces or in vacuum
- Frictional wear or fatigue
- Shrinkage and cracking in plastics

Replacing components prior to reaching the wearout period through a preventive maintenance program can prevent wearout failures.

1.5.2   MECHANICAL RELIABILITY

Mechanical reliability (Figure 1-2) differs considerably from electronic reliability in its reaction to the aging of a component or assembly. Mechanical components or assemblies begin their life cycle at a failure rate of zero and experience a rapidly increasing failure rate. This curve approximates the wearout portion of the electronics life curve.

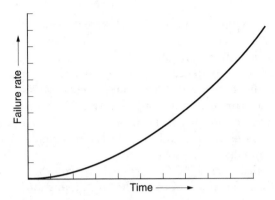

FIGURE 1-2 Mechanical reliability curve

Mechanical failures are due primarily to deterioration of the design strength of the component or assembly. Such deterioration may result from:

- Frictional wear
- Shrinkage and/or cracking in plastics
- Fatigue
- Surface erosion
- Corrosion
- Creep
- Material strength deterioration

Optimization of mechanical reliability occurs with timely replacement of components or assemblies through preventive maintenance, before the failure rate reaches unacceptably high levels.

1.5.3 SOFTWARE RELIABILITY

The following definition of reliability is given by the *IEEE Standard Glossary of Software Engineering Terminology:*

> The ability of a system or component to perform its required functions under stated conditions for a specified period of time.

In the case of medical device software, that definition should be expanded to include the concepts of safety and efficacy as follows:

> The ability of a system or component to perform its required functions in a safe and effective manner, under stated conditions, for a specified period of time.

The main point of this definition is that reliability, safety, and efficacy are inseparable requirements for medical device software.

In order to apply this definition, the software developer must know exactly what the "required functions" of the particular medical device are. Sometimes such functional definitions are obvious, but in general they are not. Such knowledge requires the existence of a formal software specification.

In addition, the software developer must know the "stated conditions." This means the environment in which the software is to operate must be fully defined. This may include whether the software will be operated during a stressful situation, the lighting and noise levels in the area of operation, and the technical knowledge of the user.

"For a specified period of time" indicates that the reliability is being measured for a specific period of time, known as a mission time. This may be the length of a surgical case, the warranty period for the device, or the total operational life of the device.

Software reliability differs considerably from both electronic and mechanical reliability in that software is not subject to the physical constraints of electronic and mechanical components. Software reliability consists of the process of preventing failures through structured design and detecting and removing errors in the coding. Once all "bugs" are removed, the program will operate without failure forever (Figure 1-3). However, practically, the software reliability curve may be as shown in Figure 1-4, with early failures as the software is first used and a long period of constant failures as bugs are fixed.

Software failures are due primarily to:

- Specification errors
- Design errors
- Typographical errors
- Omission of symbols

These are discussed in detail in Chapter 2.

1.5.4 Device reliability

The life cycle of any medical device may be represented by a graph known as the reliability bathtub curve (Figure 1-5). This is a graph of failure rate versus the age of the device.

The graph is identical to that for electronics described above. As with the electronics life curve, there are three distinct time periods:

- Infant mortality
- Useful life
- Wearout

The discussion of the three life periods contained in the section on electronic reliability applies to device reliability as well.

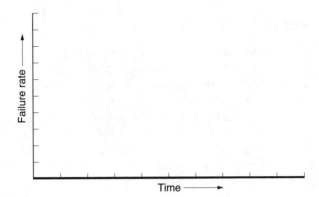

FIGURE 1-3 Ideal software reliability curve

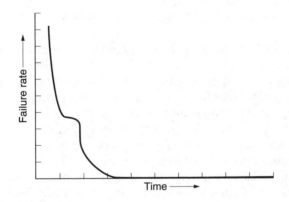

FIGURE 1-4 Practical software reliability curve

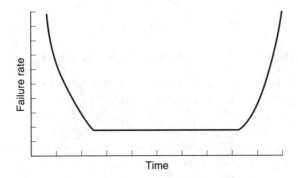

FIGURE 1-5 Reliability bathtub curve

1.6   OPTIMIZING RELIABILITY

Reliability optimization involves consideration of each of the life cycle periods. Major factors that influence and degrade a system's operational reliability must be addressed during design in order to control and maximize system reliability. Thus, early failures may be eliminated by a systematic process of controlled screening and burn-in of components, assemblies and/or the device. Stress-related failures are minimized by providing adequate design margins for each component and the device. Wearout failures may be eliminated by conducting timely preventive maintenance on the device, with appropriate replacement of affected components.

1.7   RELIABILITY ASSURANCE

Reliability assurance is the science that provides the theoretical and practical tools whereby the functionality of a component or device may be evaluated with a certain confidence. Reliability assurance includes:

- Establishing reliability in design by use of failure-free or failure-tolerant principles
- Verifying reliability by well-designed test procedures
- Producing reliability by proper manufacturing processes
- Assuring reliability by good-quality control and inspection
- Maintaining reliability by proper packaging and shipping practices
- Assuring operational reliability by proper field service and appropriate operations and maintenance manuals
- Improving reliability throughout the life of the device by information feedback on field problems and a system to address these issues

These functions of reliability assurance form a structured approach to the life cycle of a medical device. They are discussed in detail, in relation to their optimum location within the product development cycle, in subsequent chapters.

1.8   RELIABILITY'S EFFECT ON MEDICAL DEVICES

Subjecting a medical device to a reliability program provides a structured approach to the product development process. It provides techniques that improve the quality of the device over a period of time as well as reduce development and redevelopment time and cost. It yields statistical data that quantify the success, or lack of success, of the development process and predicts future performance. It also assures regulatory requirements are satisfied and gives confidence that regulatory inspections will produce no major discrepancies.

The use of the various reliability techniques results in decreased warranty costs and the resultant increase in customer acceptance. This naturally leads to an enhanced customer perception of the manufacturer and a resultant increase in market share. Reliability techniques also reduce the risk of liability by assuring safety has been the primary concern during the design and development process. By reducing up-front costs, limiting liability risks and increasing future profits, reliability is essential to the success of any company.

Most importantly, the inclusion of reliability gives development personnel a feeling of confidence that they have optimized the design to produce a device that is safe and effective for its intended use and will remain that way for a long period of time. This confidence will foster success in future products.

REFERENCES

Condra, L.W., *Reliability Improvement with Design of Experiments*, Marcel-Dekker, Inc., New York, 2001.

Dhillon, B.S., *Reliability Engineering in Systems Design and Operation*, Van Nostrand Reinhold Company, New York, 1983.

Dhillon, B.S., *Medical Device Reliability and Associated Areas*, CRC Press LLC, Boca Raton, FL, 2000.

Fries, R.C., *Reliable Design of Medical Devices*, Marcel-Dekker, Inc., New York, 1997.

Fries, R.C., *Handbook of Medical Device* Design, Marcel-Dekker, Inc., New York, 2001.

Haddar, A. and Mahadevan, S., *Probability, Reliability, and Statistical Methods in Engineering Design*, John Wiley & Sons, Inc., New York, 2000.

IEEE Std. 610.12, *Standard Glossary of Software Engineering Terminology*, Institute of Electrical and Electronics Engineers, New York, 1990.

Ireson, W.G. and Coombs, Jr. C.F., *Handbook of Reliability Engineering and Management*, McGraw-Hill Book Company, New York, 1988.

ISO 8402, *Quality Vocabulary*, International Organization for Standardization, Switzerland, 1986.

Kececioglu, D., *Reliability Engineering Handbook*, PTR Prentice Hall Inc., Englewood Cliffs, NJ, 1991.

King, P.H. and Fries, R.C., *Design of Biomedical Devices and Systems*, Marcel Dekker, Inc., New York, 2002.

Langer, E. and J. Meltroft, Eds., *Reliability in Electrical and Electronic Components and Systems*, North Holland Publishing Company, Amsterdam, 1982.

Lloyd, D.K. and Lipow M., *Reliability Management, Methods and Mathematics*, 2nd Edn, The American Society for Quality Control, Milwaukee, Wisconsin, 1984.

MIL-STD-721C, *Definition of Terms for Reliability and Maintainability*, Department of Defense, Washington, D.C., 1981.

Niehoff, K., *Designing Reliable Software*, Medical Device & Diagnostic Industry, Volume 16, Number 9, September, 1994.

O'Connor, P.D.T., *Practical Reliability Engineering*, John Wiley and Sons, New York, 1984.

Reliability Analysis Center, *Reliability Design Handbook*, ITT Research Institute, Chicago, IL, 1975.

2 The concept of failure

CONTENTS

2.1 Failure 15
2.2 Causes of failure 16
2.3 The practical aspects of failures................................... 17
2.4 Failure rate 18
2.5 Hardware failures 18
    2.5.1 Early failures 19
    2.5.2 Chance failures 19
    2.5.3 Wearout failures... 19
2.6 Software failures 20
2.7 Failures due to human error.. 21
2.8 Failures from the customer's point of view......................... 21
References.. 22

The measure of a device's reliability is the infrequency with which failures occur in time. There are many physical causes that individually or collectively may be responsible for the failure of a hardware component or device at any particular instant. It is not always possible to isolate these physical causes and mathematically account for all of them. Similarly, it is not always possible to determine the non-physical causes for failures of software components or devices. However, in both cases, it is not only possible, but of utmost importance, to define what constitutes a failure for a particular device. This definition will depend not only on the architecture of the device but on the environment in which it is used and the intended application as well.

2.1 FAILURE

The term *failure* refers to the degradation of the performance of a device outside a specified value. It may be defined as:

> The non-performance or inability of a component or system to perform its intended function for a specified time under specified environmental conditions.

15

This definition contains several interesting concepts. It assumes the normal function of the device has been defined. If the function of the device has not been specified, then a failure, or deviation from that intended function, cannot be established. The definition also assumes that the environmental conditions under which the system or component will operate have been specified. This includes environmental parameters such as temperature, lighting, ambient noise, stress level under which the user is operating, interference from other equipment in the area, and interference to other equipment in the area. Some or all may play an important part in determining when the system or component is experiencing a failure and when it is not.

Note that a failure is defined as an event or behavior that occurs at a particular instant in time. Failures, in fact, may occur in a variety of ways related to time. Failures may be intermittent, where an output may instantaneously go to zero and then suddenly return to within its specified performance limits. Failures may occur after a long period of performance degradation before falling outside the performance limits. A system or component may drift in and out of performance limits for some time or it may suddenly and permanently cease operation. In all cases, failures must be precisely defined so that failure criteria are not ambiguous. A failure must always be related to a measurable parameter or a clear indication.

The term failure is closely related to other terms with which it is sometimes confused:

- *Defect*: any imperfection, flaw, lack of completeness or other conditions at variance with technical requirements. It denotes such things as the unsatisfactory packaging of hardware, as well as part and equipment discrepancies, which may be responsible for failure
- *Deficiency*: a general term covering any defect, discrepancy or lack of conformance to specifications
- *Fault*: the immediate cause of a failure, such as maladjustment or misalignment. In general, all failures are faults, but not all faults are failures
- *Malfunction*: any occurrence of unsatisfactory performance. It need not constitute a failure if readjustment of operator controls can restore an acceptable operating condition

2.2 CAUSES OF FAILURE

There are as many causes of failure as there are types of failure themselves. Some causes are related to whether the failure occurs in hardware or software. Others are related to time in use, type of operation being performed, existence of a safety margin, etc. Two general categories of failures are systematic and random.

Systematic failures are due to errors (including mistakes and acts of omissions) in any life-cycle activity that cause a failure under some particular combination of inputs or under some particular environmental condition. Systematic failures are possible for hardware and/or software and can take place in any part of a product life cycle. An example of a systematic failure would be an incorrect limit value in a database that permits a hazardous condition to occur. The incorrect data may have been wrongly specified, wrongly copied during data preparation, or incorrectly changed during use. The potential of this type of event is difficult to predict. However, there is a relationship between the quality of the processes used during the life cycle and the probability of the fault being introduced.

Many failures occur in a random fashion. These are the most difficult to predict and analyze. For many events, a statistical probability can be assigned. For example, the probability of failure on an electronic assembly is often estimated from the failure probabilities of the components that make up the assembly. In this case, a numerical value can be given for the probability of failure. An essential presumption is that the failures are random in nature. This may be true for some failure mechanisms, but it is generally assumed not to be true for systematic failures. Hardware is assumed to fail either in a random or systematic manner. Software can appear to fail in a random manner; however, the cause of a software failure is always systematic.

2.3 THE PRACTICAL ASPECTS OF FAILURES

Failures are a fact of life. No device or component will ever have a perfect reliability. Devices and components fail. Therefore, we must learn to anticipate failures, take steps to minimize their occurrences, and optimize the operation of the device or component. To do this will require some mental gymnastics.

First, we must decide what constitutes a failure for our particular component or device. This decision is based on the intended application and the particular environment in which the device is to be used. For example, a monitor is part of a surgical suite. A patient's vital signs are being monitored during surgery. During the case, the surgeon uses a cautery to arrest bleeding. The monitor, situated close to the cautery device, displays scrambled data during the time the cautery is operational but immediately returns to reliable data when the cautery is stopped. Is this a failure? It depends on how the operation of the monitor has been specified. If the monitor is specified to constantly display reliable data during all forms of electromagnetic interference, then this scenario is a failure. If the device is specified to return reliable data immediately following cessation of a strong electromagnetic signal, then the monitor is operating as specified, and the scenario contains no failure.

Once a failure has been recognized, the next step is to correct the problem and place the unit back into operation as soon as possible. To accomplish this, the root cause of the failure must be the focal point for any type of failure analysis activity. Too often "band-aids" are applied to device failures in an effort to get a quick fix without determining the real cause of the failure. These quick fixes may cause a temporary return to the device's intended function, but eventually the device will fail again, because the real cause of the failure was not analyzed and corrected. Techniques such as hazard analysis, risk analysis, and fault tree analysis are methods of getting to the root cause of failures and establishing schemes to address them.

When developing a medical device it is of utmost importance to design the device to operate according to specification, without failure, for a maximum period of time. To do this failures must be analyzed as to whether their occurrence will allow the device to keep operating at a safe level, or whether the device should be shut down to avoid potential harm to the patient, user, or the machine. A system with good diagnostics will establish failure priorities and inform the user of the situation so they may make a decision, or, in extreme cases, terminate the operation of the device itself. In all cases the user should be informed of the occurrence of the failure.

2.4 FAILURE RATE

Failures in components or devices are usually listed in terms of a failure rate. The failure rate of a component or device is the probability of a failure per unit of time for the items still functioning. The best estimate of the failure rate is given by the equation:

$$\lambda = r/t \tag{2.1}$$

where λ is the failure rate, r is the number of failures, and t is the accumulated operating time of the item.

Failure rate is normally expressed in failures per million hours. For example, certain resistors have a failure rate of 0.0014 failures per million hours, a fuse a rate of 0.010 failures per million hours, and a high current relay a rate of 0.43 failures per million hours. Documents, such as MIL-HDBK-217, or data books from the Reliability Analysis Center, list all component failure rates with this notation. Such documents, in listing failure rates, make the assumption that the component is in its useful life period, where it experiences a constant failure rate, and that its failure rate over time operates according to the exponential distribution. This topic was discussed in detail in Chapter 1.

2.5 HARDWARE FAILURES

Hardware is very different from software. Thus, hardware failures are very different from software failures. Hardware components degrade, whereas software components do not. Hardware processes are constrained by the laws of physics, while software processes are not. The failure modes of hardware components differ from that of software components. As a result, hardware and software have their own distinct causes of failures.

One particular group of failures, particular to hardware, are the time-related failures. Time-related failures may be classified into three groups: early failures, chance or random failures and wearout failures.

2.5.1 EARLY FAILURES

Early failures occur usually within the first 1000 hours of operation. That is why integrated circuits, for example, may be subjected to an accelerated burn-in at high temperature, equivalent to 1000 hours of operation. This has been an industry standard for eliminating early failures.

There are several causes for early failures:

- Insufficient design debugging
- Substandard components
- Poor-quality control
- Poor manufacturing techniques
- Poor workmanship
- Insufficient burn-in
- Improper installation
- Replacing field components with non-screened ones

In general, early failures are the result of poor manufacturing processes or component quality.

2.5.2 CHANCE FAILURES

Chance or random failures occur during the useful life of the device. This is the long period in the life of a component or device where the failure rate is constant. They are usually the hardest failures to duplicate and analyze. Causes of such failures include:

- Interference or overlap of designed-in strength
- Insufficient safety factors
- Occurrence of higher than expected random loads
- Occurrence of lower than expected random strengths
- Component defects
- Errors in usage
- User or patient abuse

In general, chance failures usually result from weaknesses in the design, latent component problems, or customer misuse of the product.

2.5.3 WEAROUT FAILURES

Wearout failures occur at the end of the life cycle of a device or electronic component, or continuously throughout the life of a mechanical component. Causes of wearout failures include:

- Aging
- Wear
- Degradation in strength

- Creep
- Fatigue
- Corrosion
- Poor service or maintenance

In general, wearout failures are related to long-term usage of the product and the natural wearout tendency of the components over time.

2.6   SOFTWARE FAILURES

In order to understand how to avoid software errors, it is necessary to understand what causes failures in a software program. As stated earlier, software differs from hardware in several ways. Of prime importance is that software does not degrade like hardware and it is not constrained physically. Therefore, the causes of software failures are significantly different from those of hardware components. There are four basic causes of software failures:

- Specification errors
- Design errors
- Typographical errors
- Omissions of symbols

Specification errors are caused by a misunderstanding of the customer's real needs. Many programs have been developed with the customer's needs in mind, only to find out later that the device did not function as the customer expected it to. Therefore, there must be a genuine effort to fully understand what the customers need and what they expect the device to do.

Design errors are probably the most frequent cause of software errors. The designer, after reviewing the specification, may be more interested in starting to code, rather than spending time thinking through the design. This practice may lead to decision points within the program not addressing all conditions or the establishment of race conditions.

Typographical errors are the third cause of failures. When keying the code, it is easy to hit a wrong key or copy the code improperly. An example of such an error having a costly effect is the delay, just prior to launch, of a space shuttle flight. The software shut the system down with less than a minute until launch. Analysis traced the cause to a typographical error of a DO statement, where the DO was followed by a variable name. When keyed, the space between the DO and the variable name was omitted, causing the program to consider the whole line as a variable name. When the variable name was not recognized, the software shut the system down.

Another cause of software errors, similar to typographical errors, is the omission of symbols. When symbols are omitted, the code becomes unrecognizable and the program will fail.

As the causes of software errors are understood, methods can be employed to eliminate such causes, thus eliminating the failures. This puts the emphasis of the software quality assurance program on avoidance of errors, rather than detection of errors, making for a more reliable program, in a shorter period of development time.

2.7 FAILURES DUE TO HUMAN ERROR

Failures due to human error begin to take on an increasing importance as the design evolves, until this source of trouble frequently becomes the most significant of all. It is mandatory, therefore, that all such failures be reported in addition to those due to design inadequacy. The term human error as used here covers not only errors such as reversed wiring, wrong part installation, etc. – that is, errors due to gross carelessness – but also discrepancies produced by failures of the control procedures associated with manufacturing, inspection and operation. Standard Operating Procedures or Standard Inspection Procedures may be inadequate or incomplete, so that critical measurements are not taken or operations are performed which result in a failure at a later time. For example, a soldering iron may be set too hot, thus causing stress on a leaded component. The result may be a latent failure.

Further failures may be produced by not keeping procedures, change orders, and drawings up to date. When changes are made to documentation, failure to distribute the changes to appropriate personnel will cause devices to be assembled incorrectly, thus setting the stage for failure in the test area, or, worse, in the field.

Since it is impossible to anticipate all contingencies that might cause a failure, the best that can be done is to review all the procedural controls initially and modify them as their inadequacies become known. The only way to do the latter is to insist that all human errors be reported and prevent the natural tendency to relax once the design part of the problem appears close to solution.

2.8 FAILURES FROM THE CUSTOMER'S POINT OF VIEW

We have discussed the various types of failures. We talked of hardware versus software failures, time-related failures, and human error failures. To the customer, only one failure is important – that which occurs to their device and does not allow that device to be used as it was intended. This may mean a monitor will not display patient parameters, an anesthesia machine cannot be used for a case, or a pacemaker ceases to function. To the customer it is irrelevant whether hardware or software caused a unit to fail. It only matters that the device is not useable.

Tracking failures is important. They provide a database for future enhancements and designs. However, anticipating potential failures, even customer misuse of the device, is more important for establishing customer acceptance and satisfaction. We know devices are going to fail. Any steps taken to reduce down time and minimize customer inconvenience will only enhance the stature of a company in its customer's eyes and be a source for future sales.

REFERENCES

Dhillon, B.S., *Medical Device Reliability and Associated Areas*, CRC Press LLC, Boca Raton, 2000.

Fries, R.C., *Reliable Design of Medical Devices*, Marcel-Dekker, Inc., New York, 1997.

Fries, R.C., *Handbook of Medical Device Design*, Marcel-Dekker, Inc., New York, 2001.

Ireson, W.G. and Coombs, Jr., C.F., *Handbook of Reliability Engineering and Management*, McGraw-Hill Book Company, New York, 1988.

King, P.H. and Fries, R.C., *Design of Biomedical Devices and Systems*, Marcel Dekker, Inc., New York, 2002.

Leveson, N.G., *Safeware*, Addison-Wesley Publishing Company, Inc., Reading, MA, 1995.

Lloyd, D.K. and Lipow, M., *Reliability: Management, Methods, and Mathematics*, The American Society for Quality Control, Milwaukee, WI, 1984.

Mann, N.R., Schafer, R.E. and Singpurwalla, N.D., *Methods for Statistical Analysis of Reliability and Life Data*, John Wiley & Sons, New York, 1974.

MIL-HDBK-217, *Reliability Prediction of Electronic Equipment*, Department of Defense, Washington, DC, 1986.

MIL-STD-721C, *Definition of Terms for Reliability and Maintainability*, Department of Defense, Washington, DC, 1981.

Musa, J.D., Iannino, A. and Okumoto, K., *Software Reliability – Measurement, Prediction, Application*, McGraw Hill Book Company, New York, 1987.

Neufelder, A.M., *Ensuring Software Reliability*, Marcel Dekker, Inc., New York, 1993.

Schneidewind, N.F., Modeling fault detection and correction processes, *Reliability Review*, 23(4), 2003.

Section 2

Regulations and standards

3 The Food and Drug Administration

CONTENTS

3.1 History of device regulation 26
3.2 Device classification 28
    3.2.1 Class I devices 28
    3.2.2 Class II devices 28
    3.2.3 Class III devices 29
3.3 Registration and listing 30
3.4 The 510(k) process 31
    3.4.1 Determining substantial equivalency 31
    3.4.2 The regular 510(k) 31
        3.4.2.1 Types of 510(k)s 31
        3.4.2.2 The 510(k) format 33
    3.4.3 The Special 510(k) 35
        3.4.3.1 Special 510(k) content 38
    3.4.4 The Abbreviated 510(k) 38
        3.4.4.1 Abbreviated 510(k) content 39
3.5 Declaration of conformance to a recognized standard 40
3.6 The PMA application 40
    3.6.1 The PMA process 41
    3.6.2 Contents of a PMAA 41
3.7 Investigational Device Exemptions (IDEs) 42
    3.7.1 Institutional Review Boards (IRBs) 42
    3.7.2 IDE format 43
3.8 Good laboratory practices (GLPs) 44
3.9 Good manufacturing practices (GMPs) 44
3.10 Human factors 44
3.11 Design control 45
3.12 The FDA and software 46
3.13 Software classification 47
3.14 The FDA inspection 48
3.15 Advice on dealing with the FDA 48
References 49

When designing any device that will be used medically, it is important to consider all safety aspects, including the repercussions of design flaws and misuse of the device. Regulation of medical devices is intended to protect consumers' health and safety by attempting to ensure that marketed products are effective and safe. Prior to 1976, the FDA had limited authority over medical devices under the Food, Drug, and Cosmetic Act of 1938. Beginning in 1968, Congress established a radiation control program to authorize the establishment of standards for electronic products, including medical and dental radiology equipment. From the early 1960s to 1975, concern over devices increased and six U.S. Presidential messages were given to encourage medical device legislation.

In 1969, the Department of Health, Education, and Welfare appointed a special committee (the Cooper Committee) to review the scientific literature associated with medical devices. The Committee estimated that, over a 10-year period, 10 000 injuries were associated with medical devices, of which 731 resulted in death. The majority of problems were associated with three device types: artificial heart valves, cardiac pacemakers, and intrauterine contraceptive devices. There activities culminated in the passage of the Medical Devices Amendments of 1976.

Devices marketed after 1976 are subject to full regulation unless they are found substantially equivalent to a device already on the market in 1976. By the end of 1981, only about 300 of the 17 000 products submitted for clearance to the FDA after 1976 had been found not substantially equivalent.

3.1 HISTORY OF DEVICE REGULATION

In 1906, the Food and Drug Administration enacted its first regulations addressing public health. While these regulations did not address medical devices per se, they did establish a foundation for future regulations. It was not until 1938, with the passage of the Federal Food, Drug and Cosmetic Act (FFD&C), that the FDA was authorized, for the first time, to regulate medical devices. This act provided for regulation of adulterated or misbranded drugs, cosmetics and devices that were entered into interstate commerce. A medical device could be marketed without being federally reviewed and approved.

In the years following World War II, the FDA focused much of the attention on drugs and cosmetics. Over-the-counter drugs became regulated in 1961. In 1962, the FDA began requesting safety and efficacy data on new drugs and cosmetics.

By the mid-1960s, it became clear that the provisions of the FFD&C Act were not adequate to regulate the complex medical devices of the times to assure both patient and user safety. Thus, in 1969, the Cooper Committee was formed to examine the problems associated with medical devices and to develop concepts for new regulations.

In 1976, with input from the Cooper Committee, the FDA created the Medical Device Amendments to the FFD&C Act, which were subsequently signed into law. The purpose of the amendments was to assure that medical devices were safe, effective and properly labeled for their intended use. To accomplish this mandate, the amendments provided the FDA with the authority to regulate devices during most phases of their development, testing, production, distribution, and use. This marked the first time the FDA clearly distinguished between devices and drugs. Regulatory requirements were derived from this 1976 law.

In 1978, with the authority granted to the FDA by the amendments, the Good Manufacturing Practices (GMP) were promulgated. The GMP represents a quality assurance program intended to control the manufacturing, packaging, storage, distribution, and installation of medical devices. This regulation was intended to allow only safe and effective devices to reach the market place. It is this regulation that has had the greatest effect on the medical device industry. It allows the FDA to inspect a company's operations and take action on any noted deficiencies, including prohibition of device shipment.

In 1990, the Safe Medical Devices Act was passed by Congress. It gave the FDA authority to add "pre-production design validation controls" to the GMP regulations. The act also encouraged the FDA to work with foreign countries toward mutual recognition of GMP inspections.

On July 31, 1996, the new Medical Device Reporting (MDR) regulation became effective for user facilities and device manufacturers. The MDR regulation provides a mechanism for the Food and Drug Administration and manufacturers to identify and monitor significant adverse events involving medical devices. The goals are to detect and correct problems in a timely manner. Although the requirements of the regulation can be enforced through legal sanctions authorized by the Federal Food, Drug, and Cosmetic Act, the FDA relies on the goodwill and cooperation of all affected groups to accomplish the objectives of the regulation. The statutory authority for the MDR regulation is section 519 of the FD&C Act, as amended by the Safe Medical Devices Act (SMDA). The SMDA requires user facilities to:

- Report device-related deaths to the FDA and the device manufacturer
- Report device-related serious injuries and serious illnesses to the manufacturer, or to the FDA, if the manufacturer is not known
- Submit to the FDA on a semiannual basis a summary of all reports submitted during that period

In 1990, the FDA proposed revised GMP regulations. Almost 7 years of debate and revision followed, but finally, on October 7, 1996, the FDA issued its final rules. The new Quality System Regulations, incorporating the required design controls, went into effect on June 1, 1997. The design control provisions were not enforced until June 14, 1998. The Quality System Regulations will be discussed in detail in Chapter 5.

3.2   DEVICE CLASSIFICATION

A medical device is any article or health care product intended for use in the diagnosis of disease or other condition, or for use in the care, treatment, or prevention of disease that does not achieve any of its primary intended purposes by chemical action or by being metabolized.

From 1962, when Congress passed the last major drug law revision and first attempted to include devices, until 1976, when device laws were finally written, there were almost constant congressional hearings. Testimony was presented by medical and surgical specialty groups, industry, basic biomedical sciences, and various government agencies, including the FDA. Nearly two dozen bills were rejected as either inadequate or inappropriate.

The Cooper Committee concluded that the many inherent and important differences between drugs and devices necessitated a regulatory plan specifically adapted to devices. They recognized that some degree of risk is inherent in the development of many devices, so that all hazards cannot be eliminated, that there is often little or no prior experience on which to base judgements about safety and effectiveness, that devices undergo performance improvement modifications during the course of clinical trials, and that results also depend upon the skill of the user.

They therefore rejected the drug-based approach and created a new and different system for evaluating devices. All devices were placed into classes, based upon the degree of risk posed by each individual device and its use. The Pre-Market Notification Process (510(k)) and the Pre-Market Approval Application (PMAA) became the regulatory pathways for device approval. The Investigational Device Exemption (IDE) became the mechanism to establish safety and efficacy in clinical studies for PMAAs.

3.2.1   CLASS I DEVICES

Class I devices are defined as non-life-sustaining. Their failure poses no risk to life, and there is no need for performance standards. Basic standards, however, such as pre-market notification (510(k)), registration, device listing, good manufacturing practices (GMP), and proper record keeping are all required. Nonetheless, the FDA has exempted many of the simpler Class I devices from some or all of these requirements. For example, tongue depressors and stethoscopes are both Class I devices. Both are exempt from GMP, tongue depressors are exempt from 510(k) filing, whereas stethoscopes are not.

3.2.2   CLASS II DEVICES

Class II devices were also defined in 1976 as not life-sustaining. However, they must not only comply with the basic standards for Class I devices but must meet specific controls or performance standards. For example, sphygmomanometers, although not essential for life, must meet standards of accuracy and reproducibility.

Pre-market notification is documentation submitted by a manufacturer that notifies the FDA that a device is about to be marketed. It assists the agency in making a determination about whether a device is "substantially equivalent" to a previously marketed predecessor device. As provided for in section 510(k) of the Food, Drug, and Cosmetic Act, the FDA can clear a device for marketing on the basis of pre-market notification that the device is substantially equivalent to a pre-1976 predecessor device. The decision is based on pre-market notification information that is provided by the manufacturer and includes the intended use, physical composition, and specifications of the device. Additional data usually submitted include *in-vitro* and *in-vivo* toxicity studies.

The pre-market notification or 510(k) process was designed to give manufacturers the opportunity to obtain rapid market approval of these non-critical devices by providing evidence that their device is "substantially equivalent" to a device that is already marketed. The device must have the same intended use and the same or equally safe and effective technological characteristics as a predicate device.

Class II devices are usually exempt from the need to prove safety and efficacy. The FDA, however, may require additional clinical or laboratory studies. On occasion these may be as rigorous as for an IDE in support of a PMA, although this is rare. The FDA responds with an "order of concurrence" or non-concurrence with the manufacturer's equivalency claims.

The Safe Medical Device Act of 1990 and the Amendments of 1992 attempted to take advantage of what had been learned since 1976 to give both the FDA and manufacturers greater leeway by permitting reduction in the classification of many devices, including some life-supporting and life-sustaining devices previously in Class III, provided that reasonable assurance of safety and effectiveness can be obtained by application of "Special Controls" such as performance standards, post market surveillance, guidelines and patient and device registries.

3.2.3 CLASS III DEVICES

Class III devices were defined in 1976 as either sustaining or supporting life so that their failure is life threatening. For example, heart valves, pacemakers, and PCTA balloon catheters are all Class III devices. Class III devices almost always require a PMAA, a long and complicated task fraught with many pitfalls that has caused the greatest confusion and dissatisfaction for both industry and the FDA.

The new regulations permit the FDA to use data contained in four prior PMAAs for a specific device, that demonstrate safety and effectiveness, to approve future PMA applications by establishing performance standards or actual reclassification. Composition and manufacturing methods that companies wish to keep as proprietary secrets are excluded. Advisory medical panel review is now elective.

However, for PMAAs that continue to be required, all of the basic requirements for Class I and II devices must be provided, plus failure mode analysis, animal tests, toxicology studies, and then finally human clinical studies, directed to establish safety and efficacy under an IDE.

It is necessary that preparation of the PMAA must actually begin years before it will be submitted. It is only after the company has the results of all of the laboratory testing, pre-clinical animal testing, failure mode analysis and manufacturing standards on their final design, that their proof of safety and efficacy can begin, in the form of a clinical study under an IDE.

At this point the manufacturer must not only have settled on a specific, fixed design for their device, but their marketing and clinical consultants must also have decided on what the indications, contraindications, and warnings for use will be. The clinical study must be carefully designed to support these claims.

Section 520(g) of the Federal Food, Drug, and Cosmetic Act, as amended, authorizes the FDA to grant an IDE to a researcher using a device in studies undertaken to develop safety and effectiveness data for that device when such studies involve human subjects. An approved IDE application permits a device that would otherwise be subject to marketing clearance to be shipped lawfully for the purpose of conducting a clinical study. An approved IDE also exempts a device from certain sections of the Act. All new significant-risk devices not granted substantial equivalence under the 510(k) section of the Act must pursue clinical testing under an IDE.

An Institutional Review Board (IRB) is a group of physicians and lay people at a hospital who must approve clinical research projects prior to their initiation.

3.3 REGISTRATION AND LISTING

Under section 510 of the Act, every person engaged in the manufacture, preparation, propagation, compounding, or processing of a device shall register their name, place of business and such establishment. This includes manufacturers of devices and components, re-packers, re-labelers, as well as initial distributors of imported devices. Those not required to register include manufacturers of raw materials, licensed practitioners, manufacturers of devices for use solely in research or teaching, warehousers, manufacturers of veterinary devices, and those who only dispense devices, such as pharmacies.

Upon registration, the FDA issues a device registration number. A change in the ownership or corporate structure of the firm, the location, or person designated as the official correspondent must be communicated to the FDA device registration and listing branch within 30 days. Registration must be done when first beginning to manufacture medical devices and must be updated yearly.

Section 510 of the Act also requires all manufacturers to list the medical devices they market. Listing must be done when first beginning to manufacture a product and must be updated every 6 months. Listing includes not only informing the FDA of products manufactured, but also providing the agency with copies of labeling and advertising.

Foreign firms that market products in the U.S. are permitted, but not required, to register and are required to list. Foreign devices that are not listed are not permitted to enter the country.

Registration and listing provides the FDA with information about the identity of manufacturers and the products they make. This information enables the agency to schedule inspections of facilities and also to follow up on problems. When the FDA learns about a safety defect in a particular type of device, it can use the listing information to notify all manufacturers of those devices about that defect.

3.4   THE 510(k) PROCESS

3.4.1   DETERMINING SUBSTANTIAL EQUIVALENCY

A new device is substantially equivalent if, in comparison to a legally marketed predicate device, it has the same intended use and (1) has the same technological characteristics as the predicate device or (2) has different technological characteristics and submitted information that does not raise different questions of safety and efficacy and demonstrates that the device is as safe and effective as the legally marketed predicate device. Figure 3-1 is an overview of the substantial equivalence decision making process.

3.4.2   THE REGULAR 510(k)

3.4.2.1   Types of 510(k)s

There are several types of 510(k) submissions that require different formats for addressing the requirements. These include:

- Submissions for identical devices
- Submissions for equivalent but not identical devices
- Submissions for complex devices or for major differences in technological characteristics
- Submissions for software-controlled devices

The 510(k) for simple changes, or for identical devices, should be kept simple and straightforward. The submission should refer to one or more predicate devices. It should contain samples of labeling, it should have a brief statement of equivalence, and it may be useful to include a chart listing similarities and differences.

The group of equivalent but not identical devices includes combination devices, where the characteristics or functions of more than one predicate device are relied on to support a substantially equivalent determination. This

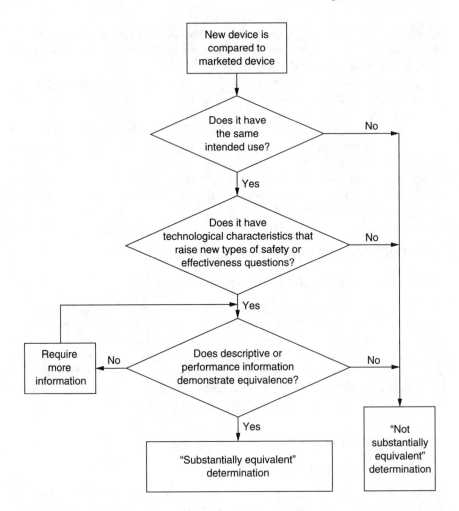

FIGURE 3-1 The substantial equivalence process

type of 510(k) should contain all of the information listed above as well as sufficient data to demonstrate why the differing characteristics or functions do not affect safety or effectiveness. Submission of some functional data may be necessary. It should not be necessary, however, to include clinical data — bench or pre-clinical testing results should be sufficient. Preparing a comparative chart showing differences and similarities with predicate devices can be particularly helpful to the success of this type of application.

Submissions for complex devices or for major differences in technological characteristics are the most difficult type of submission, since they begin to approach the point at which the FDA will need to consider whether a 510(k) is sufficient of whether a PMAA must be submitted. The key is to demonstrate that the new features or the new uses do not diminish safety or effectiveness and that there are no significant new risks posed by the device. In addition to the types of information described above, this type of submission will almost always require submission of some data, possibly including clinical data.

As a general rule, it often is a good idea to meet with the FDA to explain why the product is substantially equivalent, to discuss the data that will be submitted in support of a claim of substantial equivalence, and to learn the FDA's concerns and questions so that these may be addressed in the submission. The FDA's guidance documents can be of greatest use in preparing this type of submission.

The term software includes programs and/or data that pertain to the operation of a computer-controlled system, whether they are contained on floppy disks, hard disks, magnetic tapes, laser disks, or embedded in the hardware of a device. The depth of review by the FDA is determined by the "level of concern" for the device and the role that the software plays in the functioning of the device. Levels of concern are listed as minor, moderate, and major and are tied very closely with risk analysis.

In reviewing such submissions, the FDA maintains that end-product testing may not be sufficient to establish that the device is substantially equivalent to the predicate devices. Therefore, a firm's software development process and/or documentation should be examined for reasonable assurance of safety and effectiveness of the software-controlled functions, including incorporated safeguards. 510(k)s that are heavily software dependent will receive greater FDA scrutiny, and the questions posed must be satisfactorily addressed.

3.4.2.2   The 510(k) format

The actual 510(k) submission will vary in complexity and length according to the type of device or product change for which substantial equivalency is sought. A submission shall be in sufficient detail to provide an understanding of the basis for a determination of substantial equivalence. All submissions shall contain the following information:

- The submitter's name, address, telephone number, a contact person, and the date the submission was prepared
- The name of the device, including the trade or proprietary name, if applicable, the common or usual name, and the classification name
- An identification of the predicate or legally marketed device or devices to which substantial equivalence is being claimed
- A description of the device that is the subject of the submission, including an explanation of how the device functions, the basic scientific concepts that form the basis for the device, and the significant physical and performance characteristics of the device, such as device design, materials used, and physical properties
- A statement of the intended use of the device, including a general description of the diseases or conditions the device will diagnose, treat, prevent, cure, or mitigate, including a description, where

appropriate, of the patient population for which the device is intended. If the indication statements are different from those of the predicate or legally marketed device identified above, the submission shall contain an explanation as to why the differences are not critical to the intended therapeutic, diagnostic, prosthetic, or surgical use of the device and why the differences do not affect the safety or effectiveness of the device when used as labeled

- A statement of how the technological characteristics (design, material, chemical composition, or energy source) of the device compare to those of the predicate or legally marketed device identified above

510(k) summaries for those pre-market notification submissions in which a determination of substantial equivalence is based on an assessment of performance data shall contain the following information in addition to that listed above:

- A brief discussion of the non-clinical tests and their results submitted in the pre-market notification
- A brief discussion of the clinical tests submitted, referenced, or relied on in the pre-market notification submission for a determination of substantial equivalence. This discussion shall include, where applicable, a description of the subjects upon whom the device was tested, a discussion of the safety and/or effectiveness data obtained with specific reference to adverse effects and complications, and any other information from the clinical testing relevant to a determination of substantial equivalence
- The conclusions drawn from the non-clinical and clinical tests that demonstrate that the device is safe, effective, and performs as well as or better than the legally marketed device identified above

The summary should be in a separate section of the submission, beginning on a new page and ending on a page not shared with any other section of the pre-market notification submission, and should be clearly identified as a 501(k) summary.

A 510(k) statement submitted as part of a pre-market notification shall state as follows:

I certify that (name of person required to submit the pre-market notification) will make available all information included in this pre-market notification on safety and effectiveness that supports a finding of substantial equivalence within 30 days of request by any person. The information I agree to make available does not include confidential patient identifiers.

This statement should be made in a separate section of the pre-market notification submission and should be clearly identified as a 510(k) statement.

A Class III certification submitted as part of a pre-market notification shall state as follows:

> I certify that a reasonable search of all information known or otherwise available to (name of pre-market notification submitter) about the types and causes of reported safety and/or effectiveness problems for the (type of device) has been conducted. I further certify that the types of problems to which the (type of device) is susceptible and their potential causes are listed in the attached Class III summary, and that this Class III summary is complete and accurate.

This statement should be clearly identified as a Class III certification and should be made in the section of the pre-market notification submission that includes the Class III summary.

A 510(k) should be accompanied by a brief cover letter that clearly identifies the submission as a 510(k) pre-market notification. To facilitate prompt routing of the submission to the correct reviewing division within the FDA, the letter can mention the generic category of the product and its intended use.

When the FDA receives a 510(k) pre-market notification, it is reviewed according to a checklist to assure its completeness. A sample 510(k) checklist is shown in Figure 3-2.

3.4.3   THE SPECIAL 510(k)

Under this option, a manufacturer who is intending to modify their own legally marketed device will conduct the risk analysis and the necessary verification and validation activities to demonstrate that the design outputs of the modified device meet the design input requirements. Once the manufacturer has ensured the satisfactory completion of this process, *a Special 510(k): Device Modification* may be submitted. While the basic content requirements of the 510(k) will remain the same, this type of submission should also reference the cleared 510(k) number and contain a *Declaration of Conformity* with design control requirements.

Under the Quality System Regulation, manufacturers are responsible for performing internal audits to assess their conformance with design controls. A manufacturer could, however, use a third party to provide a supporting assessment of the conformance. In this case, the third party will perform a conformance assessment for the device manufacturer and provide the manufacturer with a statement to this effect. The marketing application should then include a declaration of conformity signed by the manufacturer, while the statement from the third party should be maintained in the Device Master Record. As always, responsibility for conformance with design control requirements rests with the manufacturer.

In order to provide an incentive for manufacturers to choose this option, the Office of Device Evaluation (ODE) intends to process Special 510(k)s within 30 days of receipt by the Document Mail Center. The Special 510(k)

	Critical elements	Yes	No
1	Is the product a device?		
2	Is the device exempt from 510(k) by regulation or policy?		
3	Is the device subject to review by CDRH?		
4	Are you aware that this device has been the subject of a previous Not Substantially Equivalent (NSE) decision? If yes, does this new 510(k) address the NSE issues?		
5	Are you aware of the submitter being the subject of an integrity investigation? If yes consult the Office of Device Evaluation (ODE) Integrity Officer		
6	Has the ODE Integrity Officer given permission to proceed with the review? (Blue Book Memo #191-2 and Federal Register 90N-0332, September 10, 1990).		
7	Does the submission contain the information required under Sections 510(k), 513(f), and 513(l) of the FFD&C Act and Subpart E of Part 807 in Title 21 of the Code of Federal Regulations?		
8	Device trade or proprietary name?		
9	Device common or usual name or classification number?		
10	Establishment registration number? (Only applies if the establishment is registered)		
11	Class into which the device is classified under 21 CFR Parts 862-892?		
12	Classification panel?		
13	Action taken to comply with section 514 of the Act?		
14	Proposed labels, labeling, and advertisements (if available) that describe the device, its intended use, and directions for use? (Blue Book Memo #G91-1)		
15	A 510(k) summary of safety and effectiveness or a 510(k) statement that safety and effectiveness information will be made available to any person upon request?		
16	For a Class III devices only, a Class III certification and a Class III summary?		
17	Photographs of the device?		
18	Engineering drawings for the device with dimensions and tolerances?		
19	The marketed device(s) to which equivalence is being claimed including labeling and description of the device?		
20	Statements of similarities and/or differences with marketed devices?		
21	Data to show consequences and effects of a modified device(s)?		

FIGURE 3-2 Sample FDA checklist

22	Additional information that is necessary under 21 CFR 807.87 (h)?		
23	Submitter's name and address?		
24	Contact person, telephone number, and fax number?		
25	Representative/consultant, if applicable?		
26	Table of contents, with pagination?		
27	Address of manufacturing facility/facilities and, if appropriate, sterilization site(s)?		
28	Additional information that may be necessary under 21 CFR 807.87 (h)?		
29	Comparison table of the new device to the marketed device?		
30	Action taken to comply with voluntary standards?		
31	Performance data:		
	Marketed device?		
	Bench testing?		
	Animal testing?		
	Clinical data?		
	New device?		
	Bench testing?		
	Animal testing?		
	Clinical data?		
32	Sterilization information?		
33	Software information?		
34	Hardware information?		
35	If this 510(k) is for a kit, has the kit certification statement been provided?		
36	Is this device subject to issues that have been addressed in specific guidance document(s)? If yes, continue review with checklist from any appropriate guidance document. If no, is 510(k) sufficiently complete to allow substantive review?		
37	Truthfulness certification?		
38	Other as required?		

FIGURE 3-2 Continued

option will allow the Agency to review modifications that do not affect the device's intended use or alter the device's fundamental scientific technology within this abbreviated time frame. The Agency does not believe that modifications that affect the intended use or alter the fundamental scientific technology of the device are appropriate for review under this type of application but rather should continue to be subject to the traditional 510(k) procedures.

To ensure the success of the Special 510(k) option, there must be a common understanding of the types of device modifications that may gain marketing clearance by this path. Therefore, it is critical that industry and Agency staff can easily determine whether a modification is appropriate for submission by this option. To optimize the chance that this option will be accepted and promptly cleared, manufacturers should evaluate each modification against the considerations described below to ensure that the particular change does not:

- Affect the intended use
- Alter the fundamental scientific technology of the device

3.4.3.1 Special 510(k) content

A Special 510(k) should include the following:

- A coversheet clearly identifying the application as a "Special 510(k): Device Modification"
- The name of the legally marketed (unmodified) device and the 510(k) number under which it was cleared
- Items required under paragraph 807.87, including a description of the modified device and a comparison to the cleared device, the intended use of the device, and the proposed labeling for the device
- A concise summary of the design control activities, including (1) an identification of the risk analysis method(s) used to assess the impact of the modification on the device and its components as well as the results of the analysis, (2) based on the risk analysis, an identification of the verification and/or validation activities required, including methods or tests used and the acceptance criteria applied, (3) a Declaration of Conformity with design controls. The Declaration of Conformity should include:
  - A statement that, as required by the risk analysis, all verification and validation activities were performed by the designated individual(s) and the results demonstrated that the predetermined acceptance criteria were met
  - A statement that the manufacturing facility is in conformance with the design control procedure requirements as specified in 21 CFR 820.30 and the records are available for review

The above two statements should be signed by the designated individual(s) responsible for those particular activities.

3.4.4 The ABBREVIATED 510(k)

Device manufacturers may choose to submit an Abbreviated 510(k) when:

- A guidance document exists
- A special control has been established, or
- The FDA has recognized a relevant consensus standard

An Abbreviated 510(k) submission must include the required elements identified in 21 CFR 807.87. In addition, manufacturers submitting an Abbreviated 510(k) that relies on a guidance document and/or special control(s) should include a summary report that describes how the guidance document and/or special control(s) were used during device development and testing. The summary report should include information regarding the manufacturer's efforts to conform with the guidance document and/or special control(s) and should outline any deviations. Persons submitting an Abbreviated 510(k) that relies on a recognized standard should provide the information described below (except for the summary report) and a declaration of conformity to the recognized standard.

In an Abbreviated 510(k), a manufacturer will also have the option of using a third party to assess conformance with the recognized standard. Under this scenario, the third party will perform a conformance assessment to the standard for the device manufacturer and should provide the manufacturer with a statement to this effect. Like a Special 510(k), the marketing application should include a declaration of conformity signed by the manufacturer, while the statement from the third party should be maintained in the Device Master Record pursuant to the Quality System Regulation. Responsibility for conformance with the recognized standard, however, rests with the manufacturer, not the third party.

The incentive for manufacturers to elect to provide summary reports on the use of guidance documents and/or special controls or declarations of conformity to recognized standards will be an expedited review of their submissions. While abbreviated submissions will compete with traditional 510(k) submissions, it is anticipated that their review will be more efficient than that of traditional 510(k) submissions, which tend to be data-intensive. In addition, by allowing ODE reviewers to rely on a manufacturer's summary report on the use of a guidance document and/or special controls and declarations of conformity with recognized standards, review resources can be directed at more complicated issues and thus should expedite the process.

3.4.4.1 Abbreviated 510(k) content

An Abbreviated 510(k) should include:

- A coversheet clearly identifying the application as an Abbreviated 510(k)
- Items required under paragraph 807.87, including a description of the device, the intended use of the device, and the proposed labeling for the device
- For a submission that relies on a guidance document and/or special control(s) that were used to address the risks associated with the

particular device type and for a submission that relies on a recognized standard, a declaration of conformity to the standard

- Data/information to address issues not covered by guidance documents, special controls, and/or recognized standards
- Indications for use enclosure

3.5 DECLARATION OF CONFORMANCE TO A RECOGNIZED STANDARD

Declarations of conformity to recognized standards should include the following information:

- An identification of the applicable recognized consensus standards that were met
- A specification, for each consensus standard, that all requirements were met, except for inapplicable requirements or deviations noted below
- An identification for each consensus standard, of any manner(s) in which the standard may have been adopted for application to the device under review (e.g., an identification of an alternative series of tests that were performed)
- An identification for each consensus standard of any requirements that were not applicable to the device
- A specification of any deviations from each applicable standard that were applied
- A specification of the differences that may exist, if any, between the tested device and the device to be marketed and a justification of the test results in these areas of difference
- The name and address of any test laboratory or certification body involved in determining the conformance of the device with the applicable consensus standards and a reference to any accreditations of those organizations

3.6 THE PMA APPLICATION

Pre-Market Approval (PMA) is an approval application for a Class III medical device, including all information submitted with or incorporated by reference. The purpose of the regulation is to establish an efficient and thorough device review process to facilitate the approval of PMAs for devices that have been shown to be safe and effective for their intended use and that otherwise meet the statutory criteria for approval, while ensuring the disapproval of PMAs for devices that have not been shown to be safe and effective or that do not otherwise meet the statutory criteria for approval.

3.6.1 THE PMA PROCESS

The first step in the PMAA process is the filing of the investigational device exemption (IDE) application for significant risk devices. The IDE is reviewed by the FDA and, once accepted, the sponsor can proceed with clinical trials.

3.6.2 CONTENTS OF A PMAA

Section 814.20 of 21 CFR defines what must be included in an application, including:

- Name and address
- Application procedures and table of contents
- Summary
- Complete device description
- Reference to performance standards
- Non-clinical and clinical investigations
- Justification for single investigator
- Bibliography
- Sample of device
- Proposed labeling
- Environmental assessment
- Other information

The summary should include indications for use, a device description, a description of alternative practices and procedures, a brief description of the marketing history, and a summary of studies. This summary should be of sufficient detail to enable the reader to gain a general understanding of the application. The PMAA must also include the applicant's foreign and domestic marketing history as well as any marketing history of a third party marketing the same product.

The description of the device should include a complete description of the device, including pictorial presentations. Each of the functional components or ingredients should be described, as well as the properties of the device relevant to the diagnosis, treatment, prevention, cure, or mitigation of a disease or condition. The principles of the device's operation should also be explained. Information regarding the methods used in, and the facilities and controls used for, the manufacture, processing, packing, storage, and installation of the device should be explained in sufficient detail so that a person generally familiar with current good manufacturing practices can make a knowledgeable judgement about the quality control used in the manufacture of the device.

To clarify which performance standards must be addressed, applicants may ask members of the appropriate reviewing division of the Office of Device Evaluation (ODE), or consult the FDA's list of relevant voluntary standards or the Medical Device Standards Activities Report.

3.7   INVESTIGATIONAL DEVICE EXEMPTIONS (IDEs)

The purpose of the Investigational Device Exemption regulation is to encourage the discovery and development of useful devices intended for human use while protecting the public health. It provides the procedures for the conduct of clinical investigations of devices. An approved IDE permits a device to be shipped lawfully for the purpose of conducting investigations of the device without complying with a performance standard or having marketing clearance.

3.7.1   INSTITUTIONAL REVIEW BOARDS (IRBs)

Any human research covered by Federal regulation will not be funded unless it has been reviewed by an IRB. The fundamental purpose of an IRB is to ensure that research activities are conducted in an ethical and legal manner. Specifically, IRBs are expected to ensure that each of the basic elements of informed consent, as defined by regulation, are included in the document presented to the research participant for signature or verbal approval.

The deliberations of the IRB must determine that:

- The risks to subjects are equitable
- The selection of subjects is equitable
- Informed consent will be sought from each prospective subject or their legally authorized representative
- Informed consent will be appropriately documented
- Where appropriate, the research plan makes adequate provision for monitoring the data collected to assure the safety of the subjects
- Where appropriate, there are adequate provisions to protect the privacy of subjects and to maintain the confidentiality of data

It is axiomatic that the IRB should ensure that the risks of participation in a research study should be minimized. The IRB must determine that this objective is to be achieved by ensuring that investigators use procedures that are consistent with sound research design and that they do not necessarily expose subjects to excessive risk. In addition, the IRB needs to assure that the investigators, whenever appropriate, minimize risk and discomfort to the research participants by using, where possible, procedures already performed on the subjects as part of routine diagnosis or treatment.

The Institutional Review Board is any board, committee, or other group formally designated by an institution to review, to approve the initiation of, and to conduct periodic review of biomedical research involving human subjects. The primary purpose of such review is to assure the protection of the rights and welfare of human subjects.

An IRB must comply with all applicable requirements of the IRB regulation and the IDE regulation in reviewing and approving device investigations involving human testing. An IRB has the authority to review and approve, require modification, or disapprove an investigation. If no IRB exists, or if the FDA finds an IRB's review to be inadequate, a sponsor may submit an application directly to the FDA.

An investigator is responsible for:

- Ensuring that the investigation is conducted according to the signed agreement, the investigational plan, and applicable FDA regulations
- Protecting the rights, safety, and welfare of subjects
- Control of the devices under investigation

An investigator is also responsible for obtaining informed consent and maintaining and making reports.

3.7.2 IDE FORMAT

There is no preprinted form for an IDE application, but the following information must be included in an IDE application for a significant risk device investigation. Generally, an IDE application should contain the following:

- Name and address of sponsor
- A complete report of prior investigations
- A description of the methods, facilities, and controls used for the manufacture, processing, packing, storage, and installation of the device
- An example of the agreements to be signed by the investigators and a list of the names and addresses of all investigators
- Certification that all investigators have signed the agreement, that the list of investigators includes all investigators participating in the study, and that new investigators will sign the agreement before being added to the study
- A list of the names, addresses, and chairpersons of all IRBs that have or will be asked to review the investigation and a certification of IRB action concerning the investigation
- The name and address of any institution (other than those above) where a part of the investigation may be conducted
- The amount, if any, charged for the device and an explanation of why sale does not constitute commercialization
- A claim for categorical exclusion or an environmental assessment
- Copies of all labeling for device
- Copies of all informed consent forms and all related information materials provided to subjects
- Any other relevant information that the FDA requests for review of the IDE application

3.8 GOOD LABORATORY PRACTICES (GLPs)

In 1978, the FDA adopted Good Laboratory Practices rules and implemented a laboratory audit and inspection procedure covering every regulated entity that conducts non-clinical laboratory studies for product safety and effectiveness. The GLPs were amended in 1984.

The GLP standard addresses all areas of laboratory operations, including requirements for a Quality Assurance Unit to conduct periodic internal inspections and keep records for audit and reporting purposes, Standard Operating Procedures (SOPs) for all aspects of each study and for all phases of laboratory maintenance, a formal mechanism for evaluation and approval of study protocols and their amendments, and reports of data in sufficient detail to support conclusions drawn from them. The FDA inspection program includes GLP compliance, and a data audit to verify that information submitted to the agency accurately reflects the raw data. Good Laboratory Practices are further discussed in Chapter 8.

3.9 GOOD MANUFACTURING PRACTICES (GMPs)

The FDA is authorized, under section 520(f) of the Act, to promulgate regulations detailing compliance with current good manufacturing practices. GMPs include the methods used in, and the facilities and controls used for, the manufacture, packing, storage and installation of a device. The GMP regulations were established as manufacturing safeguards to ensure the production of a safe and effective device and include all of the essential elements of a quality assurance program. Because manufacturers cannot test every device, the GMPs were established as a minimum standard of manufacturing to ensure that each device produced would be safe. If a product is not manufactured according to GMPs, even if it is later shown not to be a health risk, it is in violation of the Act and subject to FDA enforcement action.

The general objectives of the GMPs, not specific manufacturing methods, are found in Part 820 of the Code of Federal Regulations. The GMPs apply to the manufacture of every medical device. The GMP regulations give the FDA the authority to examine the design area of the product development cycle for the first time. The regulation also parallels very closely the ISO 9000 set of standards. GMPs are discussed in detail in Chapter 24.

3.10 HUMAN FACTORS

In April 1996, the FDA issued a draft primer on the use of human factors in medical device design, entitled *Do It By Design*. The purpose of the document was to improve the safety of medical devices by minimizing the likelihood of user error by systematic, careful design of the user interface, i.e., the hardware and software features that define the interaction between the users and the equipment. The document contains background information about human factors as a discipline, descriptions and illustrations of device problems, and a discussion of human factors methods. It also contains recommendations for manufacturers and health facilities.

As the source for this document, the FDA extensively used the guideline *Human Factors Engineering Guidelines and Preferred Practices for the Design of Medical Devices*, published by the Association for the Advancement of Medical Instrumentation, as well as interfacing with human factors consultants. It is expected that human factors requirements will become part of the product submission as well as the GMP inspection. Human factors engineering is discussed in detail in Chapter 19.

3.11 DESIGN CONTROL

With the publication of the new GMP regulations, the FDA will have the authority to cover design controls in their inspections. The FDA issued a draft guidance document in March, 1996, entitled *Design Control Guidance for Medical Device Manufacturers*. The purpose of the document was to provide readers with an understanding of what is meant by "control" in the context of the requirements. By providing an understanding of what constitutes control of a design process, readers could determine how to apply the concepts in a way that was both consistent with the requirements and best suited for their particular situation.

Three underlying concepts served as a foundation for the development of this guidance:

- The nature of the application of design controls for any device should be proportional to both the complexity of and the risks associated with that device
- The design process is a multifunctional one that involves other departments besides design and development if it is to work properly, thus involving senior management as an active participant in the process
- The product life cycle concept serves throughout the document as the framework for introducing and describing the design control activities and techniques

Design control concepts are applicable to process development as well as product development. The extent is dependent upon the nature of the product and processes used to manufacture the product. The safety and performance of a new product is also dependent on an intimate relationship between product design robustness and process capability.

The document covers the areas of:

* Risk management
* Design and development planning
* Organizational and technical interfaces
* Design input
* Design output
* Design review
* Design verification
* Design validation
* Design changes
* Design transfer

These topics are covered in detail in Sections 3, 4, 5, and 6.

3.12   THE FDA AND SOFTWARE

The subject of software in and as a medical device has become an important topic for the FDA. This interest began in 1985 when software in a radiation treatment therapy device is alleged to have resulted in a lethal overdose. The FDA then analyzed recalls by fiscal year (FY) to determine how many were caused by software problems. In FY 1985, for example, 20% of all neurology device recalls were attributable to software problems, while 8% of cardiovascular problems had the same cause. This type of analysis, along with the results of various corporate inspections, led the FDA to conclude that some type of regulation was required.

Since there are many types of software in use in the medical arena, the problem of the best way to regulate it has become an issue for the FDA. Discussions have centered on what type of software is a medical device, the type of regulation required for such software, and what could be inspected under current regulations. Agency concerns fall into three major categories: medical device software, software used in manufacturing, and software information systems used for clinical decision making.

For medical device software, the FDA is responsible for assuring that the device utilizing the software is safe and effective. It only takes a few alleged serious injuries or deaths to sensitize the Agency to a particular product or generic component that deserves attention. The Agency's review of medical device reporting (MDR) incidents and analysis of product recalls has convinced the Agency that software is a factor contributing to practical problems within devices.

When software is used during manufacturing, the FDA is concerned with whether or not the software controlling a tool or automatic tester is performing as expected. The FDA's perceptions are rooted in experiences with GMP inspections of pharmaceutical manufacturers, where computers are heavily depended upon for control of manufacturing processes. Although there are few incidents of device or manufacturing problems traceable to flaws in manufacturing software, GMP inspections have focused intensively on validation of software programs used in industry for the control of manufacturing operations.

With regard to stand-alone software used to aid clinical decision making, the FDA is concerned with hypothetical problems rather than extensive records of adverse incidents. While most commercially available health care information systems replace manual systems that had a far higher potential for errors, the FDA believes that regulations should apply to the kinds of systems that may influence clinical treatment or diagnoses. The FDA has observed academic work of "expert systems" used by medical professionals and is concerned that such systems may be commercialized without sufficient controls.

The FDA has published guidelines for developing quality software, off-the-shelf software, the requirements for product approval submissions 510(k) and the inspection of software-controlled test fixtures as a part of GMP inspections. They have also conducted training courses for their inspectors and submission reviewers on the subject of software and computer basics.

3.13 SOFTWARE CLASSIFICATION

When a computer product is a component, part, or accessory of a product recognized as a medical device in its own right, the computer component is regulated according to the requirements for the parent device unless the component of the device is separately classified. Computer products that are medical devices and not components, parts or accessories of other products that are themselves medical devices, are subject to one of three degrees of regulatory control depending on their characteristics. These products are regulated with the least degree of control necessary to provide reasonable assurance of safety and effectiveness. Computer products that are substantially equivalent to a device previously classified will be regulated to the same degree as the equivalent device. Those devices that are not substantially equivalent to a pre-amendment device or that are substantially equivalent to a Class III device are regulated as Class III devices.

Medical software is divided into three classes with regulatory requirements specific to each:

- Class I software is subject to the Act's general controls relating to such matters as misbranding, registration of manufacturers, record keeping, and good manufacturing practices. An example of Class I software would be a program that calculates the composition of infant formula
- Class II software is that for which general controls are insufficient to provide reasonable assurance of safety and effectiveness and for which performance standards can provide assurance. This is

exemplified by a computer program designed to produce radiation therapy treatment plans

- Class III software is that for which insufficient information exists to assure that general controls and performance standards will provide reasonable assurance of safety and effectiveness. Generally, these devices are represented to be life-sustaining or life-supporting and may be intended for a use that is of substantial importance in preventing impairment to health. They may be implanted in the body or present a potential unreasonable risk of illness or injury. A program that measures glucose levels and calculates and dispenses insulin based upon those calculations without physician intervention would be a Class III device

3.14 THE FDA INSPECTION

The FDA's power to inspect originates in Section 704 of the Federal Food, Drug, and Cosmetic Act. This provision allow FDA officials to inspect any factory, warehouse, or establishment in which devices are manufactured, processed, packed or held, for introduction into interstate commerce after such introduction. In addition to the "establishments" specification, FDA is permitted to enter any vehicle used to transport or hold regulated products for export or in interstate commerce. The inspection power is specifically extended to medical device manufacturers by Sections 519 and 520 of the Federal Food, Drug, and Cosmetic Act.

Every FDA inspector is authorized by law to inspect all equipment that is used in the manufacturing process. Furthermore, investigators may examine finished and unfinished devices and device components, containers, labeling for regulated products, and all documents that are required to be kept by the regulations, such as device master records and device history records.

Despite the broad inspectional authority over restricted devices, the statute provides that, regardless of the device's unrestricted status, certain information is excluded from the FDA's inspectional gambit. The kind of information to which the FDA does not have access includes financial data, sales data, and pricing data. The new GMPs give the FDA authority to inspect the design area and the qualifications of personnel in all aspects of the product development process.

3.15 ADVICE ON DEALING WITH THE FDA

Several recommendations can be made regarding how to deal with the FDA and its regulatory process. None of these bits of advice is dramatic or new, but in the course of observing a firm's interaction with the agency, it is amazing how many times the failure to think of these steps can result in significant difficulties.

Know your district office. This may not be an easy thing to accomplish, since, understandably, there is a great reluctance to walk into a regulatory agency and indicate you are there to get acquainted. As opportunities arise, however, they should not be overlooked. Situations such as responding to a notice of an investigator's observations at the conclusion of an inspection or a notice of adverse findings letter are excellent opportunities to hand deliver a reply instead of simply mailing it. The verbal discussion with the reply may make the content much more meaningful and will allow both sides to learn more about the intent and seriousness with which the subject is being approached.

Prepare for inspections. When the FDA investigator walks into your manufacturing facility or corporate offices, there should be a procedure established that everyone is familiar with as to who is called, who escorts the investigator through the facility, who is available to make copies of records requested, etc. A corollary to this suggestion is to be prepared to deal with adverse inspectional findings or other communications from the agency that indicate the FDA has found violations, a serious health hazard, or other information that requires high-level company knowledge and decision making.

Take seriously 483's and letters. Many regulatory actions are processed with no apparent indication that a firm seriously considered the violations noted by the agency.

Keep up with current events and procedures of the FDA. This will minimize the changes or surprise interpretations that could have an effect on a firm's operations and will allow for advance planning for new FDA requirements. The Agency publishes much of its new program information in bulletins and other broad distribution documents, but much more can be learned from obtaining copies of the FDA Compliance Policy Guides and Compliance Programs.

Let the FDA know of your firm's opinions on issues, whether they are in the development state at the Agency or are policies or programs established and in operation. The Agency does recognize that the firms it regulates are the true experts in device manufacturing and distribution, and their views are important. The Agency also recognizes that the regulation of manufacturers in not the only bottom line – solving public health problems is equally or more important, and there are generally many ways to solve those problems.

REFERENCES

Banta, H.D., The regulation of medical devices, *Preventive Medicine*, 19(6), 1990.

Basile, E., Overview of current FDA requirements for medical devices, in *The Medical Device Industry: Science, Technology, and Regulation in a Competitive Environment*, Marcel Dekker, Inc., New York, 1990.

Basile, E.M. and Prease A.J., Compiling a successful PMA application, in *The Medical Device Industry: Science, Technology, and Regulation in a Competitive Environment*, Marcel Dekker, Inc., New York, 1990.

Bureau of Medical Devices, Office of Small Manufacturers Assistance, *Regulatory Requirements for Marketing a Device*, U.S. Department of Health and Human Services, Washington, DC, 1982.

Center for Devices and Radiological Health, *Device Good Manufacturing Practices Manual*, U.S. Department of Health and Human Services, Washington, DC, 1987.

Food and Drug Administration, *Federal Food, Drug and Cosmetic Act, as amended January, 1979*, U.S. Government Printing Office, Washington, DC, 1979.

Food and Drug Administration, *Guide to the Inspection of Computerized Systems in Drug Processing*, Food and Drug Administration, Washington, DC, 1983.

Food and Drug Administration, *FDA Policy for the Regulation of Computer Products (Draft)*, Federal Register, Washington, DC, 1987.

Food and Drug Administration, *Software Development Activities*, Food and Drug Administration, Washington, DC, 1987.

Food and Drug Administration, *Medical Devices GMP Guidance for FDA Inspectors*, Food and Drug Administration, Washington, DC, 1987.

Food and Drug Administration, *Reviewer Guidance for Computer-Controlled Medical Devices (Draft)*, Food and Drug Administration, Washington, DC, 1988.

Food and Drug Administration, *Investigational Device Exemptions Manual*, Center for Devices and Radiological Health, Rockville, MD, 1992.

Food and Drug Administration, *Premarket Notification 510(k): Regulatory Requirements for Medical Devices*, Center for Devices and Radiological Health, Rockville, MD, 1992.

Food and Drug Administration, *Premarket Approval (PMA) Manual*, Center for Devices and Radiological Health, Rockville, MD, 1993.

Food and Drug Administration, *Design Control Guidance for Medical Device Manufacturers*, Draft, Center for Devices and Radiological Health, Rockville, MD, 1996.

Food and Drug Administration, *Do It By Design: An Introduction to Human Factors in Medical Devices, Draft*, Center for Devices and Radiological Health, Rockville, MD, 1996.

Fries, R.C., *Reliable Design of Medical Devices*, Marcel-Dekker, Inc., New York, 1997.

Fries, R.C., *Medical Device Quality Assurance and Regulatory Compliance*, Marcel-Dekker, Inc., New York, 1998.

Fries, R.C., *Handbook of Medical Device Design*, Marcel-Dekker, Inc., New York, 2001.

Fries, R.C., et al, Software regulation, in *The Medical Device Industry: Science, Technology, and Regulation in a Competitive Environment*, Marcel-Dekker, Inc., New York, 1990.

Ginzburg, H.M., Protection of research subjects in clinical research, in *Legal Aspects of Medicine*, Springer-Verlag, New York, 1989.

Gundaker, W.E., FDA's regulatory program for medical devices and diagnostics, *The Medical Device Industry: Science, Technology, and Regulation in a Competitive Environment*, Marcel-Dekker, Inc., New York, 1990.

Holstein, H.M., How to Submit a Successful 510(k), in *The Medical Device Industry: Science, Technology, and Regulation in a Competitive Environment*, Marcel-Dekker, Inc., New York, 1990.

Jorgens III, J., Computer hardware and software as medical devices, *Medical Device and Diagnostic Industry*, May, 1983.

Jorgens III, J. and Burch, C.W., FDA regulation of computerized medical devices, *Byte* 7, 1982.

Jorgens III, J. and Schneider, R., Regulation of medical software by the FDA, *Software in Health Care*, April–May, 1985.

Kahan, J.S., Regulation of computer hardware and software as medical devices, *Canadian Computer Law Reporter*, 6(3), January, 1987.

King, P.H. and Fries, R.C., *Design of Biomedical Devices and Systems*, Marcel-Dekker, Inc., New York, 2002.

Munsey, R.R. and Holstein, H.M., FDA/GMP/MDR inspections: obligations and rights, in *The Medical Device Industry: Science, Technology, and Regulation in a Competitive Environment*, Marcel-Dekker, Inc., New York, 1990.

Office of Technology Assessment, Federal Policies and the Medical Devices Industry, U.S. Government Printing Office, Washington, DC, 1984.

Sheretz, R.J. and Streed, S.A., Medical devices – significant risk vs nonsignificant risk, *Journal of the American Medical Association*, 272(12), September 28, 1994.

Trull, F.L. and Rich, B.A., The animal testing issue, in *The Medical Device Industry: Science, Technology, and Regulation in a Competitive Environment*, Marcel-Dekker, Inc., New York, 1990.

U.S. Congress, House Committee on Interstate and Foreign Commerce, *Medical Devices*, Hearings before the Subcommittee on Public Health and the Environment, October 23–24, 1973, Serial Numbers 93–61, U.S. Government Printing Office, Washington, DC, 1973.

Wholey, M.H. and Hailer, J.D., An introduction to the Food and Drug Administration and how it evaluates new devices: establishing safety and efficacy, *CardioVascular and Interventional Radiology*, 18(2), March/April, 1995.

4 The Medical Devices Directives

CONTENTS

4.1	Definition of a medical device		54
4.2	The Medical Devices Directives process		55
4.3	Choosing the appropriate directive		56
	4.3.1	Active Implantable Medical Devices Directive (AIMDD)	56
	4.3.2	Medical Devices Directive (MDD)	56
	4.3.3	*In Vitro* Diagnostic Medical Devices Directive (IVDMDD)	56
4.4	Identifying the applicable essential requirements		56
4.5	Identification of corresponding harmonized standards		58
4.6	Assurance that the device meets the essential requirements and harmonized standards and documentation of the evidence		59
	4.6.1	Essential requirement 1	59
		4.6.1.1 Hazard analysis	60
		4.6.1.2 Safety review	61
	4.6.2	Essential requirement 2	62
		4.6.2.1 Peer review	62
		4.6.2.2 Safety review	62
	4.6.3	Essential requirement 3	62
		4.6.3.1 Specification reviews	62
		4.6.3.2 Validation testing	62
	4.6.4	Essential requirement 4	63
		4.6.4.1 Environmental testing	63
		4.6.4.2 Environmental stress screening	63
		4.6.4.3 Use/misuse evaluation	64
4.7	Classification of the device		64
4.8	Decision on the appropriate conformity assessment procedure		66
	4.8.1	Medical Devices Directive	66
		4.8.1.1 Annex II	66
		4.8.1.2 Annex III	66
		4.8.1.3 Annex IV	66
		4.8.1.4 Annex V	66
		4.8.1.5 Annex VI	67

                4.8.1.6   Annex VII 67
                4.8.1.7   Class I 67
                4.8.1.8   Class IIa 67
                4.8.1.9   Class IIb 67
                4.8.1.10 Class III 67
        4.8.2   Active Implantable Medical Devices Directive 68
                4.8.2.1   Alternative 1 68
                4.8.2.2   Alternative 2 68
        4.8.3   *In Vitro* Diagnostic Medical Devices Directive 68
  4.9   Type testing 68
  4.10 Identification and choice of a Notified Body 69
  4.11 Establishing a declaration of conformity 72
  4.12 Application of the CE mark 73
  4.13 Conclusion 74
  References 74

The European Community's program on the Completion of the Internal Market has, as the primary objective for medical devices, to assure Community-wide free circulation of products. The only means to establish such free circulation, in view of quite divergent national systems, regulations governing medical devices, and existing trade barriers, was to adopt legislation for the Community, by which the health and safety of patients, users and third persons, would be ensured through a harmonized set of device related protection requirements. Devices meeting the requirements and sold to members of the Community are identified by means of a CE mark.

The Active Implantable Medical Devices Directive adopted by the Community legislator in 1990 and the Medical Devices Directive in 1993 cover more than 80% of medical devices for use with human beings. After a period of transition, i.e., a period during which the laws implementing a directive co-exist with pre-existing national laws, these directives exhaustively govern the conditions for placing medical devices on the market. Through the agreements on the European Economic Area (EEA), the relevant requirements and procedures are the same for all European Community (EC) member states and European Free Trade Association (EFTA) countries that belong to the EEA, an economic area comprising more than 380 million people.

4.1 DEFINITION OF A MEDICAL DEVICE

The various Medical Device Directives define a medical device as:

"any instrument, appliance, apparatus, material or other article, whether used alone or in combination, including the software necessary for its proper application, intended by the manufacturer to be used for human beings for the purpose of:

- Diagnosis, prevention, monitoring, treatment or alleviation of disease
- Diagnosis, monitoring, alleviation of or compensation for an injury or handicap
- Investigation, replacement or modification of the anatomy or of a physiological process
- Control of conception

and which does not achieve its principal intended action in or on the human body by pharmacological, immunological or metabolic means, but which may be assisted in its function by such means."

One important feature of the definition is that it emphasizes the "intended use" of the device and its "principal intended action." This use of the term "intended" gives manufacturers of certain products some opportunity to include or exclude their product from the scope of the particular directive.

Another important feature of the definition is the inclusion of the term "software." The software definition will probably be given further interpretation, but is currently interpreted to mean that (1) software intended to control the function of a device is a medical device, (2) software for patient records or other administrative purposes is not a device, (3) software which is built into a device, e.g., software in an electrocardiograph monitor used to drive a display, is clearly an integral part of the medical device, (4) a software update sold by the manufacturer, or a variation sold by a software house, is a medical device in its own right.

4.2   THE MEDICAL DEVICES DIRECTIVES PROCESS

The process of meeting the requirements of the Medical Devices Directives is a multi-step approach, involving the following activities:

- Analyze the device to determine which directive is applicable
- Identify the applicable Essentials Requirements List
- Identify any corresponding Harmonized Standards
- Confirm that the device meets the Essential Requirements/ Harmonized Standards and document the evidence
- Classify the device
- Decide on the appropriate conformity assessment procedure
- Identify and choose a notified body
- Obtain conformity certifications for the device
- Establish a Declaration of Conformity
- Apply for the CE mark

This process does not necessarily occur in a serial manner, but iterations may occur throughout the cycle. Each activity in the process will be examined in detail.

4.3   CHOOSING THE APPROPRIATE DIRECTIVE

Because of the diversity of current national medical device regulations, the Commission decided that totally new Community legislation covering all medical devices was needed. Software or a medical device containing software may be subject to the requirements of the Active Implantable Medical Devices Directive or the Medical Devices Directive.

Three directives are envisaged to cover the entire field of medical devices.

4.3.1   ACTIVE IMPLANTABLE MEDICAL DEVICES DIRECTIVE (AIMDD)

This directive applies to a medical device which depends on a source of electrical energy or any source of power other than that directly generated by the human body or gravity, which is intended to be totally or partially introduced, surgically or medically, into the human body or by medical intervention into a natural orifice, and which is intended to remain after the procedure.

This directive was adopted in June, 1990, implemented in January, 1993, and the transition period ended January, 1995.

4.3.2   MEDICAL DEVICES DIRECTIVE (MDD)

This directive applies to all medical devices and accessories, unless they are covered by the Active Implantable Medical Devices Directive or the *In Vitro* Diagnostic Medical Devices Directive.

This directive was adopted in June, 1993, was implemented in January, 1995, and the transition period ended June, 1998.

4.3.3   *IN VITRO* DIAGNOSTIC MEDICAL DEVICES DIRECTIVE (IVDMDD)

This directive applies to any medical device that is a reagent, reagent product, calibrator, control kit, instrument, equipment or system intended to be used in vitro for the examination of samples derived from the human body for the purpose of providing information concerning a physiological state of health or disease or congenital abnormality, or to determine the safety and compatibility with potential recipients.

4.4   IDENTIFYING THE APPLICABLE ESSENTIAL REQUIREMENTS

The major legal responsibility the directives place on the manufacturer of a medical device requires the device meet the Essential Requirements set out in Annex I of the directive which applies to them, taking into account the intended purpose of the device. The Essential Requirements are written in the form of (1) general requirements, which always apply and (2) particular requirements, only some of which apply to any particular device.

The general requirements for the Essential Requirements List take the following form:

- The device must be safe. Any risk must be acceptable in relation to the benefits offered by the device
- The device must be designed in such a manner that risk is eliminated or protected against
- The device must perform in accordance with the manufacturer's specification
- The safety and performance must be maintained throughout the indicated lifetime of the device
- The safety and performance of the device must not be affected by normal conditions of transport and storage
- Any side effects must be acceptable in relation to the benefits offered

The particular requirements for the Essential Requirements List address the following topics:

- Chemical, physical, and biological properties
- Infection and microbial contamination
- Construction and environmental properties
- Devices with a measuring function
- Protection against radiation
- Requirements for devices connected to or equipped with an energy source
- Protection against electrical risks
- Protection against mechanical and thermal risks
- Protection against the risks posed to the patient by energy supplies or substances
- Information supplied by the manufacturer

The easiest method of assuring the Essential Requirements are met is to establish a checklist of the Essential Requirements from Appendix I of the appropriate directive, which then forms the basis of the technical dossier. Figure 4-1 is an example of an Essential Requirements checklist.

The Essential Requirements checklist includes (1) a statement of the Essential Requirements, (2) an indication of the applicability of the Essential Requirements to a particular device, (3) a list of the standards used to address the Essential Requirements, (4) the activity that addresses the Essential Requirements, (5) the clause(s) in the standard detailing the applicable test for the particular Essential Requirement, (6) an indication of whether the device passed/or failed the test and (7) a statement of the location of the test documentation or certificates.

Essential requirement	A or N/A	Standards	Activity	Test clause	Pass/Fail	Document location
1. The device must be designed and manufactured in such a way that, when used under the conditions and for the purposes intended, they will not compromise the clinical condition or the safety of patients, users and, where applicable, other persons. The risks associated with devices must be reduced to an acceptable level compatible with a high level of protection for health and safety.	A	Internal	Risk analysis Safety review			Design history file Design history file
2. The solutions adopted by the manufacturer for the design and construction of the devices must comply with safety principles and also take into account the generally acknowledged state of the art.	A	Internal	Specification reviews Design reviews Safety reviews			Design history file Design history file Design history file

FIGURE 4-1 Sample Essential Requirements List

4.5 IDENTIFICATION OF CORRESPONDING HARMONIZED STANDARDS

A "harmonized" standard is a standard produced under a mandate from the European Commission by one of the European standardization organizations such as CEN (the European Committee for Standardization) and CENELEC (the European Committee for Electrotechnical Standardization), and which has its reference published in the *Official Journal of the European Communities*.

The Essential Requirements are worded such that they identify a risk and state that the device should be designed and manufactured so that the risk is avoided or minimized. The technical detail for assuring these requirements is to be found in Harmonized Standards. Manufacturers must therefore identify the Harmonized Standards corresponding to the Essential Requirements that apply to their device.

With regard to choosing such standards, the manufacturer must be aware of the hierarchy of standards that have been developed:

- *Horizontal standards* Generic standards covering fundamental requirements common to all, or a very wide range of medical devices.
- *Semi-horizontal standards* Group standards that deal with requirements applicable to a group of devices.
- *Vertical standards* Product-specific standards that give requirements to one device or a very small group of devices.

Manufacturers must give particular attention to the horizontal standards since, because of their general nature, they apply to almost all devices. As these standards come into use for almost all products, they will become extremely powerful.

TABLE 4-1
Important harmonized and EMC standards

Standard	Areas covered
EN 60 601 Series	Medical electrical equipment
EN 29000 Series	Quality systems
EN 46000 Series	Quality systems
EN 55011 (CISPR 11)	EMC/Emission
EN 60801 Series	EMC/Immunity
EN 540	Clinical investigation of medical devices
EN 980	Symbols on medical equipment
IEC 601-1-2	Medical device emission and immunity
IEC 801-2	Electrostatic discharge
IEC 801-2	Immunity to radiated radio frequency electromagnetic fields
IEC 801-4	Fast transients/burst
IEC 801-5	Voltage surge immunity

Semi-horizontal standards may be particularly important as they have virtually the same weight as horizontal standards for groups of devices, such as orthopedic implants, IVDs, or X-ray equipment.

Vertical standards might well be too narrow to cope with new technological developments when a question of a specific feature of a device arises.

Table 4-1 lists some common harmonized standards for medical devices and medical device electromagnetic compatibility standards.

4.6   ASSURANCE THAT THE DEVICE MEETS THE ESSENTIAL REQUIREMENTS AND HARMONIZED STANDARDS AND DOCUMENTATION OF THE EVIDENCE

Once the Essential Requirements List has been developed and the harmonized standards chosen, the activity necessary to address the Essential Requirements List must be conducted. Taking the activity on the Essential Requirements checklist from Figure 4-1, the following activity may be conducted to assure the requirements are met.

4.6.1   ESSENTIAL REQUIREMENT 1

This requirement is concerned with the device not compromising the clinical condition or the safety of patient, users and, where applicable, other persons.

The methods used to meet this requirement are the conduction of a hazard analysis and a safety review.

4.6.1.1 Hazard analysis

A hazard analysis is the process, continuous throughout the product development cycle, that examines the possible hazards that could occur due to equipment failure and helps the designer to eliminate the hazard through various control methods. The hazard analysis is conducted on hardware, software, and the total system during the initial specification phase and is updated throughout the development cycle. The hazard analysis is documented on a form similar to that shown in Figure 4-2.

The hazard analysis addresses the following issues:

- Potential hazard: identifies possible harm to patient, operator, or system
- Generic cause: identifies general conditions that can lead to the associated Potential Hazard
- Specific cause: identifies specific instances that can give rise to the associated Generic Cause
- Probability: classifies the likelihood of the associated Potential Hazard according to Table 4-2
- Severity: categorizes the associated Potential Hazard according to Table 4-3
- Control mode: Means of reducing the probability and/or severity of the associated Potential Hazard
- Control method: Actual implementation to achieve the associated Control Mode
- Comments: Additional information, references, etc.

When the hazard analysis is initially completed, the probability and severity refer to the potential hazard prior to its being controlled. As the device is designed to minimize or eliminate the hazard, and control methods are imposed, the probability and severity will be updated.

Potential hazard	Generic cause	Specific cause	Probability	Severity	Control mode	Control method	Comments

FIGURE 4-2 Sample Hazard Analysis Form

TABLE 4-2
Hazard Analysis Probability classification

Classification indicator	Classification rating	Classification meaning
1	Frequent	Likely to occur often
2	Occasional	Will occur several times in the life of the system
3	Reasonably remote	Likely to occur sometime in the life of the system
4	Remote	Unlikely to occur, but possible
5	Extremely remote	Probability of occurrence indistinguishable from zero
6	Physically impossible	

TABLE 4-3
Hazard Analysis Severity classification

Severity indicator	Severity rating	Severity meaning
I	Catastrophic	May cause death or system loss
II	Critical	May cause severe injury, severe occupational illness or severe system damage
III	Marginal	May cause minor injury, minor occupational illness, or minor system damage
IV	Negligible	Will not result in injury, illness, or system damage

An organization separate from R&D, such as Quality Assurance, reviews the device to assure it is safe and effective for its intended use. The device, when operated according to specification, must not cause a hazard to the user or the patient. In the conduction of this review, the following may be addressed.

4.6.1.2 Safety review

- Pertinent documentation such as drawings, test reports, and manuals
- A sample of the device
- A checklist specific to the device, which may include:
  - Voltages
  - Operating frequencies
  - Leakage currents
  - Dielectric withstand
  - Grounding impedance
  - Power cord and plug
  - Electrical insulation
  - Physical stability

- Color coding
- Circuit breakers and fuses
- Alarms, warnings and indicators
- Mechanical design integrity

The checklist is signed by the reviewing personnel following the analysis.

4.6.2 ESSENTIAL REQUIREMENT 2

This requirement is concerned with the device complying with safety principles and the generally acknowledged state of the art.

The methods used to meet this requirement are peer reviews and the safety review.

4.6.2.1 Peer review

Peer review of the Product Specification, Design Specification, Software Requirements Specification and the actual design are conducted using qualified individuals not directly involved in the development of the device. The review is attended by individuals from Design, Reliability, Quality Assurance, Regulatory Affairs, Marketing, Manufacturing, and Service. Each review is documented with issues discussed and action items. After the review, the project team assigns individuals to address each action item and a schedule for completion.

4.6.2.2 Safety review

This was discussed under Essential Requirement 1.

4.6.3 ESSENTIAL REQUIREMENT 3

This requirement is concerned with the device achieving the performance intended by the manufacturer.

The methods used to meet this requirement are the various specification reviews and the validation of the device to meet these specifications.

4.6.3.1 Specification reviews

This was discussed under Essential Requirement 2.

4.6.3.2 Validation testing

This activity involves assuring that the design and the product meet the appropriate specifications that were developed at the beginning of the development process. Testing is conducted to address each requirement in the specification and the test plan and test results documented. It is helpful to develop a requirements matrix to assist in this activity.

4.6.4 ESSENTIAL REQUIREMENT 4

This requirement is concerned with the device being adversely affected by stresses which can occur during normal conditions of use.

The methods used to meet this requirement are environmental testing, Environmental Stress Screening (ESS), and Use/Misuse Evaluation.

4.6.4.1 Environmental testing

Testing is conducted according to Environmental Specifications listed for the product. Table 4-4 lists the environmental testing to be conducted and the corresponding standards and methods employed. Test results are documented.

4.6.4.2 Environmental stress screening

The device is subjected to temperature and vibration stresses beyond that which the device may ordinarily see in order to precipitate failures. The failure may then be designed out of the device before it is produced. ESS is conducted according to a specific protocol which is developed for the particular device. Care must be taken in preparing the protocol to avoid causing failures which would not ordinarily be anticipated. Results of the ESS analysis are documented.

TABLE 4-4
List of environmental testing

Environmental test	Specification range	Applicable standard
Operating temperature	5 to 35°C	IEC 68-2-14
Storage temperature	−40 to +65°C	IEC 68-2-1-Ab
		IEC 68-2-2-Bb
Operating humidity	15 to 95% RH non-condensing	IEC 68-2-30
Operating pressure	500 to 797 mmHg	IEC 68-2-13
Storage pressure	87 to 797 mmHg	IEC 68-2-13
Radiated electrical emissions	System: 4 dB margin	CISPR 11
	Subsystem: 15 dB	
Radiated magnetic emissions	System: 4 dB margin	VDE 871
	Subsystem: 6 dB	
Linc conducted emissions	System: 2 dB margin	CISPR 11
	Subsystem: 2 dB	VDE 871
Electrostatic discharge	Contact: 7 KV	EN 60601-2
	Air: 10 KV	EN 1000-4-2
Radiated electric field immunity	5 V/m @ 1 KHz	EN 60601-2
		EN 1000-4-3
Electrical fast transient immunity	Power mains: 2.4 KV	EN 60601-2
	Cables > 3m: 1.2 KV	EN 1000-4-4
Stability		UL 2601
Transportation		NSTA Preshipment
Transportation		NSTA Overseas

4.6.4.3 Use/misuse evaluation

Whether through failure to properly read the operation manual or through improper training, medical devices are going to be misused and even abused. There are many stories of product misuse, such as the hand-held monitor that was dropped into a toilet bowl, the physician who hammered a 9-volt battery in backwards and then reported the device was not working, or the user that spilled a can of soda on and into a device.

Practically, it is impossible to make a device completely immune to misuse, but it is highly desirable to design around the misuse situations than can be anticipated. These include:

- Excess application of cleaning solutions
- Physical abuse
- Spills
- Excess weight applied to certain parts of the device
- Excess torque applied to controls or screws
- Improper voltages, frequencies, or pressures
- Interchangeable electrical or pneumatic connections

Each potential misuse situation should be evaluated for its possible result on the device and a decision made on whether the result can be designed out. Activities similar to these are carried out to complete the remainder of the Essential Requirements checklist for the device.

4.7 CLASSIFICATION OF THE DEVICE

It is necessary for the manufacturer of a medical device to have some degree of proof that a device complies with the Essential Requirements before the CE marking can be applied. This is defined as a "conformity assessment procedure." For devices applicable to the AIMDD, there are two alternatives for the conformity assessment procedure. For devices applicable to the IVDMDD, there is a single conformity assessment procedure. For devices applicable to the MDD, there is no conformity assessment procedure that is suitable for all products, as the directive covers all medical devices. Medical devices are therefore divided into four classes, which have specific conformity assessment procedures for each of the four classes.

It is crucial for manufacturers to determine the class into which each of their devices falls. This demands careful study of the Classification Rules given in Annex IX of the directive. As long as the intended purpose, the implementing rules and the definitions are clearly understood, the classification process is straightforward and the rules, which are laid out in a logical order, can be worked out in succession from Rule 1. If the device is used for more than one intended purpose, then it must be classified according to the one which gives the highest classification.

The rules for determining the appropriate classification of a medical device include:

Rule	Type of device	Class
1–4	Non-invasive devices are in Class I except:	
	use for storing body fluids connected to an active medical device in	IIa
	Class IIa or higher	IIa
	modification of body fluids	IIa/IIb
	some wound dressings	IIa/IIb
5	Devices invasive with respect to body orifices:	
	transient use	I
	short-term use	IIa
	long-term use	IIb
6–8	Surgically invasive devices:	
	re-usable surgical instruments	I
	transient or short-term use	IIa
	long-term use	IIb
	contact with CCS or CNS	III
	devices which are absorbable or have a biological effect	IIb/III
	devices which deliver medicines	IIb/III
	devices applying ionizing radiation	IIb
13	Devices incorporating medicinal products	III
14	Contraceptive devices	IIB/III
15	Chemicals used for cleaning or disinfecting:	
	medical devices	IIa
	contact lenses	IIb
16	Devices specifically intended for recording	
	X-ray images	IIa
17	Devices made from animal tissues	III
18	Blood bags	IIb

In the cases of active devices, the rules are based mainly on the purpose of the device, i.e., diagnosis or therapy, and the corresponding possibility of absorption of energy by the patient:

Rule	Type of device	Class
9	Therapeutic devices administering or exchanging energy	IIa
	if operating in a potentially hazardous way	IIb
10	Diagnostic devices:	
	supplying energy other than illumination	IIa
	imaging radiopharmaceuticals in vivo	IIa
	diagnosing/monitoring vital functions	IIa
	monitoring vital functions in critical care conditions	IIb
	emitting ionizing radiation	IIb
11	Active devices administering/removing medicines/body substances	IIa
	if operating in a potentially hazardous way	IIb
12	All other active devices	I

In order to use the classification system correctly, manufacturers must have a good understanding of the implementing rules and definitions.

The key implementing rules include:

- Application of the Classification Rules is governed by the intended purpose of the device
- If the device is intended to be used in combination with another device, the Classification Rules are applied separately to each device
- Accessories are classified in their own right, separately from the device with which they are used
- Software, which drives a device or influences the use of a device, falls automatically in the same class as the device itself

4.8   DECISION ON THE APPROPRIATE CONFORMITY ASSESSMENT PROCEDURE

4.8.1   MEDICAL DEVICES DIRECTIVE

There are six conformity assessment Annexes to the Medical Devices Directive. Their use for the different classes of devices is specified in Article 11 of the Directive.

4.8.1.1   Annex II

This Annex describes the system of full quality assurance covering both the design and manufacture of devices.

4.8.1.2   Annex III

This Annex describes the type examination procedure according to which the manufacturer submits full technical documentation of the product, together with a representative sample of the device to a Notified Body.

4.8.1.3   Annex IV

This Annex describes the examination by the Notified Body of every individual product, or one or more samples from every production batch, and the testing which may be necessary to show the conformity of the products with the approved/documented design.

4.8.1.4   Annex V

This Annex describes a production quality system which is to be verified by a Notified Body as assuring that devices are made in accordance with an approved type, or in accordance with technical documentation describing the device.

4.8.1.5 Annex VI

This Annex describes a quality system covering final inspection and testing of products to ensure that devices are made in accordance with an approved type, or in accordance with technical documentation.

4.8.1.6 Annex VII

This Annex describes the technical documentation that the manufacturer must compile in order to support a declaration of conformity for a medical device, where there is no participation of a Notified Body in the process.

The class to which the medical device is assigned has an influence on the type of conformity assessment procedure chosen.

4.8.1.7 Class I

Compliance with the Essential Requirements must be shown in technical documentation compiled according to Annex VII of the Directive.

4.8.1.8 Class IIa

The design of the device and its compliance with the Essential Requirements must be established in technical documentation described in Annex VII. However, for this Class, agreement of production units with the technical documentation must be assured by a notified Body according to one of the following alternatives:

- sample testing   Annex IV
- an audited production quality system   Annex V
- an audited product quality system   Annex VI

4.8.1.9 Class IIb

The design and manufacturing procedures must be approved by a Notified Body as satisfying Annex II, or the design must be shown to conform to the Essential Requirements by a type examination (Annex III) carried out by a Notified Body.

4.8.1.10 Class III

The procedures for this Class are similar to Class IIb, but significant differences are that, when the quality system route is used, a design dossier for each type of device must be examined by the Notified Body. Clinical data relating to safety and performance must be included in the design dossier or the documentation presented for the type examination.

4.8.2 ACTIVE IMPLANTABLE MEDICAL DEVICES DIRECTIVE

For devices following the AIMDD, Annexes II through V cover the various conformity assessment procedures available. There are two alternative procedures.

4.8.2.1 Alternative 1

A manufacturer must have in place a full quality assurance system for design and production and must submit a design dossier on each type of device to the Notified Body for review.

4.8.2.2 Alternative 2

A manufacturer submits an example of each type of his device to a Notified Body, satisfactory production must be assured by either the quality system at the manufacturing site or must comply with EN 29002 + EN 46002 and must be audited by a Notified Body, or samples of the product must be tested by a Notified Body.

4.8.3 IN VITRO DIAGNOSTIC MEDICAL DEVICES DIRECTIVE

For devices adhering to the IVDMDD, the conformity assessment procedure is a manufacturer's declaration. In vitro devices for self testing must additionally have a design examination by a Notified Body, or be designed and manufactured in accordance with a quality system.

In choosing a conformity assessment procedure it is important to remember that (1) it is essential to determine the classification of a device before deciding on a conformity assessment procedure, (2) it may be more efficient to operate one conformity assessment procedure throughout a manufacturing plant, even though this procedure may be more rigorous than strictly necessary for some products, and (3) tests and assessments carried out under current national regulations can contribute towards the assessment of conformity with the requirements of the directives.

4.9 TYPE TESTING

A manufacturer of Class IIb or Class III medical devices can choose to demonstrate that his device meets the Essential Requirements by submitting to a Notified Body for a type examination as described in Annex III of the Directive. The manufacturer is required to submit technical documentation on his device, together with an example of the device. The Notified Body will then carry out such tests as it considers necessary to satisfy itself, before issuing the EC Type Examination Certificate.

Type testing of many kinds of medical devices, particularly electromedical equipment, is required under some current national regulations. Manufacturers who are familiar with this process and who have established relations with test houses which are, or will be, appointed as Notified Bodies, are likely to find this a more attractive procedure than the design control procedures of EN29001/EN46001. Existing products which have already been type tested under current national procedures are likely to meet most of the Essential Requirements and may require little or no further testing. Testing by one of the nationally recognized test houses may also gain entitlement to national or proprietary marks which can be important in terms of market acceptance.

A major issue in type examination is the handling of design and manufacturing changes. Annex III states that the manufacturer must inform the Notified Body of any significant change made to an approved product, and that the Notified Body must give further approval if the change could affect conformity with the Essential Requirements. The meaning of *significant change* must be negotiated with the Notified Body, but clearly, for certain products or for manufacturers with a large number of products, the notification and checking of changes could impose a serious burden.

When a change could have an effect on the compliance with the Essential Requirements, the manufacturer should make his own assessment, including tests, to determine that the device still complies and submit up-dated drawings and documentation, together with the test results. The Notified Body must be informed of all changes made as a result of an adverse incident.

When the assessment is that the changes are not liable to have an effect, they should be submitted to the Notified Body "for information only." The manufacturer must, in such cases, keep records of the change and of the rationale for the conclusion that the change could not have an effect.

4.10   IDENTIFICATION AND CHOICE OF A NOTIFIED BODY

Identifying and choosing a Notified Body is one of the most critical issues facing a manufacturer. A long-term and close relationship should be developed and time and care spent in making a careful choice of a Notified Body should be viewed as an investment in the future of the company.

Notified bodies must satisfy the criteria given in Annex XI of the Medical Device Directive, namely:

- Independence from the design, manufacture or supply of the devices in question
- Integrity
- Competence
- Staff who are trained, experienced, and able to report
- Impartiality of the staff
- Possession of liability insurance
- Professional secrecy

In addition, the bodies must satisfy the criteria fixed by the relevant Harmonized Standards. The relevant Harmonized Standards include those of the EN 45000 series dealing with the accreditation and operation of certification bodies.

The tasks to be carried out by Notified Bodies include:

- Audit manufacturers; quality systems for compliance with Annexes II, V and VI
- Examine any modifications to an approved quality system
- Carry out periodic surveillance of approved quality systems
- Examine design dossiers and issue EC Design Examination Certificates
- Examine modifications to an approved design
- Carry out type examinations and issue EC Type Examination Certificates
- Examine modifications to an approved type
- Carry out EC verification
- Take measures to prevent rejected batches from reaching the market
- Agree with the manufacturer time limits for the conformity assessment procedures
- Take into account the results of tests or verifications already carried out
- Communicate to other Notified Bodies (on request) all relevant information about approvals of quality systems issued, refused, and withdrawn
- Communicate to other Notified Bodies (on request) all relevant information about EC Type Approval Certificates issued, refused, and withdrawn

Notified bodies must be located within the European Community in order that effective control may be applied by the Competent Authorities that appointed them, but certain operations may be carried out on behalf of Notified Bodies by subcontractors who may be based outside the European Community. Competent Authorities will generally notify bodies on their own territory, but they may notify bodies based in another Member State provided that they have already been notified by their parent Competent Authority.

There are several factors to be taken into account by a manufacturer in choosing a Notified Body, including:

- Experience with medical devices
- Range of medical devices for which the Notified Body has skills
- Possession of specific skills, e.g., EMC or software
- Links with subcontractors and subcontractor skills
- Conformity assessment procedures for which the body is notified
- Plans for handling issues, such as clinical evaluation
- Attitude to existing certifications

- Queue times/processing times
- Costs
- Location and working languages

Experience with medical devices is limited to a small number of test houses and their experience is largely confined to electromedical equipment. Manufacturers should probe carefully the competence of the certification body to assess their device. Actual experience with a product of a similar nature would be reassuring. The certification body should be pressed to demonstrate sufficient understanding of the requirements, particularly where special processes are involved (e.g., sterilization) and/or previous experience.

Certain devices demand specific skills that may not be found in every Notified Body. Clearly, the Notified Body must have, or be able to obtain, the skills required for the manufacturer's devices.

Many Notified Bodies will supplement their in-house skills by the use of specialist subcontractors. This is perfectly acceptable as long as all the rules of subcontracting are followed. Manufacturers should verify for themselves the reputation of the subcontractor and the degree of supervision applied by the Notified Body.

The main choice open to manufacturers is full Quality System certification or Type Examination combined with one of the less rigorous Quality System certifications. Some Notified Bodies have a tradition of either product testing or systems evaluation and it therefore makes sense to select a Notified Body with experience in the route chosen.

A clinical evaluation is required for some medical devices, especially Class III devices and implants. Although this will be a key aspect of demonstrating conformity, it will be important for manufacturers to know how the Notified Body intends to perform this function.

In preparing the Medical Device Directives, the need to avoid re-inventing the wheel has been recognized. In order to maximize this need, companies whose products have already been certified by test houses that are likely to become Notified Bodies may wish to make use of the organizations with whom they have previously worked. It will be important to verify with the Notified Body the extent to which the testing previously performed is sufficient to meeting the Essential Requirements.

At the time of this writing, most Notified Bodies seem to be able to offer fairly short lead times. The time for actually carrying out the examination or audit should be questioned.

It must be remembered that manufacturers will have to pay Notified Bodies for carrying out the conformity assessment procedures. There will certainly be competition and this may offer some control over costs. Although it will always be a factor, the choice of a Notified Body should not be governed by cost alone, bearing in mind the importance of the exercise.

For obvious reasons of expense, culture, convenience, and language there will be a tendency for European manufacturers to use a Notified Body situated in their own country. Nevertheless, this should not be the principal reason for selection and account should be taken of the other criteria discussed here. For manufacturers outside the European Community, the geographical location is less important. Of greater significance to them, particularly U.S. companies, is the existence of overseas subsidiaries or subcontractors of some of the Notified Bodies. Manufacturers should understand that the Notified Body must be a legal entity established within the Member State which has notified it. This does not prevent the Notified Body subcontracting quite significant tasks to a subsidiary.

Article 11.12 states that the correspondence relating to the conformity assessment procedures must be in the language of the Member State in which the procedures are carried out and/or in another Community language acceptable to the Notified Body. Language may thus be another factor affecting the choice of Notified Body, although most of the major certification bodies will accept English and other languages.

The most significant factor of all is likely to be existing good relations with a particular body. Notified Bodies will be drawn from existing test and certification bodies and many manufacturers already use such bodies, either as part of a national approval procedure, or as part of their own policy for ensuring the satisfactory quality of their products and processes.

Another consideration which could become significant is that of variations in the national laws implementing the directives. Notified Bodies will have to apply the law of the country in which they are situated and some differences in operation could be introduced by this means.

4.11   ESTABLISHING A DECLARATION OF CONFORMITY

Of all documents prepared for the Medical Device Directives, the most important may be the declaration of conformity. Every device, other than a custom-made or clinical investigation device, must be covered by a declaration of conformity.

The general requirement is that the manufacturer shall draw up a written declaration that the products concerned meet the provisions of the directive that applies to them. The declaration must cover a given number of the products manufactured. A strictly literal interpretation of this wording would suggest that the preparation of a declaration of conformity is not a one-and-for-all event with an indefinite coverage, but rather a formal statement that products which have been manufactured and verified in accordance with the particular conformity assessment procedure chosen by the manufacturer do meet the requirements of the directive. Such an interpretation would impose severe burdens on manufacturers, and the Commission is understood to be moving to a position where a declaration of conformity can be prepared in respect of future production of a model of device for which the conformity assessment procedures have been carried out. The CE marking of individual devices after manufacture can then be regarded as a short-form expression of

DECLARATION OF CONFORMITY

We: *Company Name*
                       Company Address

Declare that the product(s) listed below:

Product(s) to be declared

hereby conform(s) to the European Council Directive 93/42/EEC, Medical Device Directive, Annex II, Article 3. This declaration is based on the Certification of the Full Quality Assurance System by *name of Notified Body*, Notified Body # XXXX

Name (print or type): _____
Title: _____
Signature: _____
Date: _____

FIGURE 4-3 Sample declaration of conformity

the declaration of conformity in respect of that individual device. This position is likely to form part of future Commission guidance.

Even so, the declaration remains a very formal statement from the manufacturer and, accordingly, must be drawn up with care. The declaration must include the serial numbers or batch numbers of the products it covers and manufacturers should give careful thought to the appropriate coverage of a declaration. In the extreme, it may be that a separate declaration should be prepared individually for each product or batch.

A practical approach is probably to draw up one basic declaration which is stated to apply to the products whose serial (batch) numbers are listed in an Appendix. The Appendix can then be added to at sensible intervals. A suggested format is shown in Figure 4-3.

4.12 APPLICATION OF THE CE MARK

The CE marking (Figure 4-4) is the symbol used to indicate that a particular product complies with the relevant Essential Requirements of the appropriate

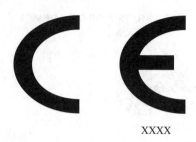

XXXX

FIGURE 4-4 Example of CE mark

directive and, as such, that the product has achieved a satisfactory level of safety and thus may circulate freely throughout the Community.

It is important to note that it is the manufacturer or his authorized representative who applies the CE marking to the product, and not the Notified Body. The responsibility for ensuring that each and every product conforms to the requirements of the Directive is that of the manufacturer and the affixing of the CE marking constitutes the manufacturer's statement that an individual device conforms.

The CE marking should appear on the device itself, if practicable, on the instructions for use, and on the shipping packaging. It should be accompanied by the identification number of the Notified Body that has been involved in the verification of the production of the device. It is prohibited to add other marks which could confuse or obscure the meaning of the CE marking.

The XXXX noted in Figure 4-4 is the identification number of the notified body.

4.13   CONCLUSION

Compliance with the new EC Directives will imply major changes for medical device manufacturers. Such changes relate to the requirements to be met in view of the design and manufacture of medical devices as well as to the procedures to be followed by manufacturers prior to and after placing medical devices on the European market. Manufacturers who wish to market medical devices in western Europe are therefore faced with a quite far-reaching and rather complex decision-making process.

REFERENCES

The Active Implantable Medical Devices Directive, 90/385/EEC, 20 June, 1990.
The Medical Devices Directive, 93/42/EEC, 14 June, 1993.
Draft Proposal for a Council Directive on In Vitro Diagnostic Medical Devices, Working Document, III/D/4181/93, April, 1993.
Fries, R.C., *Reliable Design of Medical Devices*, Marcel-Dekker, Inc., New York, 1997.
Fries, R.C., *Medical Device Quality Assurance and Regulatory Compliance*, Marcel-Dekker, Inc., New York, 1998.

Fries, R.C., *Handbook of Medical Device Design*, Marcel-Dekker, Inc., New York, 2001.

Fries, R.C. and Graber, M., Designing medical devices for conformance with harmonized standards, *Biomedical Instrumentation & Technology*, 29(4), 1995.

Higson, G.R., *The Medical Devices Directive – A Manufacturer's Handbook*, Medical Technology Consultants Europe Ltd., Brussels, 1993.

Higson, G.R., *Medical Device Safety: The Regulation of Medical Devices for Public Health and Safety*, Institute of Physics Publishing, Bristol, UK, 2002.

King, P.H. and Fries, R.C., *Design of Biomedical Devices and Systems*, Marcel-Dekker, Inc., New York, 2002.

SWBC, Organization for the European Conformity of Products, *CE-Mark: The New European Legislation for Products*, ASQC Quality Press, Milwaukee, WI, 1996.

5 Quality system regulation

CONTENTS

5.1 History of the quality system regulations 78
5.2 Scope 79
5.3 General provisions 79
5.4 Quality system 81
5.5 Design controls 81
5.6 Document controls 83
5.7 Purchasing controls 84
5.8 Identification and traceability................................... 85
5.9 Production and process controls................................. 85
5.10 Acceptance activities 88
5.11 Non-conforming product 89
5.12 Corrective and preventive action............................... 89
5.13 Labeling and packaging controls................................ 90
5.14 Handling, storage, distribution, and installation.................. 91
5.15 Records... 92
5.16 Servicing requirements... 93
References.. 94

Nearly 20 years ago the U.S. Food and Drug Administration established its Good Manufacturing Practices (GMP) for both domestic and foreign manufacturers of medical devices intended for human use. The agency took the position that the failure of manufacturers to follow good manufacturing practices was responsible for a substantial number of device failures and recalls.

The philosophy behind the FDA's requirement that manufacturers adopt GMPs is simple. While the agency's premarket review of devices serves as a check of their safety and effectiveness, it was felt that only compliance with GMPs could ensure that devices were produced in a reliable and consistent manner. At that time, the original GMPs did not in themselves guarantee that a product that was once shown to be safe and effective could be reliably produced.

Recently, spurred by an act of Congress, the FDA has changed its regulations, adding a requirement for design controls and bringing U.S. GMPs into substantive harmony with international requirements. The addition of design controls changes the very nature of the GMP requirements, which now seek to increase the chances that devices will be designed in such a manner as to be safe, effective, and reliable. Further, with the agency embracing the goal of international harmonization, the day may not be far off when manufacturers will be able to establish a single set of manufacturing practices that will satisfy regulatory requirements from New Zealand to Norway. Indeed, the agency has already spoken publicly about the mutual recognition of inspection results among industrialized countries, and has even raised the possibility of third-party audits to replace the need for some FDA inspections.

5.1 HISTORY OF THE QUALITY SYSTEM REGULATIONS

Like most U.S. medical device law, the current Good Manufacturing Practices requirements trace their genesis to the medical device amendments of 1976. Section 520(f) of the Federal Food, Drug, and Cosmetic Act authorized the FDA to establish GMPs. On July 21, 1978, the agency issued its original GMP regulations, which described the facilities and methods to be used in the manufacture, packaging, storage, and installation of medical devices. Aside from some editorial comments, these requirements would remain unchanged for nearly 20 years.

In 1990 Congress passed the Safe Medical Device Act, which gave the FDA authority to add "preproduction design validation controls" to the GMP regulations. The act also encouraged the FDA to work with foreign countries toward mutual recognition of GMP inspections.

The agency went right to work on this and in June, 1990, proposed revised GMPs. Almost 7 years of debate and revision followed, but finally, on October 7, 1996, the FDA issued its final rules. The new Quality System Regulations, incorporating the required design controls, went into effect on June 1, 1997. The design control provisions, however, would not be enforced until June 14, 1998.

The design controls embodied in the new regulations were necessary, the FDA stated, because the lack of such controls had been a major cause of device recalls in the past. A 1990 study suggested that approximately 44% of the quality problems that had led to voluntary recall actions in the previous 6 years were attributable to errors or deficiencies designed into particular devices, deficiencies that might have been prevented had design controls been in place. With respect to design flaws in software, the data were even more alarming: one study of software-related recalls indicated that more than 90% were due to design errors.

Like their predecessors, the new rules are broadly stated. "Because this regulation must apply to so many different types of devices, the regulation does not prescribe in detail how a manufacturer must produce a specific device," explained the FDA. The rules apply to all Class II and Class III devices and to some Class I devices. Failure to comply with the provisions will automatically render any device produced "adulterated" and subject to FDA sanction.

5.2 SCOPE

On October 7, 1996, the FDA published the long-awaited revision of its medical device good manufacturing practices (GMP) regulation in the Federal Register. Manufacturers that had not remained current with the changes in the regulation that the agency had proposed over the previous 6 years were in for a major surprise. And even those that kept current with the agency's proposals up through the working draft of July 1995 were to find a few new twists.

Now renamed as a quality system regulation, FDA's new revision differs significantly from the previous GMP regulation of 1978. It also adds a number of requirements not present in the agency's proposed rule of November 1993, and introduces a number of changes developed since publication of the July 1995 working draft. Specifically, the new quality system regulation contains major additional requirements in the areas of design, management responsibility, purchasing, and servicing.

It is clear that the new regulation has been greatly influenced by the work of the Global Harmonization Task Force. In slightly different wording, the regulation now incorporates all the requirements of the fullest of the quality systems standards compiled by the International Organization for Standardization (ISO). For example, there are now requirements for quality planning, for a quality manual, and for an outline of the general quality procedure. All these new requirements were added in order to bring the regulation into harmony with the quality systems standards currently accepted in the member nations of the European Union (EU), and there is certainly a benefit to their inclusion in the new regulation.

But the regulation also adds documentation requirements that would not have been included if harmonization were not an agency goal, and these requirements must now be met by all U.S. device manufacturers – even if they do not intend to export to the EU. On the up side, the language of the new regulation allows manufacturers much more flexibility than either the November 1993 proposal or July 1995 working draft would have allowed. Section 22.3 reviews the changes that the agency has incorporated into the sections of its newest regulation and discusses how those changes are likely to affect device manufacturers.

5.3 GENERAL PROVISIONS

As mentioned above, the FDA has changed the title of its revised regulation from "Good Manufacturing Practice for Medical Devices" to "Quality System Regulation." This change is more than just a matter of nomenclature; it is intended to reflect the expanded scope of the new regulation as well as to bring its terminology into harmony with that of the ISO 9000 family of quality systems standards. While the 1978 GMP regulation focused almost exclusively on production practices, the new regulation encompasses quality system requirements that apply to the entire life cycle of a device. The new rule is therefore properly referred to as a quality system regulation, into which the agency's revised requirements for good manufacturing practices have been incorporated.

The 1978 GMP regulation was a two-tier regulation that included general requirements applicable to all devices and additional requirements that applied only to critical ones. In the new quality system regulation, the notion of a critical device has been removed, and the term is no longer used. However, the new regulation's section on traceability (820.65) makes use of the same general concept, and the definition of traceable device found there is the same as the definition of critical device as presented in the 1978 GMP regulation (820.3(f)). Other critical-device requirements of the 1978 GMP regulation have been melded into appropriate sections of the quality system regulation; for instance, the critical operation requirements are now included in the section on process validation (820.75).

The new regulation's section on scope makes it clear that manufacturers need only comply with those parts of the regulation that apply to them. Thus, for example, only manufacturers who service devices need comply with the servicing requirements. Like the 1978 GMP regulation, the quality system regulation does not apply to component manufacturers, but they are encouraged to use it for guidance.

One important statement in the new regulation's section on scope is the definition of the phrase "where appropriate," which is used in reference to a number of requirements. Contrary to what manufacturers might hope, this phrase does not limit application of the regulation's requirements to times when manufacturers believe they are appropriate. Instead, the FDA means that a requirement should be considered appropriate "if nonimplementation could reasonably be expected to result in the product not meeting its specified requirements or the manufacturer not being able to carry out any necessary corrective action." In short, a requirement is considered appropriate unless the manufacturer can document justification to the contrary. Unfortunately, industry was not provided an opportunity to comment on the agency's use of this phrase.

Another important issue covered under the scope of the new regulation relates to foreign firms that export devices to the U.S. The agency has routinely inspected such firms to determine whether they are complying with GMPs although it has no authority to do so, and must rely on an invitation from the company in question. Some foreign manufacturers have refused to allow the FDA to inspect their facilities. The new regulation's section on scope addresses this situation by stating that devices produced by foreign manufacturers that refuse to permit FDA inspections will be considered adulterated and will be detained by U.S. Customs. The FDA is basing its authority to impose this penalty on the Federal Food, Drug, and Cosmetic Act (Section 801(a)).

It will be interesting to see what occurs if a foreign manufacturer chooses to challenge this position.

5.4 QUALITY SYSTEM

Each manufacturer must establish and maintain a quality system that is appropriate for the specific medical devices designed or manufactured.

The regulations make it clear that it is the responsibility of executive management to establish a quality system and to ensure that it is both implemented and understood at all levels of the organization. A member of management must be appointed whose assigned role is to ensure that the quality system requirements are effectively established and maintained, and to report to management on the system. The use of the term *establish* indicates that the requirements must be documented, either in writing or electronically, and then implemented.

Management will need to establish a procedure for auditing the quality system. The requirements provide that quality audits must be conducted by individuals who do not have direct responsibility for the area being audited. Corrective actions, including a re-audit of deficient matters, must be taken when necessary. Although the frequency of the audits is not specified, it should be determined by the organization and documented.

Manufacturers must have sufficient personnel and must establish procedures by which they may identify training needs. Training must be documented. All personnel, not just those involved in the quality system, must be made aware of the device defects that could result from the improper performance of their job. Those involved with verification and validation activities must additionally be familiarized with the particular defects and errors they may encounter.

All personnel must have the necessary background, education, and training to perform their tasks. Formal training programs are not always required. For most operations, on-the-job training is sufficient. The agency is likely, however, to require formal training for persons involved in those areas that may be especially prone to problems.

5.5 DESIGN CONTROLS

Each manufacturer of any Class II or Class III device, and the Class I devices listed in the regulations, must establish and maintain procedures to control the design of the device in order to ensure that specified design requirements are met.

Each manufacturer must establish and maintain plans that describe or reference the design and development activities and define responsibility.

Each manufacturer must establish and maintain procedures to ensure that design requirements address the intended use of the device, including the needs of the user and the patient.

Each manufacturer must establish and maintain procedures for defining and documenting design output in terms that allow an adequate evaluation of conformance to design input requirements. Design output procedures must contain or make reference to acceptance criteria.

Each manufacturer must establish and maintain procedures to ensure that formal documented reviews of the design results are planned and conducted at appropriate stages.

Design verification must confirm that the design output meets the design input requirements.

Design validation must be performed under defined operating conditions on initial production units. Design validation must ensure that devices conform to defined user needs and intended uses and must include testing of production units under actual or simulated use conditions.

Each manufacturer must establish and maintain procedures to ensure that the device is correctly translated into production specifications.

Each manufacturer must establish and maintain procedures for the identification, documentation, validation, or where appropriate, verification, review, and approval of design changes.

Records demonstrating that the device has been developed in accordance with these requirements must be kept in a Design History File (DHF). The Design History File is defined as: compilation of records that describe the design history of a finished device. It should be distinguished from other, similarly named, records required elsewhere in the regulations, such as the Device Master Record and the Device History Record.

The Design and Development Plan serves as a road map for the development process. It describes the kinds of activities that are to be undertaken and identifies who is responsible for each. One of these activities will be the establishment of design inputs, which will require interfacing with other groups, including users and patients. Such interfaces must be documented and the entire plan updated and approved as the design and development evolve. The FDA expects the Design and Development Plan to be explicit enough that employees can determine how inputs are to be gathered, what they are to do, and who is to be responsible for oversight, yet not so detailed as to dictate, for example, what kinds of tools must be used.

Design and Development Plans need not be established when an organization is purely in the research phase of a project, and development is still uncertain. However, once a company has decided to go forward with the product, a Design and Development Plan must be drawn up.

By requiring manufacturers to control the mechanism by which they obtain input for designs, the FDA is requiring that there be an established procedure for identifying precisely how design input is obtained and documented.

The result of the design effort will be the design output, consisting of the design itself, its packaging, labeling, and the Device Master Record, which includes the specifications for the device and the procedures used to build, verify, and validate it. Design output must be documented and approved with the approval bearing the date and signature of the individual responsible.

Design reviews must be performed at appropriate stages in the development process. Present at such reviews should be representatives familiar with each function involved, as well as an individual who does not have direct responsibility for the design stage being reviewed. The FDA has indicated that persons involved in one aspect of a design may serve as independent reviewers for other aspects that they are not involved in, thereby satisfying the independence requirement in even the smallest of companies. The FDA also recommends that functions far removed from the actual design process be represented. The results of the design review, annotated with the date and a list of the individuals present and their titles, must be included in the Design History File.

Design verification and validation are two different things. Verification can be thought of as the measurement of a physical parameter. Validation, by contrast, is a more complex procedure in which a total assessment of the product is undertaken to determine whether it satisfies its intended use, including the needs of users and patients. Verification is a check against an organization's internal standards. Validation reaches out to the product's consumers.

In defining design validation, the international standards upon which the new regulations are based refer to the need to perform clinical evaluations. The similarity of this term to the term "clinical trials" at first raised some alarm, but the FDA has assured the industry that clinical trials need not necessarily be part of design validation. Validation can be performed using historical data, data extracted from literature, or an evaluation of the product conducted by the company's own staff of registered nurses and doctors. An external check through an investigational-device exemption may also be used to validate a product. All of these make up what is referred to as the clinical evaluation.

When all this activity has been completed, the finished product is ready to be transferred from design and development to manufacturing. Written procedures are required that address this transfer. Written procedures are likewise required for the approval, validation, and verification of design changes.

5.6 DOCUMENT CONTROLS

Each manufacturer must establish and maintain procedures to control all documents.

Each manufacturer must designate an individual(s) to review all documents for adequacy and approval, prior to their issuance.

Documents must be available at all locations.

All obsolete documents must be promptly removed.

Changes to documents must be reviewed and approved. Approved changes must be communicated to the appropriate personnel in a timely manner.

The FDA views document control as a critical element in maintaining the quality of a product. All change records must include a description of the change, identification of all affected documents, signature of all approving individuals, date of approval, and date when the change became or will become effective. Increasingly, document control is being facilitated electronically. The FDA has proposed a regulation defining the kind of electronic signature to be used (59 FR 45160). This document is to be used only as guidance until the agency makes a final determination.

Changes must be approved by an individual serving in the same function as the one who performed the original review and approval, to ensure that the original approver will have the opportunity to review the change. Where such an arrangement is not possible, another individual may be designated, provided that the designation is documented.

5.7 PURCHASING CONTROLS

Each manufacturer must establish and maintain procedures to ensure that all purchased or otherwise received product and services conform to specified requirements.

Each manufacturer must establish and maintain the requirements that must be met by suppliers, contractors, and consultants. Each manufacturer must (1) evaluate and select on the basis of their ability to meet the specified requirements, (2) define the type and extent of control to be exercised, and (3) establish and maintain records of acceptable suppliers, contractors, and consultants.

Each manufacturer must establish and maintain data that clearly describe or reference the specified requirements for purchased or otherwise received product and services.

Components that are incorporated into finished devices, and materials that are used in their manufacture, must also be properly tested or inspected to determine that they meet documented standards. They must then be identified in such a way as to ensure that only acceptable components or materials will be used in manufacturing.

Well-known, industry-standard components may need only a minimum of testing and inspection, while newer and critical components will require more detailed examination. In either case, a record of qualification should be maintained, specifying the component's identity, the particular test/inspection method used, and the result obtained. Component specifications may include dimensions, materials, viscosity, and other features, though for routine standard components a catalog description may be enough. Quality levels should also be noted, especially for components that are available in several variants, such as industrial, reagent, or military grade.

All components will need to undergo at least a visual inspection. As for testing, it is left to the manufacturer's discretion to decide which components should be individually tested and which should be sampled. In general, some form of testing should be performed if deviations could cause the product to be unfit for its intended use. Manufacturers that decided not to sample or test components should be prepared to justify their decisions, whether on the basis of the supplier's previous performance, a component's known performance history, its application, or other criteria.

Rejected, obsolete, or deteriorated components should be placed in a separate, quarantined area. Records should be kept to document their disposition, stating whether the components were returned or scrapped. In smaller firms, the disposition can be noted directly on the purchase order.

Those components that are accepted should also have their own quarantine area. Components that are liable to be affected by moisture, dirt, or insects should be protected, and those that might degrade should be stored in such a way as to facilitate first-in, first-out (FIFO) use.

Suppliers, consultants, and contractors must also meet specified requirements that should be stated or referenced in the Device Master Record. All evaluations should be documented.

Purchasing documents must include, whenever possible, an agreement that the supplier, contractor, and consultant will notify the manufacturer of any changes so that it may be determined whether or not these will affect the quality of the finished product.

All purchasing data are subject to the document controls outlined in that section.

5.8   IDENTIFICATION AND TRACEABILITY

Each manufacturer must establish and maintain procedures for identifying product during all stages of receipt, production, distribution, and installation to prevent mix-ups.

Each manufacturer of a device that is intended for surgical implant or to support or sustain life, and whose failure can be reasonably expected to result in significant injury to the user, must establish and maintain procedures for identifying with a control number each unit, lot, or batch.

The purpose of the first requirement is to ensure that all products, including components and manufacturing materials, are properly identified so as to prevent mix-ups. The traceability provision applies to the kinds of devices categorized as critical devices in earlier GMPs.

Traceability, as referred to in this section, is held to apply from the manufacturing facility to the initial consignee. It should be distinguished from FDA tracking requirements, which are used to trace a product all the way to the patient. The tracing of critical components should make up part of the Device History Record.

5.9   PRODUCTION AND PROCESS CONTROLS

Each manufacturer must develop, conduct, control, and monitor production processes. Where deviation from device specifications could occur as a result of the manufacturing process, the manufacturer must establish and maintain process control procedures. Process controls must include:

- Documented instructions
- Monitoring and control of process parameters and components and device characteristics during production
- Compliance to specified reference standards or codes
- The approval of process and process equipment
- Criteria for workmanship which must be expressed in documented standards or by means of identified and approved representative samples

Changes must be verified or, where appropriate, validated.

Where environmental conditions could reasonably be expected to have an adverse effect, the manufacturer must establish and maintain procedures to adequately control these environmental conditions.

Each manufacturer must establish and maintain requirements for health, cleanliness, personal practices, and clothing of personnel, if contact could reasonably be expected to have an adverse effect.

Each manufacturer must establish and maintain procedures to prevent contamination.

Buildings must be of suitable design.

Each manufacturer must ensure that all equipment is appropriately designed, constructed, placed, and installed.

Each manufacturer must establish and maintain schedules for the adjustment, cleaning, and other maintenance of equipment.

Each manufacturer must conduct periodic inspections of equipment.

Each manufacturer must ensure that any inherent limitations or allowable tolerances are visibly posted or are readily available.

Where a manufacturing material could reasonably be expected to have an adverse effect, each manufacturer must establish and maintain procedures for the use and removal of such manufacturing material.

When computers or automated data processing systems are used as part of production, the manufacturer must validate the computer software.

Each manufacturer must ensure that all inspection, measuring, and test equipment is suitable for its use and is routinely calibrated, inspected, checked, and maintained.

Calibration procedures must include specific directions and limits for accuracy and precision. When accuracy and precision limits are not met, there must be provisions for remedial action. Calibration must be traceable to national or international standards. Calibration dates, the individual performing each calibration, and the next calibration date must be documented. Calibration records must be displayed on or near each piece of equipment, or shall be readily available.

Where the results of a process cannot be fully verified, the process must be validated.

No provision of the regulations is more central to the maintenance of quality standards, or more likely to occupy large amounts of the manufacturer's time, money, and attention than this one. The basic philosophy is simple: any possible deviation in the manufacturing process that could affect the quality of the final product must be documented, monitored, and controlled.

Most manufacturers find it helpful to establish standard operating procedures to produce the documents required by this section. Changes to the standard operating procedures must be made in accordance with the section on Document controls.

Provisions relating to buildings, environment, and personnel have been augmented in the FDA's guidance documents. Buildings should contain sufficient space to allow for proper cleaning, maintenance, and other operations, and should be designed with contamination control in mind. Elements such as humidity, temperature, and static electricity, as well as foreign substances such as paint chips, rust, and microorganisms, should be controlled if they are likely to affect the product adversely. Because overcrowded environments are susceptible to mix-ups, facilities should be laid out with designated, discrete areas for receiving, inspection, testing, manufacturing, labeling, packaging, and record keeping, with different operations delineated by walls or partitions. Where separate labeling operations are undertaken, each should be treated as a distinct operation, and physically isolated from all other labeling operations.

Even such mundane processes as cleaning should be documented. A record of cleanings should be kept and posted in a convenient location. A notation of mark, an initial, or the signature of the person who performed the cleaning should be entered in this log after each cleanup. Bathrooms and dressing areas should be clean and of adequate size. The use of pesticides in a facility should always be carried out with written procedures. If equipment can be affected by particulates caused by smoking, it is recommended that workers who smoke do not enter sensitive portions of the facilities for 15 minutes after smoking.

The regulations also require that equipment used in production be periodically inspected in accordance with a written plan. Inspections need to be documented. Manufacturing materials must be removed if they are likely to have an adverse effect. The removal procedures must be documented, along with the fact of the material's removal. Manufacturing materials do not have to be eradicated completely. They must, however, be eliminated to the extent that the amount that remains will not adversely affect the device's quality.

Software used to control manufacturing processes must be validated to the greatest extent possible. This applies even to off-the-shelf software purchased by the manufacturer, for which assurances must be provided that its performance will match expectations.

Those features of a product that cannot be verified must be controlled through process validation. The FDA defines process validation as:

> establishing documented evidence that provides a high degree of assurance that specific processes will consistently produce product meeting its predetermined specifications and quality characteristics.

Documented evidence is compiled by challenging the process, that is, by varying input parameters to create worst-case conditions. Parameters include not only component specifications, but also air and water quality and equipment tolerance levels. Changes to the end product are then measured. Whether or not a product is deemed acceptable will depend on its predetermined specifications. In the case of something simple such as tubing, this could mean the internal and external diameters. Other predetermined specifications could include biocompatibility, durability, and tensile strength.

Validation activities, including the date and signature of the individuals approving the validation, need to be documented. Monitoring methods, data obtained, date and, where appropriate, names of the validating individuals must all be provided. All persons involved must be qualified for their tasks. If and when changes are made to the process, revalidation will be required unless the manufacturer can show why it was not needed.

5.10 ACCEPTANCE ACTIVITIES

Each manufacturer shall establish and maintain procedures for acceptance activities.

Incoming products must be inspected, tested, or otherwise verified. Acceptance or rejection must be documented.

Procedures must ensure that in-process product is controlled.

Each manufacturer must ensure that each production run, lot, or batch of finished devices meets acceptance criteria. Finished devices must be held in quarantine or otherwise adequately controlled until release.

Finished devices must not be released for distribution until:

- The activities required in the Device Master Record are completed
- The associated data and documentation are reviewed
- The release is authorized by signature of a designated individual
- The authorization is dated

Acceptance records must include:

- The acceptance activities performed
- The date acceptance activities were performed
- The results
- The signature of the individual(s) conducting the acceptance activities
- Where appropriate, equipment used

These records must be part of the Device History Record.

Each manufacturer must identify, by suitable means, the acceptance status of product. Acceptance status must be maintained throughout manufacturing, packaging, labeling, installation, and servicing of the product.

This section of the regulations is specific to the manufacturer's own acceptance program. The criteria for determining what is acceptable are left to the manufacturer's discretion and may depend, in part, on reasonable reliance on the seller's quality control programs. However, the FDA has indicated that it considers it essential for manufacturers to maintain records of the assessments they perform, with clear indications of pass and fail criteria. All non-conforming product must be dealt with in a specific fashion (see next section).

5.11 NON-CONFORMING PRODUCT

Each manufacturer shall establish and maintain procedures to control product that does not conform to specified requirements. The procedure must address the identification, documentation, evaluation, segregation, and disposition of non-conforming product. The evaluation of non-conformance must include a determination of the need for an investigation and notification of the persons or organizations responsible.

Disposition of non-conforming product must be documented.

Each manufacturer shall establish and maintain procedures for rework including testing and reevaluation.

This section requires four things of a manufacturer. First, it must set up a program to control the disposition of all non-conforming product. Second, it must ensure that the program addresses the identification, documentation, evaluation, segregation, and disposition of non-conforming product. Third, it must provide for investigations, when necessary. Fourth, it must ensure that such investigations are documented. When an investigation is not undertaken, the rationale for the decision must be documented.

5.12 CORRECTIVE AND PREVENTIVE ACTION

Each manufacturer shall establish and maintain procedures for corrective and preventive action that include:

- Analyzing processes, quality audit reports, service records, complaints, and any other sources of quality data to identify existing and potential causes of non-conforming product
- Use of appropriate statistical methodology
- Investigating the cause of the non-conformity
- Identifying the actions required
- Verifying or validating the corrective and preventive action
- Implementing and recording changes in methods and procedures
- Ensuring information related to quality problems or non-conforming product is disseminated to those directly responsible
- Submitting relevant information for management review

All activities required in this section and their results must be documented.

Field failures, as well as customer complaints relating to the possible failure of a device to meet any of its specifications, must be reviewed, evaluated, and investigated, unless a similar investigation has already been performed. A person or unit needs to be formally designated to carry out this task. The FDA defines a complaint as any expression of dissatisfaction regarding the product's identity, quality, durability, reliability, safety, effectiveness, or performance.

The FDA requires that complaint files be reasonably accessible to investigators and readily available at the manufacturing site. Re-labelers, importers, and other entities that distribute products under their own name must forward complaints to the actual manufacturer.

Complaints for a particular product should be grouped in such a way as to enable trends to be identified. According to the FDA, if a manufacturer cannot readily identify defect trends, the firm's management is not complying with the intent of the GMP.

In describing the written procedure that must be followed in the investigation of any outright failure of a device or its components to meet performance specifications, the FDA stipulates that such guidelines must specify that the defective device not be destroyed.

Any deaths related to a device, even those attributable to user error, must also be investigated. Although it is obviously not possible for manufacturers to foresee all conceivable types of misuses, once a potential misuse has come to light, the manufacturer should consider taking corrective and preventative action.

Investigation may be called for even where there is no external complaint. The FDA is of the opinion, for example, that changes in yields mandate the need for investigation.

5.13   LABELING AND PACKAGING CONTROLS

Each manufacturer shall establish and maintain procedures to control labeling activities.

Labels must be printed and applied so as to remain legible and affixed during customary conditions.

Labeling must not be released for storage or use until a designated individual(s) has examined the labeling. The release, including the date and signature of the individual(s) performing the examination, must be documented in the Device History Record.

Each manufacturer must store labeling in a manner that provides proper identification and is designed to prevent mix-ups.

The label and labeling used must be documented in the Device History Record.

Each manufacturer must ensure that containers are designed and constructed to protect the device from alteration or damage during the customary conditions of processing, storage, handling, and distribution.

The precise definitions of the various terms are important here. The term labels is defined as those things that appear on the device itself. Labeling refers to virtually everything else, including dispenser carton labels, case labels, package labels, and directions for use.

The content and design of the labels should be specified or referenced in the Device Master Record, with the specifications to include artwork for each label as well as appropriate inspection and control procedures. The artwork should be accompanied by the name of the preparer, an approval signature, and the approval date. Labels on printed packaging should be treated as components. As such, purchase specifications should define label dimensions, ink, and finish to help ensure that the label and labeling will remain legible throughout the life of the product.

Labels and labeling that have been accepted from vendors should be stored in segregated areas and a documented procedure should be followed when they are released for use. This procedure will need to include a check for any lot numbers or expiration dates. Inspection of the label should be documented on a form that provides the name of the person performing the inspection and its date. Further, since labeling is to be included in the Device Master Record, all changes therein should be performed under the document change control system. Automated label readers, backed up by human oversight, may be used to inspect labels.

Packaging, too, must be evaluated for suitability, with special attention paid to devices that must remain sterile, for which some form of validation is usually required. Where products are labeled *sterile* but have not yet been sterilized, a high level of control is required and specific FDA regulations apply (21 CFR 801.150(e)).

Intentional tampering is not one of the customary conditions that manufacturers are required to anticipate.

5.14 HANDLING, STORAGE, DISTRIBUTION, AND INSTALLATION

Each manufacturer must establish and maintain procedures to ensure that mix-ups, damage, deterioration, contamination, or other adverse effects to product do not occur during handling.

Each manufacturer must establish and maintain procedures for the control of storage areas and stock rooms. When the quality of a product deteriorates over time, it must be stored in a manner to facilitate proper stock rotation.

Each manufacturer must describe the methods for authorizing receipt from and dispatch to storage areas.

Each manufacturer must ensure that only those devices approved for release are distributed and that purchase orders are reviewed to ensure that ambiguities and errors are resolved.

Each manufacturer must maintain distribution records which include:

- The name and address of the initial consignee
- The identification and quantity of devices shipped
- The date shipped
- Any control number(s) used

Each manufacturer of a device requiring installation must establish and maintain adequate installation and inspection instructions and, where appropriate, test procedures.

The person installing the device must document the inspection and any test results to demonstrate proper installation.

Where needed, instructions must be supplied with the product so it can be properly installed. Installers must be trained to perform any tests that may be required upon installation. These requirements apply regardless of whether the installer is an employee of the manufacturer or a contractor.

When an installer is affiliated with the manufacturer, records of the installation should be left by the manufacturer, but the FDA does not expect manufacturers to retain copies of records when installations are performed by third parties. In such cases, the third party is obligated to keep the necessary records.

5.15   RECORDS

All records required by this section must be maintained at the manufacturing establishment or other location that is reasonably accessible to the responsible officials of the manufacturer and to employees of the FDA.

Any records stored in automated data processing systems must be backed up.

Records deemed confidential by the manufacturer may be marked to aid the FDA in determining whether information in those records may be disclosed.

All records must be retained for a period of time equivalent to the design and expected life of the device.

The Device Master Record for each type of device must include or refer to the location of the following information:

- Device specifications, including appropriate drawings, composition, formulation, component specifications, and software specifications
- Production process specifications, including the appropriate equipment specifications, production methods, production procedures, and production environment specifications
- Quality assurance procedures and specifications, including acceptance criteria and the quality assurance equipment used
- Packaging and labeling specifications, including methods and processes used
- Installation, maintenance, and servicing procedures and methods

The Device History Record must include or refer to the location of the following information:

- The dates of manufacture
- The quantity manufactured
- The quantity released for distribution

- The acceptance records which demonstrate that the device is manufactured in accordance with the Device Master Record
- The primary identification label and labeling used for each production unit
- Any device identification(s) and control number(s) used

Each manufacturer must establish and maintain procedures for receiving, reviewing, and evaluating complaints by a formally designated unit. Such procedures must ensure that:

- All complaints are processed in a uniform and timely manner
- Oral complaints are documented

Each manufacturer must review and evaluate all complaints to determine whether investigation is necessary.

Any complaint involving possible failure of a device to meet any of its specifications must be reviewed, evaluated, and investigated, unless such an investigation has already been performed for a similar complaint.

Any complaint which represents an event that must be reported to the FDA must be promptly reviewed, evaluated, and investigated and must be maintained in a separate portion of the complaint files.

The regulations clearly state that the FDA may review and copy any records required to be kept by the Quality System Regulations, with the exception of records documenting management review, internal audits, or supplier audits. Manufacturers may mark such records as confidential, but the FDA will make its own determination as to whether confidentiality may be maintained.

The precise contents of the Device Master Record, Device History Record, and Quality System Record are also laid out in this section. It is important to note that the required documents do not themselves have to be contained in such records. An index referring to their actual location will suffice. All such records must be maintained at the manufacturing establishment or other location that is reasonably accessible to responsible officials of the manufacturers and to the FDA.

Foreign manufacturers must store all complaints received about their products, either at some location within the U.S. where they regularly keep records, or at a location of their initial distributor.

5.16 SERVICING REQUIREMENTS

Each manufacturer must establish and maintain instructions and procedures for servicing.

Each manufacturer must analyze service reports with appropriate statistical methodology.

Each manufacturer who receives a service report that represents an event which must be reported to the FDA must automatically consider the report a complaint.

Service reports must be documented.

All service reports must include:

- The name of the device serviced
- Any device identification
- The date the service was performed
- The individual(s) servicing the device
- The service performed
- The test and inspection data

REFERENCES

Dash, G., CGMPs for medical device manufacturers, *Compliance Engineering*, 14(2), March–April, 1997.

Dash, G., Current good manufacturing practices for medical device manufacturers, *Compliance Engineering*, 14(3), May–June, 1997.

European Committee for Standardization, Quality systems – medical devices – particular requirements for the application of EN 29001, *European Norm 46001*, European Committee for Standardization, Brussels, 1996.

Food and Drug Administration, Quality System Regulation, *Federal Register*, October 7, 1996.

Food and Drug Administration, Medical Devices; Current Good Manufacturing Practice (CGMP) Final Rule; Quality System Regulation, *Federal Register*, October 7, 1996.

Food and Drug Administration, Code of Federal Regulations, 21 CFR 820, Good Manufacturing Practice for Medical Devices, *Federal Register*, July 21, 1997.

Food and Drug Administration, Medical Devices; Current Good Manufacturing Practice (CGMP) Regulations; Proposed Revisions; Request for Comments, *Federal Register*, November 23, 1993.

Food and Drug Administration, Medical Devices; Working Draft of the Current Good Manufacturing Practice (CGMP) Final Rule; Notice of Availability; Request for Comments; Public Meeting, *Federal Register*, July 24, 1995.

Fries, R.C., *Reliable Design of Medical Devices*, Marcel-Dekker, Inc., New York, 1997.

Fries, R.C., *Medical Device Quality Assurance and Regulatory Compliance*, Marcel-Dekker, Inc., New York, 1998.

Fries, R.C., *Handbook of Medical Device Design*, Marcel-Dekker, Inc., New York, 2001.

Global Harmonization Task Force, *Guidance on Quality Systems for the Design and Manufacture of Medical Devices*, Issue 7, August 1994.

International Organization for Standardization, Quality Systems – Model for Quality Assurance in Design, Development, Production, Installation, and Servicing, *ISO 9001:1994*, International Organization for Standardization (ISO), Geneva, 1994.

King, P.H. and Fries, R.C., *Design of Biomedical Devices and Systems*, Marcel-Dekker, Inc., New York, 2002.

6 Domestic standards

CONTENTS

6.1   Domestic standards organizations...................................... 95
      6.1.1   AAMI... 95
      6.1.2   ANSI 96
      6.1.3   ASQC... 96
      6.1.4   ASTM 96
      6.1.5   IEEE.. 96
      6.1.6   IES... 96
      6.1.7   IPC 97
      6.1.8   NEMA.. 97
      6.1.9   NFPA... 97
      6.1.10 OSHA.. 97
      6.1.11 UL... 97
6.2   Software standards and regulations 98
References... 99

The degree to which formal standards and procedures are applied to product development varies from company to company. In many cases, standards are dictated by customers or regulatory mandate. In other situations, standards are self-imposed. If formal standards do exist, assurance activity must be established to assure that they are being followed. An assessment of compliance to standards may be conducted as part of a formal technical review or by audit.

Standards simplify communication, promote consistency and uniformity, and eliminate the need to invent yet another solution to the same problem. They also provide vital continuity so that we are not forever reinventing the wheel. They are a way of preserving proven practices above and beyond the inevitable staff changes within organizations. Standards, whether official or merely agreed upon, are especially important when talking to customers and suppliers, but it is easy to underestimate their importance when dealing with different departments and disciplines within our own organization.

6.1 DOMESTIC STANDARDS ORGANIZATIONS

6.1.1 AAMI

The Association for the Advancement of Medical Instrumentation is an alliance of health care professionals, united by the common goal of increasing the understanding and beneficial use of medical devices and instrumentation. In meeting this goal, the AAMI distributes information in the form of various publications, including voluntary standards. The AAMI is a highly respected and widely recognized national and international consensus standards organization. The AAMI is accredited by the American National Standards Institute (ANSI) and is one of the principal voluntary standards organizations in the world.

6.1.2   ANSI

The American National Standards Institute not only creates standards, but also is responsible for U.S. representation at the International Electrotechnical Commission and is the U.S. representative for the International Organization for Standards.

6.1.3   ASQC

The American Society for Quality Control is a worldwide network of more than 83 000 individual members and over 600 sustaining members in the quality field. Coverage ranges from the fundamentals of quality technology to total quality management.

6.1.4   ASTM

The American Society for Testing and Materials is a scientific and technical organization formed for the development of standards on characteristics and performance of materials, products, systems, and services. The ASTM is the world's largest source of voluntary concensus standards.

6.1.5   IEEE

The Institute of Electrical and Electronic Engineers was founded in 1884 and is one of the oldest societies in the U.S. It is an organization that develops standards on a variety of topics relating to electrical and electronic equipment. In recent years, a primary focus for the standards organization has been the areas of software development and software quality assurance. Some of their software standards have been accredited by the American National Standards Institute and have been primarily used for the development and validation of military software. Recently, these standards have been referenced by the FDA in the development of guidelines on medical software.

6.1.6   IES

The Institute of Environmental Sciences is a technical society that covers space simulation, contamination control practices, solar and nuclear energy, military environmental testing, reliability testing, and environmental stress screening of components and systems.

6.1.7 IPC

The Institute for Interconnecting and Packaging Electronic Circuits is known for work on printed circuit boards, specifications, and standards, including general requirements for soldered connections, component packaging, inter-connecting and mounting, surface-mount land patterns, and studies such as the Impact of Moisture on Plastic IC Packaging Cracking (IPC-SM-786).

6.1.8 NEMA

The National Electrical Manufacturers Association publishes standards including power circuits, plugs, receptacles, and sockets.

6.1.9 NFPA

The National Fire Protection Association is organized to assure the appointment of technically competent committees, with balanced representation, to establish criteria to minimize the hazards of fire, explosion and electricity in health care facilities. These criteria include:

- Performance
- Maintenance
- Testing
- Safe practices
- Material
- Equipment
- Appliances

The NFPA does not approve, inspect or certify any installation, procedure, equipment, or material. The NFPA has no authority to police or enforce compliance to their standards. However, installations may base acceptance of a device on compliance with their standards.

6.1.10 OSHA

The Occupational Safety and Health Administration was established in 1970 and is responsible for regulating workplace health and safety.

6.1.11 UL

Underwriters Laboratory is an independent, not-for-profit testing laboratory organized for the purpose of investigating materials, devices, products, equipment construction, methods and systems with respect to hazards affecting life and property. It tests devices in six different areas:

- Burglary protection and signaling
- Casualty and chemical hazards
- Electrical
- Fire protection
- Heating, air conditioning and refrigeration
- Marine

UL inspection services personnel visit companies unannounced to verify that products that bear the UL mark comply with applicable UL safety requirements. The registered UL mark on a device is a means by which a manufacturer, distributor or importer can show that samples of the product have been verified for compliance with safety standards.

Many hospitals require that the medical devices they purchase comply with applicable UL standards.

6.2   SOFTWARE STANDARDS AND REGULATIONS

There are a myriad of software standards to assist the developer in designing and documenting his program. IEEE standards cover documentation through all phases of design. Military standards describe how software is to be designed and developed for military use. There are also standards on software quality and reliability to assist developers in preparing a quality program. The international community has produced standards, primarily dealing with software safety. In each case, the standard is a voluntary document that has been developed to provide guidelines for designing, developing, testing, and documenting a software program.

In the U.S., the FDA is responsible for assuring the device utilizing software or the software as a device is safe and effective for its intended use. The FDA has produced several drafts of reviewer guidelines, auditor guidelines, software policy, and GMP regulations addressing both device and process software. In addition, guidelines for FDA reviewers have been prepared as well as training programs for inspectors and reviewers. The new version of the GMP regulation addresses software as part of the design phase.

The U.S. is ahead of other countries in establishing guidelines for medical software development. There is, however, movement within several international organizations to develop regulations and guidelines for software and software-controlled devices. For example, ISO 9000-3 specifically addresses software development in addition to what is contained in ISO 9001. CSA addresses software issues in four standards covering new and previously developed software in critical and non-critical applications. IEC has a software document currently in development.

REFERENCES

ECRI, *Health Care Standards: 1995*, Plymouth Meeting, PA, ECRI, 1995.

Fries, R.C., *Reliable Design of Medical Devices*, Marcel-Dekker, Inc., New York, 1997.

Fries, R.C., *Handbook of Medical Device Design*, Marcel-Dekker, Inc., New York, 2001.

Jorgens III, J., Computer hardware and software as medical devices, *Medical Device and Diagnostic Industry*, May, 1983.

Jorgens III, J. and Burch, C.W., FDA Regulation of Computerized Medical Devices, *Byte* 7, 1982.

Jorgens III, J. and Schneider, R., Regulation of medical software by the FDA, *Software in Health Care*, April-May, 1985.

Kahan, J.S., Regulation of computer hardware and software as medical devices, *Canadian Computer Law Reporter*, 6(3), January, 1987.

King, P.H. and Fries, R.C., *Design of Biomedical Devices and Systems*, Marcel-Dekker, Inc., New York, 2002.

Meeldijk, V., *Electronic Components: Selection and Application Guidelines*, John Wiley & Sons, Inc., New York, 1996.

Shaw, R., Safety critical software and current standards initiatives, *Computer Methods and Programs in Biomedicine*, 44(1), July, 1994.

7 International standards

CONTENTS

7.1 The international notion of standards............................ 102
7.2 The international regulatory scene 103
    7.2.1 BSI.. 103
    7.2.2 CEN 103
    7.2.3 CENELAC... 103
    7.2.4 CISPR 104
    7.2.5 CSA.. 104
    7.2.6 DIN.. 104
    7.2.7 DoH 104
    7.2.8 IEC 105
    7.2.9 IEE 105
    7.2.10 ISO 105
    7.2.11 JSA 105
    7.2.12 Other Japanese standards organizations.................. 105
7.3 The TickIT program... 106
7.4 The Software Quality System Registration program 106
7.5 The ISO guidance documents for ISO 9001 and 9002 107
7.6 Proposed regulatory requirements for Canada.................... 108
7.7 ISO 14000 series.. 108
7.8 Medical informatics 110
References.. 111

No country regulates medical devices as consistently and thoroughly as the U.S. However, there is a trend toward regulation in other industrialized countries, especially in Europe. France requires registration and evaluation of medical devices for public hospitals. Germany passed a law in 1987 that requires the registration of all medical devices linked to approval by defined testing organizations. The U.K.'s Department of Health and Social Security is active in evaluating selected devices. And Italy also has a law, passed in 1986, that requires registration of all medical devices marketed in that country.

In Europe, an important international organization working in the area of devices is the European Commission (EC). The EC has directives dealing with medical equipment. For example, under EC directives, all governments are required to develop standards for X-ray machines and X-ray therapy. Under another EC directive, issued by the International Electrotechnical Committee

(IEC), member states are required to set standards for electrical safety. An EC working group on Biomedical Engineering focuses on the safety of medical equipment. At present, the group is examining such technologies as perinatal monitoring, chromosome analysis, technology for sensory impairment, aids to the disabled, replacement of body function, quantitative electrocardiography, imaging (especially NMR), blood flow measurement by ultrasound, medical telemetry, and accelerated fracture healing.

The World Health Organization, especially the European Office in Copenhagen, has become increasingly involved in medical devices, especially promoting the idea of international exchange of information. International cooperation and communication could make much more information on medical equipment available and save evaluation resources of all countries.

7.1 THE INTERNATIONAL NOTION OF STANDARDS

The British Standards Institute defines a standard as:

> A technical specification or other document available to the public, drawn up with the cooperation and consensus or general approval of all interests affected by it, based on the consolidated results of science, technology and experience, aimed at the promotion of optimum community benefits and approved by a body on the national, regional or international level.

While this definition goes some way to saying what a standard is, it says nothing about the subject matter or purpose, apart from stating that the objectives of the standard must in some way be tied to community benefits.

Standards, however, have a definite subject matter. They include:

- To standardize particular processes
- To provide a consistent and complete definition of a commodity or process
- To record good practice regarding the development process associated with the production of commodities
- To encode good practice for the specification, design, manufacture, testing, maintenance, and operation of commodities

One of the primary requirements of a standard is that it be produced in such a way that conformance to the standard can be unambiguously determined. A standard is devalued if conformance can not be easily determined or if the standard is so loosely worded that it becomes a matter of debate and conjecture as to whether the standard has been complied with.

Standards also exist in various types:

- De facto and de jure standards. These are usually associated with the prevailing commercial interests in the market place. These de facto standards are often eventually subject to the standardization process

- Reference models. These provide a framework within which standards can be formulated
- Product versus process standards. Some standards relate to specific products while others relate to the process used to produce products
- Codes of practice, guidelines and specifications. These terms relate to the manner in which a standard may be enforced. Codes of practice and guidelines reflect ways of working that are deemed to be *good* or *desirable*, but for which conformance is difficult to determine. Specifications are far more precise and conformance can be determined by analysis or test
- Prospective and retrospective standards. It is clearly undesirable to develop a standard before the subject matter is well understood scientifically, technically and through practice. However, it may be desirable to develop a standard alongside the evolving technology

7.2   THE INTERNATIONAL REGULATORY SCENE

The production and adoption of software standards is very much the responsibility of international and national standards organizations and, in the case of the European context, bodies set up to represent a number of national organizations. Progressively, it is becoming the case that standards are developed by the international bodies and then adopted by the national bodies. Some of the international bodies include the following.

7.2.1   BSI

The British Standards Institute is the U.K.'s national standards-making organization. In performing its duties, it collaborates with industry, government agencies, other standard bodies, professional organizations, etc.

7.2.2   CEN

The Comite Europeen de Normalisation (European Committee for Standardization) is composed of members drawn from the European Union (EU) and the European Free Trade Association (EFTA). The role of the CEN is to produce standards for use within Europe and effectively covers the area addressed by the ISO.

7.2.3   CENELAC

The Comite Europeen de Normalisation Electronique (European Committee for Electrotechnical Standardization) is made up of representatives from the national electrotechnical committees, the majority of whom are represented on the IEC. Its responsibilities are for electrical and electronic standards within Europe and it has close links with the activities of the IEC.

7.2.4 CISPR

The International Special Committee on Radio Interference is a committee under the auspices of the IEC and run through a Plenary Assembly consisting of delegates from all the member bodies, including the U.S. The committee is headquartered in Geneva, Switzerland and is composed of seven sub-committees, including:

- Radio Interference Measurement and Statistical Methods
- Interference from Industrial, Scientific and Medical Radio Frequency Apparatus
- Interference from Overhead Power Lines, High Voltage Equipment and Electric Traction Systems
- Interference Related to Motor Vehicles and Internal Combustion Engines
- Interference Characteristics of Radio Receivers
- Interference from Motor, Household Appliances, Lighting Apparatus and the like
- Interference from Information Technology Equipment

7.2.5 CSA

The Canadian Standards Association is a membership association that brings people and ideas together to develop services that meet the needs of businesses, industry, governments, and consumers. Among the many services available are standards development, testing and application of the CSA mark to certified products, testing to international standards, worldwide inspection and related services.

7.2.6 DIN

The Deutsches Institut für Normung (German Standardization Institute) is the committee that sets German standards.

7.2.7 DoH

The Department of Health has the same responsibility in the U.K. that the FDA has in the U.S. The DoH sets forth standards for medical devices and has established a Good Manufacturing Practice for Medical Equipment, similar to that of the FDA. The DoH is headquartered in London. The DoH currently has reciprocity with the FDA, meaning the FDA will accept DoH inspection data as their own and the DoH will accept FDA inspection data. This is particularly applicable for companies with facilities in both the U.K. and the U.S.

7.2.8 IEC

The International Electrotechnical Commission was established in 1906 with the responsibility for developing international standards within the electrical and electronics field. By agreement with the International Standards Organization, the IEC has sole responsibility for these standards.

7.2.9 IEE

The Institution of Electrical Engineers is the main U.K. professional body responsible for electrical and electronic engineering. It is responsible for the production of a wide range of standards in the electrical engineering field and is progressively widening its interests to include software engineering.

7.2.10 ISO

The International Standards Organization was established in 1947 and its members are drawn from the national standards bodies of its members. The ISO is responsible for standardization in general, but with the exception of electrical and electronic standards which are the responsibility of the IEC.

7.2.11 JSA

The Japanese Standards Association was established as a public institution for the promotion of industrial standardization on December 6, 1945, under government authorization. The JSA has no true performance standards, but tends to follow IEC 601-1. The JSA does have a complicated approval process that can be very lengthy (up to 9 months). This process can delay the distribution of products in Japan. JSA activities include:

- Standards and document publishing
- Seminars and consulting services
- Research on standardization
- National sales agent for foreign national standard bodies

7.2.12 OTHER JAPANESE STANDARDS ORGANIZATIONS

The unified national system of industrial standardization began to function by the setup of the Japanese Engineering Standards Committee (JESC) in 1921. This group undertook the establishment of national standards. In 1949 the Industrial Standardization Law was promulgated and the Japanese Industrial Standards Committee (JISC) was established under the law as an advisory organization of competent ministers in charge of the elaboration of Japanese Industrial Standards (JIS) and the designation of the JIS mark to products.

7.3   THE TICKIT PROGRAM

The TickIT project came from two studies commissioned by the Department of Trade and Industry (DTI) which showed that the cost of poor quality in software in the U.K. was very considerable and that quality system certification was desired by the market. The studies undertook extensive research into the respective subjects and included a broad consultative process with users, suppliers, in-house developers and purchasers, with a primary task being to identify options for harmonization. The reports made a number of significant recommendations, including:

- All Quality Management System standards in common use were generically very similar
- The best harmonization route was through ISO 9001
- Action was required to improve market confidence in third party certifications of Quality Management Systems
- There was an urgent need to establish an accredited certification body or bodies for the software sector

These principal recommendations were accepted by the DTI and further work was commissioned with the British Computer Society (BCS) to set up an acceptable means to gain accredited certification of Quality Management Systems by auditors with necessary expertise. Draft guidance material for an acceptable certification scheme was developed. The onward development from this draft material has become known as the TickIT project.

TickIT is principally a certification scheme, but this is not its primary purpose. The main objectives are to stimulate developers to think about what quality really is and how it may be achieved. Unless certification is purely a by-product of these more fundamental aims, much of the effort will be wasted. To stimulate thinking, TickIT includes some quality themes that give direction to the setting up of a quality management system (QMS) and the context of certification.

Generally, TickIT certification applies for information technology (IT) systems supply where software development forms a significant or critical part. The main focus of TickIT is software development because this is the component that gives an information system its power and flexibility. It is also the source of many of the problems.

7.4   THE SOFTWARE QUALITY SYSTEM
REGISTRATION PROGRAM

The Software Quality System Registration Committee was established in 1992. The Committee's charter was to determine whether a program should be created in the U.S. for ISO 9001 registration of software design, production, and supply. A comparable program, TickIT, had been operational in the U.K.

for over one year and was gaining European acceptance. To ensure mutual recognition and to leverage the experience of the world-wide software industry, the SQSR program preserves ISO 9001 as the sole source for requirements and ISO 9000-3 as a source of official guidance for software registrants.

The Software Quality System Registration (SQSR) program is designed for ISO 9001 registration of suppliers who design and develop software as a significant or crucial element in the products they offer. The SQSR program addresses the unique requirements of software engineering and provides a credible technical basis to allow the Registrar Accreditation Board (RAB) to extend its current programs for accrediting ISO 9000 registrars, certifying auditors, and accrediting specific courses and course providers.

The program is intended to ensure that ISO registration is an effective, enduring indicator of a software supplier's capability. The effectiveness of the SQSR program is based on three factors: mutual recognition, guidance, and an administrative infrastructure tailored to the U.S. marketplace.

7.5   THE ISO GUIDANCE DOCUMENTS FOR ISO 9001 AND 9002

ISO Technical Committee 210 has recently developed two guidelines relating ISO 9001 and 9002 to medical devices. The 1994 versions of ISO 9001 and 9002 are intended to be general standards defining quality system requirements. ISO 13485 provides particular requirements for suppliers of medical devices that are more specific than the general requirements of ISO 9001. ISO 13488 provides particular requirements for suppliers of medical devices that are more specific than the general requirements of ISO 9002.

In conjunction with ISO 9001 and 9002, these International Standards define requirements for quality systems relating to the design, development, production, installation and servicing of medical devices. They embrace all the principles of the good manufacturing practices (GMPs) used in the production of medical devices. They can only be used in conjunction with ISO 9001 and 9002 and are not stand-alone standards.

They specify the quality system requirements for the production and, where relevant, installation of medical devices. They are applicable when there is a need to assess a medical device supplier's quality system or when a regulatory requirement specifies that this standard shall be used for such assessment. As part of an assessment by a third party for the purpose of regulatory requirements, the supplier may be required to provide access to confidential data in order to demonstrate compliance with one of these standards. The supplier may be required to exhibit these data, but is not obliged by the standard to provide copies for retention.

Particular requirements in a number of clauses of these standards are covered in detail in other International Standards. Suppliers should review the requirements and consider using the relevant International Standards in these areas.

To assist in the understanding of the requirements of ISO 9001, 9002, ISO 13485, and 13488, an international guidance standard is being prepared. The document provides general guidance on the implementation of quality systems for medical devices based on ISO 13485. Such quality systems include those of the EU Medical Device Directives and the GMP requirements currently in preparation in Canada, Japan, and the U.S. It may be used for systems based on ISO 13488 by the omission of sub-clause 4.4.

The guidance given in this document is applicable to the design, development, production, installation and servicing of medical devices of all kinds. The document describes concepts and methods to be considered by medical device manufacturers who are establishing and maintaining quality systems. This document describes examples of ways in which the quality system requirements can be met, and it is recognized that there may be alternative ways that are better suited to a particular device/manufacturer. It is not intended to be directly used for assessment of quality systems.

7.6   PROPOSED REGULATORY REQUIREMENTS FOR CANADA

In February, 1991, a review of the Medical Devices Regulatory Program was initiated when the Minister of National Health and Welfare established the Medical Devices Review Committee to formulate recommendations concerning the regulation of medical devices and associated activities. This Committee was established in recognition of the increased volume and complexity of new medical devices used in health care and the need for timely availability of safe and effective devices in the next decade.

In May 1993, a Development Plan for an Improved Medical Devices Regulatory Program was published. The plan is based on two principles. First, the level of scrutiny afforded a device is dependent upon the risk the device presents. Secondly, the safety and effectiveness of medical devices can best be assessed through a balance of quality systems, pre-market scrutiny and post-market surveillance. In order to enshrine these two principles into the Medical Device Regulatory Program, it was evident that a reengineering of the Program was necessary. This reengineering activity is currently ongoing.

The document describes a plan to establish a regulatory mark for Canada, similar to the CE mark currently being used in the European Union. A manufacturer would need to be audited by a Canadian third party for the successful implementation of a quality system as well as meeting the requirements for the regulatory mark.

7.7   ISO 14000 SERIES

The ISO formed Technical Committee 207 in 1993 to develop standards in the field of environmental management tools and systems. The work of

ISO TC 207 encompasses seven areas:

- Management systems
- Audits
- Labeling
- Environmental performance evaluation
- Life cycle assessment
- Terms and definitions
- Environmental aspects in product standards

The ISO 14000 standards are not product standards, nor do they specify performance or pollutant/effluent levels. They specifically exclude test methods for pollutants and do not set limit values regarding pollutants or effluents.

The 14000 standards are intended to promote the broad interests of the public and users, be cost-effective, non-prescriptive and flexible, and be more easily accepted and implemented. The goal is to improve environmental protection and quality of life.

ISO 14000 provides for the basic tenets of an environmental management system (EMS). An environmental management system is the management system which addresses the environmental impact of a company's processes and product on the environment. The EMS provides a formalized structure for ensuring that environmental concerns are addressed and met, and works to both control a company's significant environmental effects and achieve regulatory compliance.

The certification process for ISO 14000 has six steps:

- Quality documentation review
- Initial visit, preassessment or checklist
- On-site audit
- Follow-up audits to document corrective action
- Periodic audits to document compliance
- Renewal audit every 3 to 5 years

Currently, there is limited correlation between ISO 14000 and ISO 9000, but the requirements of the two series may become more harmonized in the future. Under certain conditions, the ISO 14000 audit and the ISO 9000 audit can be combined into one. It has been estimated that the cost of complying to ISO 14000 would be comparable to that for certification to ISO 9000. The registration process itself could take up to 18 months to complete.

In the U.S., ANSI has established a national program to accredit ISO 14000 registrars, auditor certifiers, and training providers. The ISO 14000 registrars are likely to come from the registrars currently performing certifications in ISO 9000.

The creation of a universal single set of EMS standards will help companies and organizations to better manage their environmental affairs, and show a commitment to environmental protection. It should also help them avoid multiple registrations, inspections, permits, and certifications of products exchanged among countries. In addition, it should concentrate worldwide attention on environmental management. The World Bank and other financial institutions may qualify their loans to less-developed countries and begin to use the 14000 standards as an indicator of commitment to environmental protection.

In the U.S., implementation of ISO 14000 could become a condition of business loans to companies that are not even involved in international trade. Insurance companies may lower premiums for those who have implemented the standard. It may become a condition of some supplier transactions, especially in Europe and with the U.S. government. Evidence of compliance could become a factor in regulatory relief programs, the exercise of prosecutorial and sentencing discretion, consent decrees and other legal instruments, and multilateral trade agreements. U.S. government agencies considering the ISO 14000 standards include:

- The Environmental Protection Agency
- The Department of Defense
- The Department of Energy
- The Food and Drug Administration
- The National Institute of Standards and Technology
- The Office of the U.S. Trade Representative
- The Office of Science, Technology and Policy

7.8 MEDICAL INFORMATICS

The real world is perceived as a complex system characterized by the existence of various parallel autonomous processes evolving in a number of separate locations, loosely coupled, cooperating by the interchange of mutually understandable messages. Due to the fact that medical specialties, functional areas, and institutions create, use and rely on interchanged information, they should share a common basic understanding in order to cooperate in accordance with a logical process constrained under an administrative organization, a medical heuristics and approach to care.

A health care framework is a logical mapping between the real world, in particular the health care environment, and its health care information systems architecture. This framework, representing the main health care subsystems, their connections, rules, etc., is the basis for an evolutionary development of heterogeneous computer-supported health care information and communications systems. A key feature of the framework is its reliance on the use of abstractions. In this way, the framework, at its most abstract level, reflects the fundamental and essential features of health care processes and information, and can be seen as applicable to all health care entities. It defines the general information structure and enables the exchangeability of the information.

The European health care framework will maintain and build upon the diversity of national health care systems in the European countries. A harmonized description/structure of planning documentation will be provided to ensure comparisons between European countries.

The main rationale for a standardized health care information framework is:

- To act as a contract between the users and procurers on the one hand and the developers and providers of information systems on the other
- To ensure that all applications and databases are developed to support the health care organization as a whole, as opposed to just a single organization or department
- To obtain economies of scale, originating from enhanced portability, as health care information systems are expensive to develop and to maintain, and tend to be installed on an international basis
- To define a common basic understanding that allows all health care information systems to interchange data

To this end, CEN/CENELAC has tasked a committee with creating the Health Care Framework model.

REFERENCES

Association for the Advancement of Medical Instrumentation, *ISO/DIS 13485, Medical Devices – Particular Requirements for the Application of ISO 9001*, Association for the Advancement of Medical Instrumentation, Arlington, VA, 1995.

Association for the Advancement of Medical Instrumentation, *ISO/DIS 13488, Medical Devices – Particular Requirements for the Application of ISO 9002*, Association for the Advancement of Medical Instrumentation, Arlington, VA, 1995.

Association for the Advancement of Medical Instrumentation, *First Draft of Quality Systems – Medical Devices – Guidance on the Application of ISO 13485 and ISO 13488*, Association for the Advancement of Medical Instrumentation, Arlington, VA, 1995.

Banta, H.D, The regulation of medical devices, *Preventive Medicine*, 19(6), November, 1990.

Cascio, J. (ed.) *The ISO 114000 Handbook*, The American Society for Quality Control, Milwaukee, WI, 1996.

CEN/CENELAC, *Directory of the European Standardization Requirements for Health Care Informatics and Programme for the Development of Standards*, European Committee for Standardization, Brussels, Belgium, 1992.

CEN/CENELAC, *EN 46001*, European Committee for Standardization, Brussels, Belgium, 1995.

CEN/CENELAC, *EN 46002*, European Committee for Standardization, Brussels, Belgium, 1995.

Department of Trade and Industry, *Guide to Software Quality Management System Construction and Certification Using EN 29001*, DISC TickIT Office, London, 1987.

Donaldson, J., U.S. companies gear up for ISO 14001 certification, *In Tech* 43(5), May, 1996.

Fries, R.C., *Reliability Assurance for Medical Devices, Equipment and Software*, Interfirm Press, Buffalo Grove, IL, 1991.

Fries, R.C., *Reliability Assurance for Medical Devices, Equipment and Software*, Interfirm Press, Buffalo Grove, IL, 1997.

Fries, R.C., *Handbook of Medical Device Design*, Marcel-Decker, Inc., New York, 2001.

International Standard Organization, *Quality Management and Quality Assurance Standards – Part 3: Guidelines for the Application of ISO 9001 to the Development, Supply and Maintenance of Software*, International Organization for Standardization, Geneva, Switzerland, 1991.

King, P.H. and Fries, R.C., *Design of Biomedical Devices and Systems*, Marcel Dekker, Inc., New York, 2002.

Meeldijk, V., *Electronic Components: Selection and Application Guidelines*, John Wiley & Sons, Inc., New York, 1996.

Shaw, R. Safety critical software and current standards initiatives, *Computer Methods and Programs in Biomedicine*, 44(1), July, 1994.

Tabor, T. and Feldman, I., *ISO 14000: A Guide to the New Environmental Management Standards*, The American Society for Quality Control, Milwaukee, WI, 1996.

Working Group #4, *Draft of Proposed Regulatory Requirements for Medical Devices Sold in Canada*, Environmental Health Directorate, Ottawa, Ontario, 1995.

Section 3

Specifying the product

8 The medical device as an entity

CONTENTS

8.1 What is a medical device?.. 115
    8.1.1 Food and Drug Administration 116
    8.1.2 The Medical Device Directives........................... 116
8.2 A brief history of medical devices................................ 117
8.3 Current medical devices 117
References.. 119

Medical devices are an important part of health care. Yet they are an extraordinarily heterogeneous category of products. The term "medical device" includes such technologically simple articles as ice bags and tongue depressors on one end of the continuum and very sophisticated articles such as pacemakers and surgical lasers on the other. Perhaps it is this diversity of products, coupled with the sheer number of different devices, that makes the development of an effective and efficient regulatory scheme a unique challenge for domestic and international regulatory bodies.

The patient is the ultimate consumer of medical devices, from the simplest cotton swab to the most sophisticated monitoring devices. However, with the exception of some over-the counter products, the medical device manufacturer rarely has a direct relationship with the patient in the marketplace. Unlike many other consumer products, a host of intermediaries influence the demand for medical devices. These intermediaries include policy makers, providers, and payers of health care services.

8.1 WHAT IS A MEDICAL DEVICE?

There are as many different definitions for a medical device as there are regulatory and standards organizations. Though the definitions may differ in verbiage, they have a common thread of content. Two of the more popular definitions are reviewed below.

8.1.1   FOOD AND DRUG ADMINISTRATION

Section 201(h) of the Federal Food, Drug, and Cosmetic Act defines a medical device as:

> an instrument, apparatus, implement, machine, contrivance, implant, in vitro reagent, or other similar or related article, including any component, part, or accessory, which is:
>
> - Recognized in the official National Formulary, or the United States Pharmacopeia, or any supplement to them
> - Intended for use in the diagnosis of disease or other conditions, or in the cure, mitigation, treatment, or prevention of disease, in man or other animals, or
> - Intended to affect the structure or any function of the body of man or other animals, and
>
> which does not achieve any of its principal intended purposes through chemical action within or in the body of man or other animals and which is not dependent upon being metabolized for the achievement of any of its principal intended purposes.

The Medical Device Amendments of 1976 expanded the definition to include:

- Devices intended for use in the diagnosis of conditions other than disease, such as pregnancy, and
- In vitro diagnostic products, including those previously regulated as drugs

A significant risk device is a device that presents a potential for serious risk to the health, safety, or welfare of a subject and (1) is intended as an implant, (2) is used in supporting or sustaining human life, and/or (3) is of substantial importance in diagnosing, curing, mitigating, or treating disease or otherwise preventing impairment of human health.

A non-significant risk device is a device that does not pose a significant risk.

8.1.2   THE MEDICAL DEVICE DIRECTIVES

The various Medical Device Directives define a medical device as:

> any instrument, appliance, apparatus, material or other article, whether used alone or in combination, including the software necessary for its proper application, intended by the manufacturer to be used for human beings for the purpose of:
>
> - Diagnosis, prevention, monitoring, treatment or alleviation of disease
> - Diagnosis, monitoring, alleviation of or compensation for an injury or handicap

- Investigation, replacement or modification of the anatomy or of a physiological process
- Control of conception

and which does not achieve its principal intended action in or on the human body by pharmacological, immunological, or metabolic means, but which may be assisted in its function by such means.

One important feature of the definition is that it emphasizes the "intended use" of the device and its "principal intended action." This use of the term *intended* gives manufacturers of certain products some opportunity to include or exclude their product from the scope of the particular Directive.

Another important feature of the definition is the inclusion of the term *software*. The software definition will probably be given further interpretation, but is currently interpreted to mean that (1) software intended to control the function of a device is a medical device, (2) software for patient records or other administrative purposes is not a device, (3) software which is built into a device, e.g., software in an electrocardiographic monitor used to drive a display, is clearly an integral part of the medical device, (4) a software update sold by the manufacturer, or a variation sold by a software house, is a medical device in its own right.

8.2   A BRIEF HISTORY OF MEDICAL DEVICES

The diagnosis and treatment of disease experienced relatively few break-throughs until the 17th century. One major contribution to modern medicine was the invention of the thermometer. In 1603, Galileo invented a device to measure temperature and Sanatoria Santonio made improvements to the device, allowing him to measure the temperature of the human body. A second important contribution occurred in 1819, when the French physician Laennec is attributed with refining the "hearing tube" or stethoscope. These inventions helped physicians diagnose and treat patients with more confidence and better accuracy.

The real breakthrough in medical diagnostic equipment came in 1895 with the discovery of X-rays by the German physicist Wilhelm Roentgen. Roentgen's discovery helped usher in the equipment age of medicine. The practice of medicine has grown tremendously since 1900. Wilhelm Einthoven's invention of the electrocardiograph in 1903 started the wave of physiological measuring instrumentation that is used in every hospital and doctor's office today.

8.3   CURRENT MEDICAL DEVICES

Current medical devices may be composed entirely of hardware, entirely of software, or a combination of the two.

Medical devices composed strictly of hardware range from tongue depressors to CO_2 absorbers. Hardware devices have improved significantly as new materials have become available that make the devices lighter, autoclavable, and more reliable. Some typical hardware medical devices include:

- Tongue depressor
- Ice bag
- Tracheal tube
- Intra-aortic balloon
- Replacement heart valve
- Absorbable surgical sutures
- Implantable staple
- Aneurysm clip
- Intraocular lens
- Bone cap
- Various protheses

During the first three decades of the computing era, the primary challenge was to develop computer hardware that reduced the cost of processing and storing data. Throughout the decade of the 1980s, advances in microelectronics have resulted in more computing power at increasingly lower cost. Today, the primary challenge is to reduce the cost and improve the quality of computer-based solutions – solutions that are implemented with software. The power of yesterday's mainframe computer is available on a single integrated circuit. The awesome processing and storage capabilities of modern hardware represent computing potential. Software is the mechanism that enables us to harness and tap this potential.

With the evolution of software engineering, the number of medical devices composed strictly of software has increased. Some typical software medical devices include:

- Blood analyzers
- EKG interpretation
- Diagnostic software

Most modern medical devices are a combination of electrical and mechanical hardware as well as software. Devices such as patient monitors, EKG machines, pacemakers and surgical lasers are examples of combining hardware and software into a system that provides a significant benefit to the patient. Some typical medical devices composed of hardware and software include:

- Ventilators
- Anesthesia machines
- Infant radiant warmers
- Incubators

- Cardiac pacemakers
- Pacemaker programmers
- Neuromuscular stimulators
- Infusion pumps
- X-ray machines
- Surgical lasers
- Patient monitors
- Oximeters

Although medical devices may vary in size, weight, complexity,and functionality, they have one thing in common. All must be safe and effective for their intended uses. If the company producing the device is to be a success the devices must also be highly reliable. Making devices safe, effective, and reliable begins in the earliest stages of product design and is a continuous process through production and maintenance.

REFERENCES

Aston, R., *Principles of Biomedical Instrumentation and Measurement*, Merrill, Columbus, OH, 1990.

Banta, H.D., The regulation of medical devices, *Preventive Medicine*, 19(6), November, 1990.

Croswell, D.W., The evolution of biomedical equipment technology, *Journal of Clinical Engineering*, 20(3), May–June, 1995.

Food and Drug Administration, *Medical Device Good Manufacturing, Practices Manual*, U.S. Department of Health and Human Services, Washington, DC, 1991.

Fries, R.C., *Reliability Assurance for Medical Devices, Equipment and Software*, Interpharm Press, Inc., Buffalo Grove, IL, 1991.

Fries, R.C., *Reliable Design of Medical Devices*, Marcel-Dekker, Inc., New York, 1997.

Fries, R.C., *Handbook of Medical Device Design*, Marcel-Dekker, Inc., New York, 2001.

Fries, R.C., et al., Software Regulation, In *The Medical Device Industry – Science, Technology, and Regulation in a Competitive Environment*, Marcel Dekker, Inc., New York, 1990.

Hamrell, M.R., The history of the United States Food, Drug and Cosmetic Act and the development of medicine, *Biochemical Medicine*, 33(2), April, 1985.

Jorgens, J. III., Computer hardware and software as medical devices, *Medical Device and Diagnostic Industry*, May, 1983.

King, P.H. and Fries, R.C., *Design of Biomedical Devices and Systems*, Marcel Dekker, Inc., New York, 2002.

Pressman, R.S., *Software Engineering, A Practitioner's Approach*, 2nd Edition, McGraw-Hill Book Company, New York, 1987.

Sheretz, R.J. and Streed S.A., Medical devices: significant risk vs nonsignificant risk, *The Journal of the American Medical Association*, 272(12), September, 1994.

9 Defining the device

CONTENTS

9.1 The product definition process..................................... 122
    9.1.1 Surveying the customer 123
    9.1.2 Defining the company's needs............................. 123
    9.1.3 What are the company's competencies?.................... 123
    9.1.4 What are the outside competencies?...................... 124
    9.1.5 Completing the product definition 124
9.2 Overview of quality function deployment 124
9.3 The QFD process 125
    9.3.1 The voice of the customer 125
    9.3.2 The technical portion of the matrix 126
    9.3.3 Overview of the QFD process............................ 127
9.4 Summary of QFD.. 131
9.5 The business proposal 133
    9.5.1 Project overview, objectives, major milestones,
           and schedule... 134
    9.5.2 Market need and market potential 134
    9.5.3 Product proposal 135
    9.5.4 Strategic fit... 135
    9.5.5 Risk analysis and research plan 135
    9.5.6 Economic analysis 137
    9.5.7 Core project team 137
References.. 138

New product ideas are not simply born. New product ideas come from examining the needs of hospitals, nurses, respiratory therapists, physicians, and other medical professionals, as well as from sales and marketing personnel. It is also important to talk with physicians and nurses and determine what their problems are and how they can be addressed. These problems generally represent product opportunities. A successful new product demands that it meet the end user's needs. It must have the features and provide the benefits the customer expects.

The multiphased process of defining a product involves the customer, the company, potential vendors, and current technologies (Figure 9-1). The result is a clear definition of what the product is and is expected to do, included in

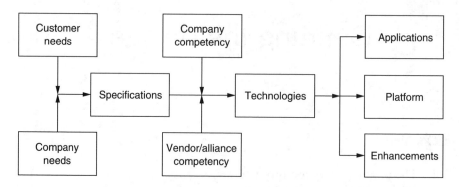

FIGURE 9-1 The product definition process

a business proposal. The first inputs to the process are the needs of the customer and the needs of the company.

The customer's needs and expectations are the primary source of information when defining a device. If the new product does not meet the customer's needs or expectations, there is no market for the device. In addition, the needs of the company are important in defining the device. Issues such as market need, product niche, etc., must be considered in the definition process.

The company's competencies must be taken into consideration. What are they, how do they match the customer's and company's needs, what is required outside of the company's competencies, and is it easily available? In addition, the competencies of potential vendors or other companies in alliance or partnership with the original company must be considered.

Once a rough idea of the potential device is taking shape, the next consideration is technologies. What technologies are appropriate for the proposed device, how available are they, are they within the company's competency, are resources readily available?

Finally, the type of proposed device must be decided. Is it a new application for older devices, is it a new platform, or is it an enhancement to an older device?

Establishing answers in these areas leads to the definition of a device which leads to the development of a product specification. Let's look at each area in more detail.

9.1   THE PRODUCT DEFINITION PROCESS

Numerous methods of obtaining new product information exist. They include various ways of collecting data, such as internal sources, industry analysis, and technology analysis. Then the information is screened and a business analysis is conducted. Regardless of the method of obtaining the information, there are certain key questions:

- Where are we in the market now?
- Where do we want to go?

- How big is the potential market?
- What does the customer really want?
- How feasible is technical development?
- How do we get where we want to go?
- What are the chances of success?

9.1.1 SURVEYING THE CUSTOMER

The customer survey is an important tool in changing an idea into a product. The criticality of the survey is exhibited by an estimate that, on the average, it takes 58 initial ideas to get one commercially successful new product to market. It is therefore necessary to talk with various leaders in potential markets to build a credible database of product ideas.

The goal of the customer survey is to match the needs of the customer with the product concept. Quality has been defined as meeting the customer needs. So a quality product is one that does what the customer wants it to do. The objective of consumer analysis is to identify segments or groups within a population with similar needs so that marketing efforts can be directly targeted to them. Several important questions must be asked to find that market which will unlock untold marketing riches:

- What is the *need* category?
- Who is buying and who is using the product?
- What is the *buying* process?
- Is what I'm selling a high- or low-involvement product?
- How can the market be segmented?

9.1.2 DEFINING THE COMPANY'S NEEDS

While segmentation analysis focuses on consumers as individuals, market analysis takes a broader view of potential consumers to include market sizes and trends. Market analysis also includes a review of the competitive and regulatory environment. Three questions are important in evaluating a market:

- What is the *relevant* market?
- Where is the product in its product life cycle?
- What are the key *competitive* factors in the industry?

9.1.3 WHAT ARE THE COMPANY'S COMPETENCIES?

Once a market segment has been chosen, a plan to beat the competition must be chosen. To accomplish this, a company must look at itself with the same level of objectivity it looks at its competitors. Important questions to assist in this analysis include:

- What are our core competencies?
- What are our weaknesses?

- How can we capitalize on our strengths?
- How can we exploit the weaknesses of our competitors?
- Who are we in the marketplace?
- How does my product map against the competition?

9.1.4 WHAT ARE THE OUTSIDE COMPETENCIES?

Once a company has objectively looked at itself, it must then look at others in the marketplace:

- What are the strengths of the competition?
- What are their weaknesses?
- What are the resources of the competition?
- What are the market shares of the industry players?

9.1.5 COMPLETING THE PRODUCT DEFINITION

There are many other questions that need to be answered in order to complete the product definition. In addition to those mentioned above, an organization needs to determine:

- How does the potential product fit with our other products?
- Do our current technologies match the potential product?
- How will we differentiate the new product?
- How does the product life cycle affect our plans?

It is also important to consider the marketing mix of products, distribution networks, pricing structure, and the overall economics of the product plan. These are all important pieces of the overall product plan as developed in a business proposal. However, the needs and wants of the customer remain the most important information to be collected. One method of obtaining the required customer requirements is quality function deployment.

9.2 OVERVIEW OF QUALITY FUNCTION DEPLOYMENT

Quality function deployment (QFD) is a process in which the "voice of the customer" is first heard and then deployed through an orderly, four-phase process in which a product is planned, designed, made, and then made consistently. It is a well-defined process that begins with customer requirements and keeps them evident throughout the four phases. The process is analytical enough to provide a means of prioritizing design trade-offs, to track product features against competitive products, and to select the best manufacturing process to optimize product features. Moreover, once in production, the process affords a means of working backwards to determine what a prospective change in the manufacturing process or in the product's components may do to the overall product attributes.

The fundamental insight of QFD from an engineering perspective is that customer wants and technical solutions do not exist in a one-to-one correspondence. Though this sounds simplistic, the implications are profound. It means that product "features" are not what customers want; instead, they want the "benefits" provided by those features. To make this distinction clear, QFD explicitly distinguishes between customer attributes that the product may have and technical characteristics that may provide some of the attributes the customer is looking for. Taking a pacemaker as an example, the customer attribute might be that the patient wants to extend their life, while the technical characteristic is that the pacemaker reduces arrhythmias.

9.3   THE QFD PROCESS

The QFD process begins with the wants of the customer, since meeting these is essential to the success of the product. Product features should not be defined by what the developers think their customers want. For clear product definition that will lead to market acceptance, manufacturers must spend both time and money learning about their customers' environments, their constraints, and the obstacles they face in using the product. By fully understanding these influencers, a manufacturer can develop products that are not obvious to its customers or competitors at the outset, but will have high customer appeal.

Quality function deployment should be viewed from a very global perspective as a methodology that will link a company with its customers and assist the organization in its planning processes. Often, an organization's introduction to QFD takes the form of building matrices. A common result is that building the matrix becomes the main objective of the process. The purpose of QFD is to get in touch with the customer and use this knowledge to develop products that satisfy the customer, not to build matrices.

QFD uses a matrix format to capture a number of issues pertinent and vital to the planning process. The matrix represents these issues in an outline form that permits the organization to examine the information in a multi-dimensional manner. This encourages effective decisions based on a team's examination and integration of the pertinent data.

The QFD matrix has two principal parts. The horizontal portion of the matrix contains information relative to the customer (Figure 9-2). The vertical portion of the matrix contains technical information that responds to the customer inputs (Figure 9-3).

9.3.1   THE VOICE OF THE CUSTOMER

The voice of the customer is the basic input required to begin a QFD project. The customer's importance rating is a measure of the relative importance that customers assign to each of the voices. The customer's competitive evaluation

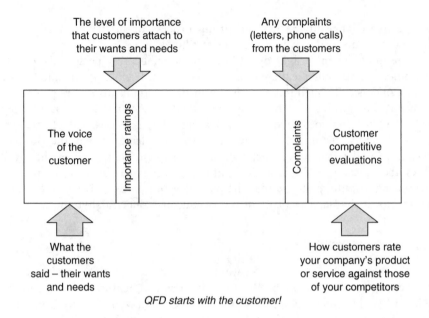

FIGURE 9-2 The customer information portion of the matrix

of the company's products or services permits a company to observe how its customers rate its products or services on a numerical scale. Any complaints that customers have personally registered with the company serve as an indication of dissatisfaction.

9.3.2 THE TECHNICAL PORTION OF THE MATRIX

The first step in developing the technical portion of the matrix is to determine how the company will respond to each voice. The technical or design requirements that the company will use to describe and measure each customer's voice are placed across the top of the matrix. For example, if the voice of the customer stated "want the control to be easy to operate," the technical requirement might be "operating effort." The technical requirements represent how the company will respond to its customer's wants and needs.

The center of the matrix, where the customer and technical portion intersect, provides an opportunity to record the presence and strength of relationships between these inputs and action items. Symbols may be used to indicate the strength of these relationships. The information in the matrix can be examined and weighed by the appropriate team. Goals or targets can be established for each technical requirement. Trade-offs can be examined and recorded in the triangular matrix at the top of Figure 9-3. This is accomplished by comparing each technical requirement against the other technical requirements. Each relationship is examined to determine the net result that changing one requirement has on the others.

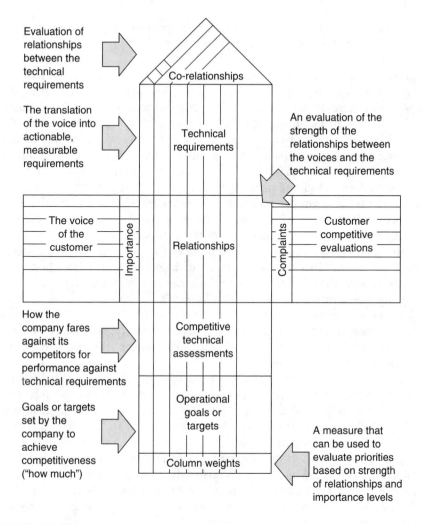

FIGURE 9-3 The technical portion of the matrix

9.3.3 OVERVIEW OF THE QFD PROCESS

The quality function deployment process is a nine step process consisting of:

- Determining the voice of the customer
- Customer surveys for importance ratings and competitive evaluation
- Develop the customer portion of the matrix
- Develop the technical portion of the matrix
- Analyze the matrix and choose priority items
- Compare proposed design concepts and synthesize the best
- Develop a part planning matrix for priority design requirements

- Develop a process-planning matrix for priority process requirements
- Develop a manufacturing planning chart

In planning a new project or revisions to an old one, organizations need to be in touch with the people who buy and use their products and services. This is vital for hard issues, such as a product whose sales are dependent on the customer's evaluation of how well their needs and wants are satisfied. It is equally crucial for softer issues, such as site selection and business planning.

Once the customers' wants and needs are known, the organization can obtain other pertinent customer information. Through surveys, it can establish how its customers feel about the relative importance of the various wants and needs. It can also sample a number of customers who use its products and competitors' products. This provides the customers' evaluation of both the organization's performance and that of its chief competitors.

Records can be examined to determine the presence of any customer complaint issues. This can be the result of letters of complaint, phone complaints, reports to the FDA, or other inquiries and comments.

Once this information is available, it can be organized and placed in the horizontal customer information portion of the QFD matrix. The voices of the customers represent their wants and needs – their requirements. These are the inputs to the matrix, along with importance ratings, competitive evaluations, and complaints.

The appropriate team can then begin developing the technical information portion of the matrix. The customers' voices must be translated into items that are measurable and actionable within the organization. Companies use a variety of names to describe these measurable items, such as design requirements, technical requirements, product characteristics, and product criteria.

The relationship between the inputs and the actionable items can then be examined. Each technical requirement is analyzed to determine if action on the item will affect the customers' requirements. A typical question would be: "Would the organization work on this technical requirement to respond favorably to the customers' requirements?"

For those items in which a relationship is determined to exist, the team then must decide on the strength of the relationship. Symbols are normally used to denote a strong, moderate, or weak relationship. Some of the symbols commonly used are a double circle, single circle, and a triangle, respectively. The symbols provide a quick visual impression of the overall relationship strengths of the technical requirements and the customers' wants and needs.

The team must instigate testing to develop technical data showing the performance of the parent company and its competitors for each of the technical requirements. Once this information is available, the team can begin a study to determine the target value that should be established for each technical requirement. The objective is to ensure that the next-generation product will be truly competitive and satisfy its customers' wants and needs. A comparison of the customers' competitive ranges and the competitive technical assessments helps the organization determine these targets.

Additional information can be added to the matrix depending on the team's judgement of value. Significant internal and regulatory requirements may be added. A measure of organizational difficulty can be added. Column weights can be calculated. These can serve as an index for highlighting those technical requirements that have the largest relative effect on the product.

Once this matrix is complete, the analysis stage begins. The chief focus should be on the customer portion of the matrix. It should be examined to determine which customer requirements need the most attention. This is an integrated decision involving the customers' competitive evaluation, their importance ratings, and their complaint histories. The number of priority items selected will be a balance between their importance and the resources available within the company.

Items selected for action can be treated as a special project or can be handled by use of the QFD matrix at the next level of detail. Any items so selected can become the input to the new matrix. Whereas the first matrix was a planning matrix for the complete product, this new matrix is at a lower level. It concerns the subsystem or assembly that affects the requirement.

The challenge in the second-level matrix (Figure 9-4) is to determine the concept that best satisfies the deployed requirement. This requires evaluation of some design concept alternatives. Several techniques are available for this type of comparative review. The criteria or requirements for the product or service are listed at the left of the matrix. Concept alternatives are listed across the top. The results of the evaluation of each concept versus the criteria can be entered in the center portion.

Once the best concept alternative is selected, a QFD part planning matrix can be generated for the component level (Figure 9-5). The development of this matrix follows the same sequence as that of the prior matrix. Generally, less competitive information is available at this level and the matrix is simpler. The technical requirements from the prior matrix are the inputs. Each component in the selected design concept is examined to determine its critical part requirements. These are listed in the upper portion. Relationships are examined and symbols are entered in the center portion. The specifications are then entered for these selected critical part requirements in the lower portion of the matrix.

The part planning matrix should then be examined. Experience with similar parts and assemblies should be a major factor in this review. The analysis should involve the issue of which of the critical part requirements listed are the most difficult to control or ensure continually. This review will likely lead to the selection of certain critical part requirements that the team believes deserve specific follow up attention.

If a team believes the selected critical part characteristics are best handled through the QFD process, a matrix should be developed (Figure 9-6) for process planning. The critical part concerns from the part planning matrix should be used as inputs in the left area of the matrix. The critical process requirements are listed across the top. Relationships are developed and examined in the central area. The specification for operating levels for each

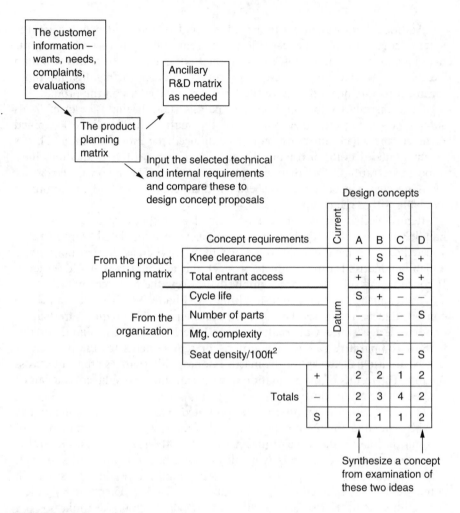

The customer information – wants, needs, complaints, evaluations

Ancillary R&D matrix as needed

The product planning matrix

Input the selected technical and internal requirements and compare these to design concept proposals

Design concepts

	Concept requirements	Current	A	B	C	D
From the product planning matrix	Knee clearance			+	S	+	+
	Total entrant access			+	+	S	+
	Cycle life	Datum		S	+	–	–
From the organization	Number of parts			–	–	–	S
	Mfg. complexity			–	–	–	–
	Seat density/100ft^2			S	–	–	S
Totals	+		2	2	1	2
	–		2	3	4	2
	S		2	1	1	2

Synthesize a concept from examination of these two ideas

FIGURE 9-4 Second-level matrix

process requirement are recorded in the lower area of the matrix. For example, if a critical part requirement was spot-weld strength, one critical process parameter would be weld current. The amount of current would be a critical process parameter to ensure proper spot weld strength. The specification for this critical process requirement would be the amperes of current required to ensure the weld strength.

Upon completion of the planning at the part and process levels, the key concerns should be deployed to the manufacturing level. Most organizations have detailed planning at this level and have developed spreadsheets and forms for recording their planning decisions. The determinations from the prior matrices should become inputs to these documents. Often, the primary document at this level is a basic planning chart (Figure 9-7). Items of concern are entered in the area farthest left. The risk associated with these items is

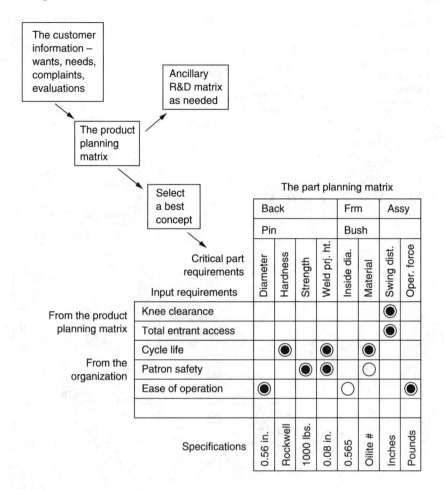

FIGURE 9-5 Part planning matrix

assessed and recorded in the next column. In typical risk assessments, the level of the concern and the probability of its occurrence are listed, as are the severity of any developing problems and the probability of detection. These items, along with other concerns, can be used to develop an index to highlight items of significant concern. Other areas in the chart can be use to indicate issues such as the general types of controls, frequency of checking, measuring devices, responsibility, and timing.

9.4   SUMMARY OF QFD

The input to the QFD planning matrix is the voice of the customer. The matrix cannot be started until the customers' requirements are known This applies to internal planning projects as well as products and services that will be sold to marketplace customers. Use of the QFD process leads an organization to develop a vital customer focus.

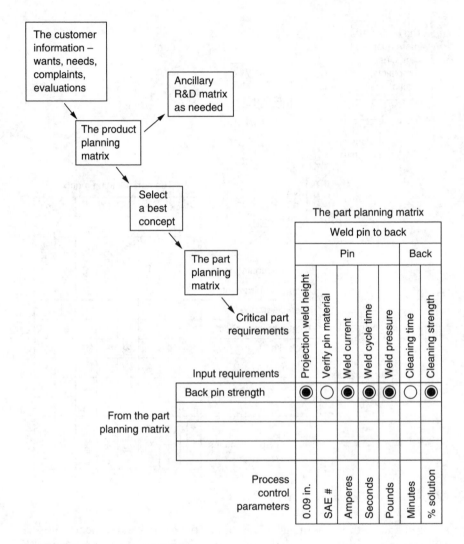

FIGURE 9-6 Process planning matrix

The initial matrix is usually the planning matrix. The customers' requirements are inputs. Subsequent matrices may be used to deploy or flow down selected requirements from the product planning matrix for part planning and process planning. Some forms of a manufacturing chart or matrix can be used to enter critical product and process requirements from prior matrices.

The principal objective of the QFD process is to help a company organize and analyze all the pertinent information associated with a project and to use the process to help it select the items demanding priority attention. All companies do many things right. The QFD process will help them focus on the areas that need special attention.

• The following are typical tools that should be considered
to assist analysis of key issues in the matrix

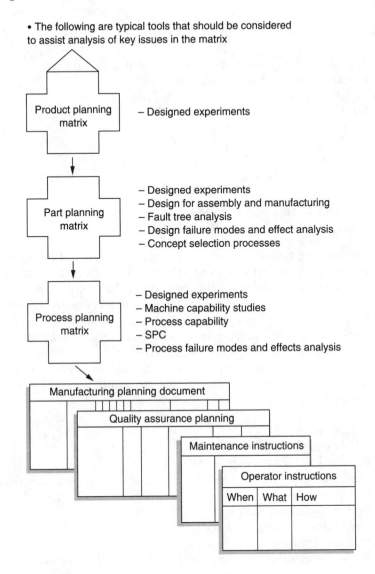

FIGURE 9-7 Manufacturing planning chart

9.5   THE BUSINESS PROPOSAL

The purpose of the business proposal is to identify and document market
needs, market potential, the proposed product, and product alternatives, risks
and unknowns, and potential financial benefits. The business proposal also
contains a proposal for further research into risks and unknowns, estimated
project costs, schedule, and a request to form a core team to carry out needed
research, to define the product and to prepare the project plan.

The business proposal usually contains:

- Project overview, objectives, major milestones, schedule
- Market need and market potential
- Product proposal
- Strategic fit
- Risk analysis and research plan
- Economic analysis
- Recommendation to form a core project team
- Supporting documentation

9.5.1 PROJECT OVERVIEW, OBJECTIVES, MAJOR MILESTONES, AND SCHEDULE

This portion of the business proposal contains a statement of overall project objectives and major milestones to be achieved. The objectives clearly define the project scope and provide specific direction to the project team.

The major milestones and schedule follow the statement of objectives. The schedule anticipates key decision points and completion of the primary deliverables throughout all phases of development and implementation. The schedule contains target completion dates; however, it must be stressed that these dates are tentative and carry an element of risk. Events contingent upon achievement of the estimated dates should be clearly stated. Examples of milestones include:

- Design feasibility
- Patent search completed
- Product specification verified by customers
- Design concept verified through completion of sub-system functional model completed
- Process validation completed
- Regulatory approval obtained
- Successful launch into territory A
- Project assessment complete, project transferred to manufacturing and sustaining engineering

9.5.2 MARKET NEED AND MARKET POTENTIAL

This section of the business proposal defines the customer and clinical need for the product or service, and identifies the potential territories to be served. Specific issues which are to be addressed include, but should not be limited to, the following:

- What is the market need for this product, i.e., what is the problem to be solved?
- What clinical value will be delivered?

- What incremental clinical value will be added over existing company or competitive offerings?
- What trends are occurring that predict this need?
- In which markets are these trends occurring?
- What markets are being considered, what is the size of the market and what are the competitive shares?
- What is the market size and the estimated growth rate for each territory to be served?
- What are the typical selling prices and margins for similar products?
- When must the product be launched to capture the market opportunity?
- If competitors plan to launch similar products, what is our assessment of their launch date?
- Have competitors announced a launch date?
- What other similar products compose the market?
- Will the same product fit in all markets served? If not, what are the anticipated gross differences and why?
- What modifications will be required?
- Is the target market broad-based and multifaceted or a focused niche?
- What are the regulatory requirements, standards, and local practices which may impact the product design for every market to be served?

9.5.3 PRODUCT PROPOSAL

The product proposal section proposes the product idea which fulfills the market need sufficiently well to differentiate its features and explain how user and/or clinical value will be derived. The product specification is not written nor does design commence during this phase. It may be necessary to perform some initial feasibility studies, construct non-working models, perform simulations and conduct research in order to have a reasonable assurance that the product can be designed, manufactured, and serviced. Additionally, models, simulations, and product descriptions will be useful to verify the idea with customers. It is also recommended that several alternative product ideas be evaluated against the "base case" idea. Such evaluation will compare risks, development timelines, costs, and success probabilities.

9.5.4 STRATEGIC FIT

This section discusses how the proposed product conforms with (or departs from) stated strategy with respect to product, market, clinical setting, technology, design, manufacturing, and service.

9.5.5 RISK ANALYSIS AND RESEARCH PLAN

This section contains an assessment of risks and unknowns, an estimate of the resources needed to reduce the risks to a level whereby the product can be designed, manufactured, and serviced with a reasonably high level of confidence. The personnel resource requirement should be accompanied by the plan and timetable for addressing, researching, and reducing the risks.

The following categories of risks and unknowns should be addressed. Not all of these categories apply for every project. Select those which could have a significant impact on achieving project objectives.

- Technical
  - Feasibility (proven, unknown, or unfamiliar?)
  - New technology
  - Design
  - Manufacturing process
  - Accessibility to technologies
  - Congruence with core competencies
  - Manufacturing process capability
  - Cost constraints
  - Component and system reliability
  - Interface compatibility
- Market
  - Perception of need in market place
  - Window of opportunity; competitive race
  - Pricing
  - Competitive positioning and reaction
  - Cannibalization of existing products
  - Customer acceptance
- Financial
  - Margins
  - Cost to develop
  - Investment required
- Regulatory
  - Filings and approvals (IDE, PMA, 510k, CE, TUV, etc.)
  - Compliance with international standards
  - Clinical studies; clinical trials
  - Clinical utility and factors, unknowns
- Intellectual property
  - Patents
  - Licensing agreements
  - Software copyrights
- Requisite skill sets available to design and develop
  - Electrical
  - Mechanical
  - Software
  - Industrial design
  - Reliability

- Manpower availability
- Vendor selection
  Quality system
  Documentation controls
  Process capability
  Component reliability
  Business stability
- Schedule
  Critical path
  Early or fixed completion date
  Resource availability
- Budget

9.5.6 ECONOMIC ANALYSIS

This section includes a rough estimate of the costs and personnel required to specify, design, develop, and launch each product variant into the market place.

9.5.7 CORE PROJECT TEAM

This section discusses the formation of a core project team to perform the research required to reduce risks and unknowns to a manageable level, to develop and verify the user specification and to prepare the project plan.

The requisite skills of the proposed team members should also be outlined. To the extent possible, the following functions should be involved in research, preparation of the user specification, and the preparation of the project plan:

- Marketing
- Engineering.
- Manufacturing
- Service
- Regulatory
- Quality assurance
- Finance

The approximate amount of time required of each participant as well as incremental expenses should also be estimated. Some examples of incremental expenses include: model development, simulation software, travel for customer verification activities, laboratory supplies, market research, and project status reviews.

REFERENCES

Day, R.G., *Quality Function Deployment – Linking a Company with its Customers*, ASQC Quality Press, Milwaukee, WI, 1993.

Fries, R.C., *Reliable Design of Medical Devices*, Marcel-Dekker, Inc., New York, 1997.

Fries, R.C., *Handbook of Medical Device Design*, Marcel-Dekker, Inc., New York, 2001.

Gause, D.C. and G.M., *Exploring Requirements: Quality Before Design*, Dorset House Publishing, New York, 1989.

Guinta, L.R. and Praizler, N.C., *The QFD Bool: The Team Approach to Solving Problems and Satisfying Customers Through Quality Function Deployment*, AMACOM Books, New York, 1993.

King, P.H. and Fries, R.C., *Design of Biomedical Devices and Systems*, Marcel Dekker, Inc., New York, 2002.

Kriewall, T.J. and Widin, G.P., An application of quality function deployment to medical device development, in *Case Studies in Medical Instrument Design*, The Institute of Electrical and Electronics Engineers, Inc., New York, 1991.

Potts, C., Takahashi, K. and Anton, A.I., Inquiry-based requirements analysis, in *IEEE Software*, 11(2), March, 1994.

Silbiger, S., *The Ten Day MBA*, William Morrow and Company, Inc., New York, 1993.

Taylor, J.W., *Planning Profitable New Product Strategies*, Chilton Book Company, Radnor, PA, 1984.

10 Requirements engineering

CONTENTS

10.1 Requirements, design, verification, and validation................. 140
    10.1.1 Refinement of requirements 141
    10.1.2 Assimilation of requirements 141
    10.1.3 Requirements versus design........................... 143
10.2 The product specification....................................... 144
10.3 The reliability goal 145
10.4 Specification review 147
10.5 The design specification 147
10.6 The software quality assurance plan (SQAP)..................... 148
    10.6.1 Purpose 149
    10.6.2 Reference documents 149
    10.6.3 Management 149
    10.6.4 Documentation....................................... 149
    10.6.5 Standards, practices, conventions, and metrics 149
    10.6.6 Review and audits.................................... 150
    10.6.7 Test... 150
    10.6.8 Problem reporting and corrective action 150
    10.6.9 Tools, techniques, and methodologies.................. 150
    10.6.10 Code control 150
    10.6.11 Media control.. 150
    10.6.12 Supplier control 150
    10.6.13 Records collection, maintenance, and retention 151
    10.6.14 Training... 151
    10.6.15 Risk management 151
    10.6.16 Additional sections as required 151
10.7 Software requirements specification (SRS) 151
    10.7.1 Purpose 151
    10.7.2 Scope 152
    10.7.3 Definitions, acronyms, and abbreviations 152
    10.7.4 References 152
    10.7.5 Overview.. 152
    10.7.6 Product perspective.................................. 152
    10.7.7 Product functions 152
    10.7.8 User characteristics.................................. 152
    10.7.9 General constraints................................... 153

          10.7.10   Assumptions and dependencies 153
          10.7.11   Specific requirements 153
10.8   The software design description (SDD) 153
          10.8.1   Decomposition description............................. 154
          10.8.2   Dependency description 154
          10.8.3   Interface description................................. 155
          10.8.4   Detailed design description 155
References 155

A widely shared piece of conventional wisdom states that requirements constitute a complete statement of what the system will do without referring to how it will do it. The resiliency of this view is indeed surprising since researchers have long argued against this simple distinction.

Clearly, requirements and design are interdependent, as practitioners surely realize. Perhaps the continuing prevalence of the "what versus how" distinction is due to the well meaning desire on the part of requirements of engineers to avoid over-constraining implementers.

10.1   REQUIREMENTS, DESIGN, VERIFICATION, AND VALIDATION

As medical products encompass more features and technology, they will grow in complexity and sophistication. The hardware and software for these products will be driven by necessity to become highly synergistic and intricate which will in turn dictate tightly coupled designs. The dilemma is whether to tolerate longer development schedules in order to achieve the features and technology, or to pursue shorter development schedules. There really is no choice given the competitive situation of the marketplace. Fortunately, there are several possible solutions to this difficulty. One solution that viably achieves shorter development schedules is a reduction of the quantity of requirements that represent the desired feature set to be implemented. By documenting requirements in a simpler way, the development effort can be reduced by lowering the overall product development complexity. This would reduce the overall hardware and software requirements which in turn reduces the overall verification and validation time.

The issue is how to reduce the number of documented requirements without sacrificing feature descriptions. This can be achieved by limiting the number of product requirements, being more judicious about how the specified requirements are defined, or by recognizing that some requirements are really design specifications. A large part of requirements definition should be geared toward providing a means to delay making decisions about product feature requirements that are not understood until further investigation is carried out.

As stated above, verification and validation must test the product to assure that the requirements have been met and that the specified design has been implemented. At worst, every requirement will necessitate at least one test to demonstrate that it has been satisfied. At best, several requirements might be grouped such that at least one test will be required to demonstrate that they all have been satisfied. The goal for the design engineer is to specify the requirements in such a manner as to achieve as few requirements as are absolutely necessary and still allow the desired feature set to be implemented. Several methods for achieving this goal are refinement of requirements, assimilation of requirements, and requirements versus design.

10.1.1 REFINEMENT OF REQUIREMENTS

As an example, suppose a mythical device has the requirement "the output of the analog to digital converter (ADC) must be accurate to within plus or minus 5%." Although conceptually this appears to be a straight-forward requirement, to the software engineer performing the testing to demonstrate satisfaction of this requirement, it is not as simple as it looks. As stated, this requirement will necessitate at least three independent tests and most likely five tests. One test will have to establish that the ADC is outputting the specified nominal value. The second and third tests will be needed to confirm that the output is within the plus or minus 5% range. Being a good software engineer, the 5% limit is not as arbitrary as it may seem due to the round off error of the percent calculation with the ADC output units. Consequently, the fourth and fifth tests will be made to ascertain the sensitivity of the round-off calculation.

A better way to specify this requirement is to state "the output of the analog to digital converter (ADC) must be between X and Y," where X and Y values correspond to the original requirement of "plus or minus 5%." This is a better requirement statement because it simplifies the testing that occurs. In this case, only two tests are required to demonstrate satisfaction of this requirement. Test one is for the X value and test two is for the Y value. The requirement statements are equivalent but the latter is more effective because it has reduced the test set size, resulting in less testing time and consequently a potential for the product to reach the market earlier.

10.1.2 ASSIMILATION OF REQUIREMENTS

Consider the situation where several requirements can be condensed into a single equivalent requirement. In this instance, the total test set can be reduced through careful analysis and an insightful design. Suppose that the user interface of a product is required to display several fields of information that indicate various parameters, states and values. It is also required that the user be able to interactively edit the fields, and that key system critical fields must flash or blink so that the user knows that a system critical field is being edited. Further assume that the software requirements document specifies that "all displayed fields can be edited. The rate field shall flash while being edited. The exposure time shall flash while being edited. The volume delivered field shall flash while being edited."

These statements are viable and suitable for the requirements specification but they may not be optimum from an implementation and test point of view. There are three possible implementation strategies for these requirements. First, a "monolithic" editor routine can be designed and implemented that handles all aspects of the field editing, including the flash function. Second, a generic field editor can be designed which is passed a parameter that indicates whether or not the field should flash during field editing. Third, an editor executive could be designed such that it selects either a non-flashing or flashing field editor routine depending on whether the field was critical or not. Conceptually, based on these requirements statements, the validation team would ensure that (1) only the correct fields can be displayed, (2) the displayed fields can be edited, (3) critical fields blink when edited, and (4) each explicitly named field blinks.

The first "monolithic" design option potentially presents the severest test case load and should be avoided. Since it is monolithic in structure and performs all editing functions, all validation tests must be performed within a single routine in order to determine whether the requirements are met. The validation testing would consist of the four test scenarios presented above.

The second design option represents an improvement over the first design. Because the flash/no flash flag is passed as a parameter into the routine, the testing internally to the routine is reduced because part of the testing burden has been shifted to the interface between the calling and called routines. This is easier to test because the flash/no flash discrimination is made at a higher level. It is an inherent part of the calling sequence of the routine and therefore can be visually verified without formal tests. The validation testing would consist of test situations 1, 2, and 4 as presented above.

The third design option represents the optimum from a test stand point because the majority of the validation testing can be accomplished with visual inspections. This is possible because the flash/no flash discrimination is also implemented at a higher level and the result of the differentiation is a flashing field or a non-flashing field. The validation testing would consist of test situations 2 and 4 as presented above.

Based on the design options, the requirements could be rewritten in order to simplify testing even further. Assume that the third design option in fact requires less testing time and is easier to test. The requirement statements can then be written in order to facilitate this situation even more. The following requirements statements are equivalent to those above and in fact tend to drive the design in the direction of the third design option. "All displayed fields can be edited. All critical items being edited shall flash to inform the user that editing is in progress." In this instance, the third design can be augmented by creating a list or look-up table of the fields required to be edited and a flag can be associated with each that indicates whether the field should flash or not. This approach allows a completely visual inspection to replace the testing because the field is either in the edit list or it is not and, if it is, then it either flashes or it does not. Testing within the routine is still required, but it now is associated with debug testing during development and not with formal validation testing after implementation.

10.1.3 REQUIREMENTS VERSUS DESIGN

There is agreement that there is a lot of overlap between requirements and design, yet the division between these two is not a hard line. Design can itself be considered a requirement. Many individuals, however, do not appreciate that the distinction between them can be used to simplify testing and consequently shorten overall software development times. Requirements and their specification concentrate on the functions that are needed by the system or product and the users. Requirements need to be discussed in terms of what has to be done, and not how it is to be done.

The requirement "hardcopy strip chart analysis shall be available" is a functional requirement. The requirement "hardcopy strip chart analysis shall be from a pull down menu" has design requirements mixed with the functional requirements. Consequently, there may be times when requirements specifications will contain information that can be construed as design. When developing a requirements specification, resist placing the "how to" design requirements in the system requirements specification and concentrate on the underlying "what" requirements.

As more "how" requirements creep into the requirements specification, more testing must occur on principally two levels. First, there is more detail to test for and second, but strategically more important, there is more validation than verification that needs to be done. Since verification is qualitative in nature and ascertains that the process and design were met, low-key activities have been transferred from the visual and inspection methods into validation testing, which is more rigorous and requires formal proof of requirements fulfillment. The distinction of design versus requirements is difficult, but a careful discrimination of what goes where is of profound benefit. As a rule of thumb, if it looks like a description of "what" needs to be implemented, then it belongs in the requirements specification. If it looks like a "how to" description, if a feature can be implemented in two or more ways and one way is preferred over another, or if it is indeterminate as to whether it is a requirement or design, then it belongs in the design specification.

There is another distinct advantage to moving as many "how" requirements to design as possible. The use of computer-aided software engineering (CASE) tools has greatly automated the generation of code from design. If a feature or function can be delayed until the design phase, it can then be implemented in an automated fashion. This simplifies the verification of the design because the automation tool has been previously verified and validated so that the demonstration that the design was implemented is simple.

10.2   THE PRODUCT SPECIFICATION

The product specification is the first step in the process of transforming product ideas into approved product development efforts. It details the results of the customer survey and subsequent interface between the marketing, design engineering, reliability assurance and regulatory affairs personnel. It specifies what the product will do, how it will do it, and how reliable it will be. To be effective, it must be as precise as possible.

The product specification should be a controlled document, that is, subject to revision level control, so that any changes that arise are subjected to review and approval prior to implementation. It prevents the all too typical habit of making verbal changes to the specification, without all concerned personnel being informed. This often leads to total confusion in later stages of development, as the current specification is only a figment of someone's imagination or a pile of handwritten papers in someone's desk.

The specification should also have joint ownership. It should only be written after all concerned departments have discussed the concept and its alternatives and have agreed on the feasibility of the design. Agreement should come from marketing, design engineering, manufacturing, customer service, reliability assurance and regulatory affairs.

The specification is a detailed review of the proposed product and includes:

- The type of product
- The market it addresses
- The function of the product
- The product parameters necessary to function effectively
- Accuracy requirements
- Tolerances necessary for function
- The anticipated environment for the device
- Cautions for anticipated misuse
- Safety issues
- Human factors issues
- The anticipated life of the product
- The reliability goal
- Requirements from applicable domestic or international standards

Each requirement should be identified with some form of notation, such as brackets and a number. For traceability purposes, each numbered subsection of the specification should start numbering its requirements with the number 1. For example:

5.3.1 Analog to Digital Converter
The output of the analog to digital converter must be between X and Y [1].

In parsing the requirements, this particular one would be referred to as 5.3.1-1. Subsequent requirements in this paragraph would be numbered in

Requirement number	Requirement	Paragraph number	Requirement number	Author	Requirement responsibility	Test type
1221	The machine shall contain no burrs or sharp edges	3.1	1	Smith	System	Visual
1222	The maximum height of the machine shall be 175 cm	3.1	2	Smith	System	Valid
1223	The maximum height of the shipping package shall be 185 cm	3.1	3	Smith	System	Valid
1224	The power supply shall have a maximum inrush current of 7.3 volts	3.2	1	Jones	Subsystem B	Verification
1225	The power supply shall provide currents of +5V, +15V, and −15V	3.2	2	Jones	Subsystem B	Verification
1226	The check valve shall withstand a pressure of 150 PSI	3.3	1	Thomas	Subsystem C	Verification

FIGURE 10-1 Example of a parsing database

consecutive order. Requirements in the next paragraph would restart the numbering with #1.

Software programs are available to assist in the parsing process. The software establishes a database of requirements for which a set of attributes are developed that help trace each requirement. Some attributes which might be established include:

- Paragraph number
- Requirement number
- Author of the requirement
- System or subsystem responsible for the requirement
- Type of verification or validation test

The database might appear as in Figure 10-1.

10.3 THE RELIABILITY GOAL

The reliability goal is a statement of how effective the product is expected to be. The reliability goal is based upon several parameters:

- The anticipated life of the device
- The anticipated usage time per year
- The complexity of the device
- The anticipated use of the device
- The technology to be used
- The failure history of similar products

The reliability goal may be defined in any of three ways:

- Reliability over a period of time
- Mean time between failure
- Warranty cost as a percentage of sales

The reliability goal may be specified as the reliability of the device over a specified period of time. For example, the reliability goal may state that the device must have a reliability of 0.99998 for an operational period of one year. This would mean 99.998% of the active units in the field would not have failed within one year. This number would be developed after analyzing the cost of repair for that number of units and whether that expense would be cost effective for the product.

The goal may be stated as a certain mean time between failure (MTBF). For example, the goal may be stated that a MTBF of 23 000 hours is desired. This would mean that 63% of the active units in the field would have failed once after 23 000 hours of operation. Again, this number would be developed from a cost analysis of the service program required to meet this goal. A review of the MTBF history of similar products is helpful in developing this number.

The third method of stating the reliability goal is warranty cost. This is defined as the expenses a company incurs in order to guarantee their product will operate without failure for a certain amount of time, usually one year. It ordinarily includes:

- The cost of replaced or repaired parts
- The cost of service's labor
- The cost of service's travel

Warranty cost directly reduces the profit from the device and may be an indicator of customer dissatisfaction. Warranty cost is typically stated as a percentage of sales.

Obviously, lower warranty cost means a more reliable device. It has been an industry standard for many years that a very successful company keeps its warranty cost at 3% of sales or less and a successful company keeps its warranty cost between 3% and 5% of sales. When the warranty cost rises above 5%, immediate action should be taken to bring it back within range, as the product expense will seriously affect profits.

Each of the three parameters can be calculated from any of the others. A detailed discussion of the mathematics involved can be found in Chapters 15 and 23.

The reliability goal is a necessary parameter for the reliability engineer to plan subsequent activities. For example, when the MTBF and reliability of the device are initially calculated from the parts list, the result will indicate whether the device will meet the reliability goal or whether the design must be revisited. As various tests are conducted, results are related to either MTBF or reliability. Again, this figure will be related to the reliability goal to determine if the design meets the specification. Finally, as field data are collected and field MTBF and reliability calculated, it ideally can be shown how the reliability has grown over time from the initial goal and has now surpassed it.

It should be apparent to the reader that it would be simple to state the reliability goal as a reliability of 1.0 or a MTBF of 1 000 000 hours or a warranty cost of 0%. This would be an ideal situation, but practically impossible. Medical devices are designed, manufactured, and serviced by human beings and, therefore, at some time, may fail. It is the responsibility of development personnel to minimize the number and reduce the effects of such failures. Thus, the reliability goal should be a practical number based on a realistic set of parameters and any history of similar types of products. Unrealistic goals result in frustration and in unnecessary activities that attempt to accomplish something impossible. It takes some research and a realistic approach to the product to develop a reliability goal that everyone can live with.

10.4 SPECIFICATION REVIEW

Once the marketing survey is complete, the reliability goal established and the product specification drafted, a review of the specification is held. The review is attended by marketing, design engineering, manufacturing, customer service, reliability engineering, and regulatory affairs. The draft of the specification is reviewed in detail. Discussion and appropriate action items are documented. Once the specification is approved, it is placed under revision level control.

With the successful completion of the review, the development process moves into the design phase, where the design specification is produced from the product specification.

10.5 THE DESIGN SPECIFICATION

The design specification is a document that is derived from the product specification. Specifically, the requirements found in the product specification are partitioned and distilled down into specific design requirements for each subassembly. The design specification should address the following areas for each subsystem:

- The reliability budget
- Service strategy
- Manufacturing strategy
- Hazard consideration
- Environmental constraints
- Safety
- Cost budgets
- Standards requirements
- Size and packaging
- The power budget

- The heat generation budget
- Industrial design/human factors
- Controls/adjustments
- Material compatibility

In addition, all electrical and mechanical inputs and outputs and their corresponding limits under all operating modes must be defined.

Each performance specification should be listed with nominal and worst-case requirements under all environmental conditions. Typical performance parameters to be considered include:

- Gain
- Span
- Linearity
- Drift
- Offset
- Noise
- Power dissipation
- Frequency response
- Leakage
- Burst pressure
- Vibration
- Long-term stability
- Operation forces/torques

As in the product specification, the requirements in the design specification should be identified by a notation such as a bracket and numbers. The parsing tool works well for focusing on these requirements.

10.6   THE SOFTWARE QUALITY ASSURANCE PLAN (SQAP)

The term *software quality assurance* is defined as a planned and systematic pattern of activities performed to assure the procedures, tools, and techniques used during software development and modification are adequate to provide the desired level of confidence in the final product. The purpose of a software quality assurance program is to assure the software is of such quality that it does not reduce the reliability of the device. Assurance that a product works reliably has been classically provided by a test of the product at the end of its development period. However, because of the nature of software, no test appears sufficiently comprehensive to adequately test all aspects of the program. Software quality assurance has thus taken the form of directing and documenting the development process itself, including checks and balances.

Specifying the software is the first step in the development process. It is a detailed summary of what the software is to do and how it will do it. The specification may consist of several documents, including the software quality assurance plan, the software requirements specification and the software design specification. These documents serve not only to define the software package, but are the main source for requirements to be used for software verification and validation.

A typical software quality assurance plan includes the following sections.

10.6.1 PURPOSE

This section delineates the specific purpose and scope of the particular SQAP. It lists the names of the software items covered by the SQAP and the intended use of the software. It states the portion of the software life cycle covered by the SQAP for each software item specified.

10.6.2 REFERENCE DOCUMENTS

This section provides a complete list of documents referenced elsewhere in the text of the SQAP.

10.6.3 MANAGEMENT

This section describes the organizational structure that influences and controls the quality of the software. It also describes that portion of the software life cycle covered by the SQAP, the tasks to be performed, with special emphasis on software quality assurance activities, and the relationships between these tasks and the planned major checkpoints. The sequence of the tasks shall be indicated as well as the specific organizational elements responsible for each task.

10.6.4 DOCUMENTATION

This section identifies the documentation governing the development, verification and validation, use, and maintenance of the software. It also states how the documents are to be checked for adequacy.

10.6.5 STANDARDS, PRACTICES, CONVENTIONS, AND METRICS

This section identifies the standards, practices, conventions, and metrics to be applied as well as how compliance with these items is to be monitored and assured.

10.6.6 REVIEW AND AUDITS

This section defines the technical and managerial reviews and audits to be conducted, states how the reviews and audits are to be accomplished, and states what further actions are required and how they are to be implemented and verified.

10.6.7 TEST

This section identifies all the tests not included in the software verification and validation plan and states how the tests are to be implemented.

10.6.8 PROBLEM REPORTING AND CORRECTIVE ACTION

This section describes the practices and procedures to be followed for reporting, tracking, and resolving problems identified in software items and the software development and maintenance processes. It also states the specific organizational responsibilities.

10.6.9 TOOLS, TECHNIQUES, AND METHODOLOGIES

This section identifies the special software tools, techniques, and methodologies that support SQA, states their purpose, and describes their use.

10.6.10 CODE CONTROL

This section defines the methods and facilities used to maintain, store, secure, and document controlled versions of the identified software during all phases of the software life cycle.

10.6.11 MEDIA CONTROL

This section states the methods and facilities used to identify the media for each computer product and the documentation required to store the media and protect computer program physical media from unauthorized access or inadvertent damage or degradation during all phases of the software life cycle.

10.6.12 SUPPLIER CONTROL

This section states the provisions for assuring that software provided by suppliers meets established requirements. It also states the methods that will be used to assure that the software supplier receives adequate and complete requirements.

10.6.13 RECORDS COLLECTION, MAINTENANCE,
AND RETENTION

This section identifies the SQA documentation to be retained, states the methods and facilities to be used to assemble, safeguard, and maintain this documentation, and designates the retention period.

10.6.14 TRAINING

This section identifies the training activities necessary to meet the needs of the SQAP.

10.6.15 RISK MANAGEMENT

This section specifies the methods and procedures employed to identify, assess, monitor, and control areas of risk arising during the portion of the software life cycle covered by the SQAP.

10.6.16 ADDITIONAL SECTIONS AS REQUIRED

Some material may appear in other documents. Reference to these documents should be made in the body of the SQAP. The contents of each section of the plan shall be specified either directly or by reference to another document.

10.7 SOFTWARE REQUIREMENTS
SPECIFICATION (SRS)

The SRS is a specification for a particular software product, program, or set of programs that perform certain functions. The SRS must correctly define all of the software requirements, but no more. It should not describe any design, verification, or project management details, except for required design constraints. A good SRS is unambiguous, complete, verifiable, consistent, modifiable, traceable, and usable during the operation and maintenance phase.

Each software requirement in an SRS is a statement of some essential capability of the software to be developed. Requirements can be expressed in a number of ways:

- Through input/output specifications
- By use of a set of representative examples
- By the specification of models

A typical software requirements specification includes the following sections.

10.7.1 PURPOSE

This section should delineate the purpose of the particular SRS and specify the intended audience.

10.7.2 SCOPE

This section should identify the software product to be produced by name, explain what the software product will, and if necessary, will not do, and describe the application of the software being specified.

10.7.3 DEFINITIONS, ACRONYMS, AND ABBREVIATIONS

This section provides the definitions of all terms, acronyms, and abbreviations required to properly interpret the SRS.

10.7.4 REFERENCES

This section should provide a complete list of all documents referenced elsewhere in the SRS or in a separate specified document. Each document should be identified by title, report number if applicable, date, and publishing organization. It is also helpful to specify the sources from which the references can be obtained.

10.7.5 OVERVIEW

This section should describe what the rest of the SRS contains and explain how the SRS is organized.

10.7.6 PRODUCT PERSPECTIVE

This section puts the product into perspective with other related products. If the product is independent and totally self-contained, it should be stated here. If the SRS defines a product that is a component of a larger system, then this section should describe the functions of each subcomponent of the system, identify internal interfaces, and identify the principal external interfaces of the software product.

10.7.7 PRODUCT FUNCTIONS

This section provides a summary of the functions that the software will perform. The functions should be organized in a way that makes the list of functions understandable to the customer or to anyone else reading the document for the first time. Block diagrams showing the different functions and their relationships can be helpful. This section should not be used to state specific requirements.

10.7.8 USER CHARACTERISTICS

This section describes those general characteristics of the eventual users of the product that will affect the specific requirements. Certain characteristics of these people, such as educational level, experience, and technical expertise impose important constraints on the system's operating environment. This section should not be used to state specific requirements or to impose specific design constraints on the solution.

10.7.9 GENERAL CONSTRAINTS

This section provides a general description of any other items that will limit the developer's options for designing the system. These can include regulatory policies, hardware limitations, interfaces to other applications, parallel operation, control functions, higher-order language requirements, criticality of the application, or safety and security considerations.

10.7.10 ASSUMPTIONS AND DEPENDENCIES

This section lists each of the factors that affect the requirements stated in the SRS. These factors are not design constraints on the software, but are any changes to them that can affect the requirements.

10.7.11 SPECIFIC REQUIREMENTS

This section contains all the details the software developer needs to create a design. The details should be defined as individual-specific requirements. Background should be provided by cross-referencing each specific requirement to any related discussion in other sections. Each requirement should be organized in a logical and readable fashion. Each requirement should be stated such that its achievement can be objectively verified by a prescribed method.

The specific requirements may be classified to aid in their logical organization. One method of classification would include:

- Functional requirements
- Performance requirements
- Design constraints
- Attributes
- External interface requirements

This section is typically the largest section within the SRS.

10.8 THE SOFTWARE DESIGN DESCRIPTION (SDD)

A software design description is a representation of a software system that is used as a medium for communicating software design information. The software design description is a document that specifies the necessary information content and recommended organization for a software design description. The SDD shows how the software system will be structured to satisfy the requirements identified in the software requirements specification. It is a translation of requirements into a description of the software structure, software components, interfaces, and data necessary for the implementation phase. In essence, the SDD becomes a detailed blueprint for the implementation activity. In a complete SDD, each requirement must be traceable to one or more design entities.

The SDD should contain the following information:

- Introduction
- References
- Decomposition description
- Dependency description
- Interface description
- Detailed design

10.8.1 DECOMPOSITION DESCRIPTION

The decomposition description records the division of the software system into design entities. It describes the way the system has been structured and the purpose and function of each entity. For each entity, it provides a reference to the detailed description via the identification attribute.

The decomposition description can be used by designers and maintainers to identify the major design entities of the system for purposes such as determining which entity is responsible for performing specific functions and tracing requirements to design entities. Design entities can be grouped into major classes to assist in locating a particular type of information and to assist in reviewing the decomposition for completeness. In addition, the information in the decomposition description can be used for planning, monitoring, and control of a software project.

10.8.2 DEPENDENCY DESCRIPTION

The dependency description specifies the relationships among entities. It identifies the dependent entities, describes their coupling, and identifies the required resources. This design view defines the strategies for interactions among design entities and provides the information needed to easily perceive how, why, where, and at what level system actions occur. It specifies the type of relationships that exist among the entities.

The dependency description provides an overall picture of how the system works in order to assess the impact of requirements and design changes. It can help maintenance personnel to isolate entities causing system failures or resource bottlenecks. It can aid in producing the system integration plan by identifying the entities that are needed by other entities and that must be developed first. This description can also be used by integration testing to aid in the production of integration test cases.

10.8.3 INTERFACE DESCRIPTION

The entity interface description provides everything designers, programmers, and testers need to know to correctly use the functions provided by an entity. This description includes the details of external and internal interfaces not provided in the software requirements specification.

The interface description serves as a binding contract among designers, programmers, customers, and testers. It provides them with an agreement needed before proceeding with the detailed design of entities. In addition, the interface description may be used by technical writers to produce customer documentation or may be used directly by customers.

10.8.4 DETAILED DESIGN DESCRIPTION

The detailed design description contains the internal details of each design entity. These details include the attribute descriptions for identification, processing, and data.

The description contains the details needed by programmers prior to implementation. The detailed design description can also be used to aid in producing unit test plans.

REFERENCES

ANSI/IEEE Standard 830, *IEEE Guide to Software Requirements Specifications*, The Institute of Electrical and Electronics Engineers, Inc., New York, 1984.

ANSI IEEE Standard 1016, *IEEE Recommended Practice for Software Design Descriptions*, The Institute of Electrical and Electronics Engineers, Inc., New York, 1987.

ANSI/IEEE Standard 730, *IEEE Standard for Software Quality Assurance Plans*, The Institute of Electrical and Electronics Engineers, Inc., New York, 1989.

Chevlin, D.H. and Jorgens III, J., Medical device software requirements: definition and specification, *Medical Instrumentation* 30(2), March/April, 1996.

Davis, A.M. and Hsia, P., Giving voice to requirements engineering, *IEEE Software*, 11(2), March, 1994.

Fairly, R.E., *Software Engineering Concepts*, McGraw-Hill Book Company, New York, 1985.

Fries, R.C., *Reliability Assurance for Medical Devices, Equipment and Software*, Interpharm Press, Buffalo Grove, IL, 1991.

Fries, R.C., *Reliable Design of Medical Devices*, Marcel-Dekker, Inc., New York, 1997.

Fries, R.C., *Handbook of Medical Device Design*, Marcel-Dekker, Inc., New York, 2001.

Gause, D.C. and Weinberg, G.M., *Exploring Requirements: Quality Before Design*, Dorset House Publishing, New York, 1989.

Keller, M. and Shumate, K., *Software Specification and Design: A Disciplined Approach for Real-Time Systems*, John Wiley & Sons, Inc., New York, 1992.

King, P.H. and Fries, R.C., *Design of Biomedical Devices and Systems*, Marcel Dekker, Inc., New York, 2002.

Potts, C., Takahashi, K. and Anton, A.I., Inquiry-based requirements analysis, *IEEE Software*, 11(2), March, 1994.

Pressman, R.S., *Software Engineering: A Practitioner's Approach*, McGraw-Hill Book Company, New York, 1987.

Siddiqi, J. and Shekaran, M.C., Requirements engineering: the emerging wisdom, *Software*, 13(2), March, 1996.

11 Safety and risk management

CONTENTS

11.1   Risk 158
11.2   Deciding on acceptable risk......................................160
11.3   Factors important to medical device risk assessment 160
    11.3.1   Device design and manufacture 160
    11.3.2   Materials 161
    11.3.3   Device users 161
    11.3.4   Human factors 162
    11.3.5   Medical device systems 162
11.4   Risk management 162
11.5   The risk management process.....................................162
    11.5.1   Identifying the risk factors 164
    11.5.2   Assessing risk probabilities and effects on the project..... 164
    11.5.3   Developing strategies to mitigate identified risks 165
    11.5.4   Monitoring risk factors 165
    11.5.5   Invoking a contingency plan 166
    11.5.6   Managing the crisis 166
    11.5.7   Recovering from the crisis 166
11.6   Tools for risk estimation 166
    11.6.1   Hazard/risk analysis 166
    11.6.2   Failure mode and effects analysis 169
        11.6.2.1   The FMEA process 169
    11.6.3   Fault tree analysis 172
        11.6.3.1   The fault tree process 172
        11.6.3.2   Example of a fault tree analysis 173
References 176

Medical devices have become a visible and dramatic part of modern medical care. The period following World War II has seen the development of a tremendous range of devices that have revolutionized medical practice and improved or prolonged millions of lives. At the same time, devices are not automatically beneficial, and they, like all technology, are associated with risk.

Recent examples include ultrasound equipment that often does not comply with electrical safety guidelines, leakage of insulin pumps, defective artificial cardiac valves, and reactions of the body to materials used in implants.

Issues of balancing risk and benefit are familiar in the field of drugs. Drugs are regulated for efficacy and safety in most countries, and many countries make concerted attempts to influence how drugs are prescribed. International organizations, such as Health Action International, continually monitor safety and efficacy with regard to drugs. Devices, however, get much less attention. It seems they are almost ignored despite their similarities to drugs: they are pervasive in medical care, they are products made and marketed by a profit-making industry, they are often taken into the body, and they are associated with demonstrable problems of efficacy and safety. In addition, they are associated with important economic effects in terms of health care expenditures and the strength of national industrial efforts.

11.1   RISK

The term risk is defined as the probable rate of occurrence of a hazard causing harm and the degree of severity of the harm. The concept has two elements: (1) the possibility of a hazardous event and (2) the severity of the consequence of that hazardous event.

The probability of occurrence may be classified into various levels as described in Table 11-1. The levels of severity may be classified as indicated in Table 11-2. The US Food and Drug Administration has rated medical devices into three levels of concern: major, moderate, and minor. The severity levels in Table 11-2 approximate the FDA levels as follows:

Major	Critical
Moderate	Marginal
Minor	Negligible

Risk may be graphed into three regions when analyzing the probabilities of occurrence and the levels of severity (Figure 11-1). The risk regions are

---

TABLE 11-1
Probability of occurrence and consequences

Probability of occurrence	Consequence
Frequent	Likely to occur often
Probable	Will occur several times in the lifetime of the device
Occasional	Likely to occur sometime in the lifetime of the device
Remote	Unlikely to occur, but possible
Improbable	Probability of occurrence indistinguishable from zero
Impossible	Probability of occurrence is zero

TABLE 11-2
Severity levels and consequences

Severity level	Consequence
Catastrophic	Potential of resulting in multiple deaths or serious injuries
Critical	Potential of resulting in death or serious injury
Marginal	Potential of resulting in injury
Negligible	Little or no potential to result in injury

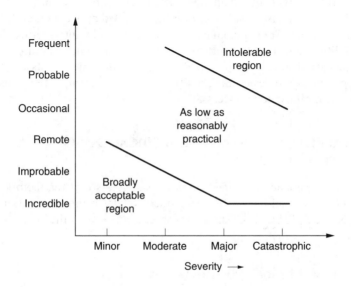

FIGURE 11-1 Risk probability regions

classified as the intolerable region, the as low as reasonably practical region, and the broadly acceptable region.

The intolerable region contains the risk of some hazards that are so bad, a system which incorporated them would not be tolerated. A risk in this region has to be reduced either by reducing the severity and/or the probability of occurrence.

The region between the intolerable and the broadly acceptable is called the as low as reasonably practical (ALARP) region. In this region, risks are reduced to the lowest practical level, bearing in mind the benefits of accepting the risk and the cost of further risk reduction. Any risk must be reduced to a level which is as low as reasonably practical. Near the limit of intolerable risk, risks would normally be reduced, even at considerable cost. Risks near the broadly acceptable region would be reduced if reasonable to do so, but the measure of reasonableness will have been raised. If the risk falls between the intolerable and broadly acceptable and if the ALARP principle has been applied, the resulting risk is the acceptable risk for that particular hazard.

In some cases, either the severity and/or the probability of occurrence is so low that the risk is negligible compared with the risk of other hazards that are accepted. Risk reduction, in this broadly acceptable region, need not be actively pursued.

11.2 DECIDING ON ACCEPTABLE RISK

There is no standard that defines acceptable risk. It is planned that particular device standards will give guidance. Often acceptable risk has to be established on a case by case basis, based on the intended application and the operating environment. Some guidance may be obtained by interpreting the single fault condition and from the performance of similar equipment already in use.

In the case of medical equipment, it may be that the risk associated with the equipment would be acceptable if the prognosis was improved. This cannot be used as an excuse for unnecessary risk.

11.3 FACTORS IMPORTANT TO MEDICAL DEVICE RISK ASSESSMENT

The FDA's experience with medical devices suggests that the factors that are important to medical device risk assessment relate to the device itself and to how it is used. Table 11-3 shows those categories and the major elements of each.

11.3.1 DEVICE DESIGN AND MANUFACTURE

A device can present a hazard if it is poorly manufactured or if insufficient attention is paid to design elements that influence performance. For example, the failure to design a structural component to resist the stress to which it will be subjected could lead to its fracture. Quality control or quality assurance

---

TABLE 11-3
Major factors considered in medical device risk assessment

For the device	For device use
Design	Adequacy of instructions
Human factors engineering	Training of users
Manufacturing of quality control and quality assurance	Interaction with other devices
Materials toxicity	Human factors engineering
Materials degradation	

during manufacturing may not correct the problem. The FDA's experience suggests strongly that good manufacturing practices do not eliminate inherently bad designs, and could simply ensure that a bad design is faithfully produced. Alternatively, inattention to manufacturing quality assurance could unintentionally cause a device defect.

Device hazards also can be considered in terms of whether the product does something that can cause harm, or whether the product fails to provide a benefit that it could. For example, patients and health professionals may be harmed by an electric shock from a supposedly insulated device. A missed diagnosis, on the other hand, could lead to inappropriate therapy or no therapy at all, each with dire consequences for the patient. It is important to the eventual management of risk to determine if the hazard arises from omission or commission.

11.3.2 Materials

Materials from which devices are made are a part of the design and manufacturing process considerations. Proper design includes selection of appropriate materials. Good manufacturing practice includes process validation to ensure that the material's properties are not compromised. It is also important to consider materials separately when the device in question is applied to or implanted in the body. In this regard, both the effect of the material on the body and the effect of the body on the material are important.

11.3.3 Device users

The FDA's experience has repeatedly and consistently been that how a device is used is a significant part of the overall safety and effectiveness of that device. From the sample collection procedures that can influence the result obtained from an in vitro diagnostic device to the poor X-ray film processing techniques that lead to the need for a retake, experience clearly indicates the importance of the user.

The user of a medical device can be a health care professional, a patient, or a family member. There is a large variability in users' skills with devices, due to factors such as education and training, health status, environment, and motivation. Whatever the capability of a particular user, circumstances occur that can be a controlling influence, such as the inattention that can result when a tired individual tries to perform a repetitive task.

The user also represents the decision point on the application of medical technology. The decision may be wrong. Patients may inappropriately rely on over-the-counter devices.

The kinds of hazards that may result from user error are not unusual in themselves. What is unusual is that the incidence of such hazards occurring can range from non-existent to frequent, depending on the influence of the user. Thus, the training of the user and the adequacy of the instructions provided with the device relate directly to assessing the above risks.

11.3.4   HUMAN FACTORS

Human factors are those device design elements and use conditions that influence how the device and the user interact. This interaction places an additional complexity on the ability to identify the hazards that might be associated with a particular device. Without considering human factors as part of the risk assessment, it would have been difficult to consider the appropriate risk management approach.

11.3.5   MEDICAL DEVICE SYSTEMS

The device-intensive nature of certain medical circumstances results in many devices used within close proximity to each other. Such configurations may have been considered by the manufacturer as part of the design, but the ingenuity of device users to devise new systems may outstrip the manufacturer's expectations. Depending on the configuration and number of devices involved, hazards to the patient can result from the interference of one device with another, for example, electromagnetic interference. Users may also attempt to interchange incompatible device components in an attempt at repair and create a risk to the patient. Even if the manufacturer intended for the device to be used in an environment with many others, patients can be at risk because of user behavior in dealing with the total amount of information that must be monitored. Again, developing appropriate problem-solving approaches depends on accurate problem identification.

11.4   RISK MANAGEMENT

Risk management is an ongoing process continually iterated throughout the life of a project. Some potential problems never materialize. Others materialize and are dealt with. New risks are identified and mitigation strategies are devised as necessary. Some potential problems submerge, only to resurface later. Following the risk management procedures described here can increase the probability that potential problems will be identified, confronted, and overcome before they become crisis situations.

11.5   THE RISK MANAGEMENT PROCESS

Many software projects fail to deliver acceptable systems within schedule and budget. Many of these failures might have been avoided had the project team properly assessed and mitigated the risk factors, yet risk management is seldom applied as an explicit project management activity. One reason risk management is not practiced is that very few guidelines are available that offer a practical, step-by-step approach to managing risk.

The risk management process is a multi-stepped process consisting of:

- Identifying the risk factors
- Assessing risk probabilities and effects on the project

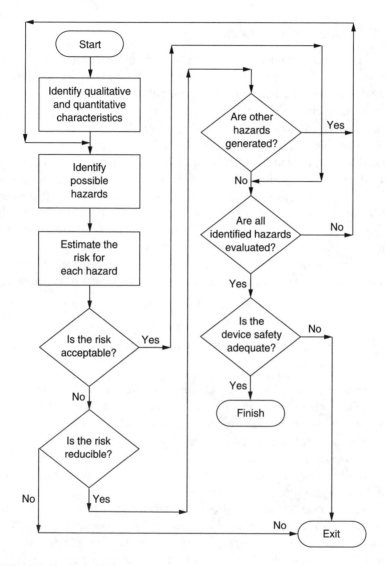

FIGURE 11-2 Typical risk management process

- Developing strategies to mitigate identified risks
- Monitoring risk factors
- Invoking a contingency plan
- Managing the crisis
- Recovering from the crisis

A risk management process should be used throughout the development life cycle. The objective of the process is to manage risk so that it is both less than the maximum tolerable risk and also is as low as reasonably practical. A typical risk management process is shown in Figure 11-2.

11.5.1 IDENTIFYING THE RISK FACTORS

A risk is a potential problem. A problem is a risk that has materialized. Exactly when the transformation takes place is somewhat subjective. A schedule delay of 1 week might not be a cause for concern, but a delay of 1 month could have serious consequences. The important thing is that all parties who may be affected by a schedule delay agree in advance on the point at which a risk will become a problem. That way, when the risk does become a problem, it is mitigated by the planned corrective actions. In identifying a risk, one must take care to distinguish symptoms from underlying risk factors. A potential delay may in fact be a symptom of difficult technical issues or inadequate resources.

Whether you identify a situation as a risk or an opportunity depends on your point of view. Is the glass half full or half empty? Situations with high potential for failure often have the potential for high payback as well. Risk management is not the same as risk aversion. Competitive pressures and the demands of modern society require that one take risks to be successful.

11.5.2 ASSESSING RISK PROBABILITIES AND EFFECTS ON THE PROJECT

Because risk implies a potential loss, one must estimate two elements of a risk: the probability that the risk will become a problem and the effect the problem would have on the project's desired outcome. For software projects, the desired outcome is an acceptable product delivered on time and within budget. Factors that influence product acceptability include delivered functionality, performance, resource use, safety, reliability, versatility, ease of learning, ease of use, and ease of modification.

Depending on the situation, failure to meet one or more of these criteria within the constraints of schedule and budget can precipitate a crisis for the developer, the customer, and/or the user community. Thus, the primary goal of risk management is to identify and confront risk factors with enough lead time to avoid a crisis.

The best approach is to assess the probability of risk by computing probability distributions for code size and complexity and use them to determine the effect of limited target memory and execution time on overall project effort. Monte Carlo simulation is then used to compute the distribution of estimated project effort as a function of size, complexity, timing, and memory, using regression based modeling. This approach uses estimated effort as the metric to assess the impact of risk factors. Because effort is the primary cost factor for most software projects, one can use it as a measure of overall project cost, especially when using loaded salaries burdened with facilities, computer time, and management, for example.

11.5.3 DEVELOPING STRATEGIES TO MITIGATE IDENTIFIED RISKS

In general, a risk becomes a problem when the value of a quantitative metric crosses a predetermined threshold. For that reason, two essential parts of risk management are setting thresholds, beyond which some corrective action is required, and determining ahead of time what that corrective action will be. Without such planning, one quickly realizes the truth in the answer to Fred Brooks' rhetorical question, "How does a project get to be a year late?" One day at a time.

Risk mitigation involves two types of strategies: action planning and contingency planning.

Action planning addresses risks that can be mitigated by immediate response. To address the risk of insufficient experience with a new hardware architecture, for example, the action plan could provide for training the development team, hiring experienced personnel, or finding a consultant to work with the project team. Of course, one should not spend more on training or hiring than would be paid back in increased productivity. If you estimate that training and hiring can increase productivity by 10%, for example, one should not spend more than 10% of the project's personnel budget in this manner.

Contingency planning, on the other hand, addresses risks that require monitoring for some future response should the need arise. To mitigate the risk of late delivery by a hardware vendor, for example, the contingency plan could provide for monitoring the vendor's progress and developing a software emulator for the target machine.

Of course, the risk of late hardware delivery must justify the added cost of preparing the contingency plan, monitoring the situation, and implementing the plan's actions. If the cost is justified, plan preparation and vendor monitoring might be implemented immediately, but the action to develop an emulator might be postponed until the risk of late delivery became a problem. This raises the issue of sufficient lead time. When does one start to develop the emulator? The answer lies in analyzing the probability of late delivery. As that probability increases, the urgency of developing the emulator becomes greater.

11.5.4 MONITORING RISK FACTORS

One must monitor the values of risk metrics, taking care that the metrics data are objective, timely, and accurate. If metrics are based on subjective factors, your project will quickly be reported as 90% complete and remain there for many months. One must avoid situations in which the first 90% of the project takes the first 90% of the schedule, while the remaining 10% of the project takes another 90% of the schedule.

11.5.5 INVOKING A CONTINGENCY PLAN

A contingency plan is invoked when a quantitative risk indicator crosses a predetermined threshold. One may find it difficult to convince the affected parties that a serious problem has developed, especially in the early stages of a project. A typical response is to plan on catching up during the next reporting period, but most projects never catch up without the explicit, planned corrective actions of a contingency plan. One must also specify the duration of each contingency plan to avoid contingent actions of interminable duration. If the team cannot solve the problem within a specified period, typically one or two weeks, they must invoke a crisis-management plan.

11.5.6 MANAGING THE CRISIS

Despite a team's best efforts, the contingency plan may fail, in which case the project enters the crisis mode. There must be some plan for seeing a project through this phase, including allocating sufficient resources and specifying a drop-dead date, at which time management must reevaluate the project for more drastic corrective action.

11.5.7 RECOVERING FROM THE CRISIS

After a crisis, certain actions are required, such as rewarding personnel who have worked in burnout mode for an extended period and reevaluating cost and schedule in light of the drain on resources from managing the crisis.

11.6 TOOLS FOR RISK ESTIMATION

Several tools are helpful in conducting a risk estimation. These include:

- Hazard/risk analysis
- Failure mode and effects analysis (FMEA)
- Fault tree analysis (FTA)

11.6.1 HAZARD/RISK ANALYSIS

A hazard/risk analysis is the process, continuous throughout the product development cycle, that examines the possible hazards that could occur due to equipment failure and helps the designer to eliminate the hazard through various control methods. The hazard analysis is conducted on hardware, software, and the total system during the initial specification phase and is updated throughout the development cycle. The hazard analysis is documented on a form similar to that shown in Figure 11-3.

Hazard/risk analysis

Device: _____   Designer: _____   Data: _____

Potential hazard	Generic cause	Specific cause	Probability of occurrence	Severity level	Risk level	Control mode	Control method	Comments

FIGURE 11-3 Hazard analysis form

The following issues are addressed on the hazard analysis form:

- Potential hazard   Identifies possible harm to patient, operator, or system
- Generic cause   Identifies general conditions that can lead to the associated potential hazard
- Specific cause   Identifies specific instances that can give rise to the associated generic cause
- Probability   Classifies the likelihood of the associated potential hazard according to Table 11.4
- Severity   Categorizes the associated potential hazard according to Table 11.5
- Control mode   Means of reducing the probability and/or severity of the associated potential hazard
- Control method   Actual implementation to achieve the associated control mode
- Comments   Additional information, references, etc.
- Review comments   Comments written down during the review meeting

---

TABLE 11-4
Probability of occurrence table

Probability	Occurrence	Details
1	Frequent	Likely to occur often
2	Occasional	Will occur several times in the lifetime of the device
3	Reasonably remote	Likely to occur sometime in the lifetime of the device
4	Remote	Unlikely to occur, but possible
5	Extremely remote	Probability of occurrence indistinguishable from zero
6	Physically impossible	Probability of occurrence is zero

TABLE 11-5
Hazard severity table

Severity	Occurrence	Details
I	Catastrophic	Potential of resulting in multiple deaths or serious injuries
II	Critical	Potential of resulting in death or serious injury
III	Marginal	Potential of resulting in non-life-threatening injury
IV	Negligible	Little or no potential to result in non-life-threatening injury

When the hazard analysis is initially completed, the probability and severity refer to the potential hazard prior to its being controlled. As the device is designed to minimize or eliminate the hazard, and control methods are imposed, the probability and severity will be updated.

11.6.2 FAILURE MODE AND EFFECTS ANALYSIS

The failure mode and effects analysis (FMEA) is a method of reliability analysis intended to identify failures which have significant consequences affecting the system performance in the application considered.

Generally, failures or failure modes of any component will affect system performance adversely. In the study of system reliability, safety, and availability, both qualitative and quantitative analyses are required and these complement one another. Quantitative analysis methods allow the calculation or prediction of performance indices of the system while fulfilling a specific task or in long term operation under specific conditions. Typical indices denote reliability, safety, availability, failure rates, etc.

The FMEA is based on that defined component or sub-assembly level where the basic failure criteria are available. Starting from the basic element failure characteristics and the functional system structure, the FMEA determines the relationship between the element failures and the system failures, malfunctions, operational constraints and degradation of performance or integrity. To evaluate secondary and higher-order system and subsystem failures, the sequences of events in time may also have to be considered.

In a narrow sense, the FMEA is limited to a qualitative analysis of failure modes of hardware, and does not include human errors and software errors, despite the fact that current systems are usually subject to both. In a wider sense, these factors could be included.

Information from the FMEA identifies priorities for process controls and inspection tests during manufacture and installation, and for qualification, approval, acceptance, and start-up tests. It provides essential information for diagnostic and maintenance procedures.

11.6.2.1 The FMEA process

The analysis is initiated by selecting the lowest level of interest (usually the part, circuit, or module level) at which sufficient information is available. At this lowest level, the various failure modes that can occur for each item at that level are tabulated. The corresponding failure effect for each, taken singly and in turn, is interpreted as a failure mode for consideration of the failure effect at the next higher functional level. Successive iterations result in the identification of the failure effects, in relation to specific failure modes, at all necessary functional levels up to the system or highest level.

Appendix 3 lists common failure modes and their frequency of occurrence.

Failure modes and effects analysis

Device: _____ Designer: _____ Date: _____

Component	Component function	Failure mode	Effect on system	Cause of failure	Severity level	Probability of occurrence	Risk level	Design control

FIGURE 11-4 Failure mode and effects analysis form

The failure mode and effects analysis is documented on a form similar to that shown in Figure 11-4. The following issues are addressed on the FMEA form:

- Component   Name of the component under analysis
- Function   Function performed by the component
                       in the system
- Failure mode   The specific failure mode
- Effect   The effect of the failure mode on the
                       system
- Cause   The specific cause of the failure mode
- Severity   Categorizes the associated potential
                       hazard according to Table 11-5
- Probability   Classifies the likelihood of the associated
                       potential hazard according to Table 11-4
- Overall risk   Categorizes the overall risk of the failure
                       according to Tables 11-6 and 11-7
- Comments   Additional information, references, etc.
- Review comments   Comments written down during the
                       review meeting

TABLE 11-6
An example of a risk table

		Consequence		
Occurrence	Negligible	Marginal	Critical	Catastrophic
Frequent	II	I	I	I
Probable	III	II	I	I
Occasional	III	III	II	I
Remote	IV	III	III	II
Improbable	IV	IV	III	III
Incredible	IV	IV	IV	IV

TABLE 11-7
An example interpretation of risk levels

Risk Level	Interpretation
I	Intolerable risk
II	Undesirable risk, tolerable only if reduction is impractical or if the costs are grossly disproportionate to the improvement gained
III	Tolerable risk if the cost of risk reduction would exceed the improvement gained
IV	Negligible risk

11.6.3 Fault tree analysis

Fault tree analysis is a "paper analysis" type of testing. Analysis starts by considering the various system modes of failures and working downward to identify the component cause of the failure and the probability of that failure.

A fault tree is a logic diagram of a system that pictorially shows all probable failure modes and the sequence in which they occur, leading to a specified system failure. Since a logic flow process is used, standard logic and event symbols are used (Figure 11-5).

11.6.3.1 The fault tree process

Fault tree analysis is a step-wise sequential process beginning with the collection of appropriate documentation for creating the fault tree. This documentation may include parts lists, operating environment requirements, user manual, etc.

Once the documentation is reviewed, a failure is chosen that becomes the top event on the tree. This is the starting point for analysis and should be well defined and measurable. Where more than one top event can be identified, a separate fault tree should be conducted for each event.

Once this top event is identified, the fault tree can be developed. Branches from the top event are drawn to the events on the next level that could

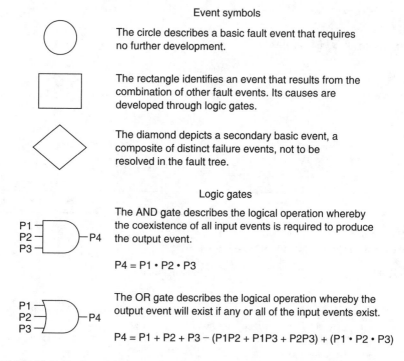

Event symbols

The circle describes a basic fault event that requires no further development.

The rectangle identifies an event that results from the combination of other fault events. Its causes are developed through logic gates.

The diamond depicts a secondary basic event, a composite of distinct failure events, not to be resolved in the fault tree.

Logic gates

The AND gate describes the logical operation whereby the coexistence of all input events is required to produce the output event.

$$P4 = P1 \cdot P2 \cdot P3$$

The OR gate describes the logical operation whereby the output event will exist if any or all of the input events exist.

$$P4 = P1 + P2 + P3 - (P1P2 + P1P3 + P2P3) + (P1 \cdot P2 \cdot P3)$$

FIGURE 11-5 Logic symbols

cause it. The secondary events are analyzed to determine if they are OR gates, AND gates, or can be represented by an event symbol. The analysis continues downward until the lowest level is composed of basic fault events.

Once the tree is drawn, probability values are assigned to each gate or event. The quantification of the basic fault events can be derived from established sources of component failure rates, e.g., MIL–HDBK–217, field use failure data, or vendor test data. Upper levels are calculated using the equations for the particular gates.

Finally, the analysis is reviewed to determine where corrective action is necessary. Once corrective action is decided upon, action items are assigned and completion dates set. Following the review, a summary test report is issued.

11.6.3.2   Example of a fault tree analysis

An alarm circuit (Figure 11-6) is to be analyzed. Components and their probability of failure are shown in Table 11-8. The top event is chosen to be the lamp (C5) failing to light. The lamp would fail to light if:

> the switches failed to close
> > or
> the source failed
> > or
> the lamp and resistor failed

The next level of failures is chosen. The source fails if:

> the source fails
> > or
> the emergency battery is ineffective

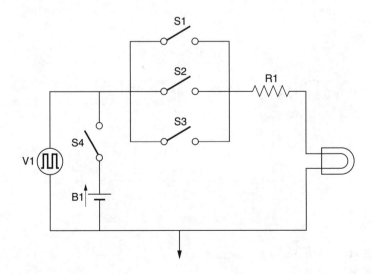

FIGURE 11-6 Alarm circuit

TABLE 11-8
Components and failure probabilities

Component	Designation	Failure probability
Voltage source	V1	0.01752
Switch	S4	0.00438
Battery	B1	0.03679
Switch	S1	0.00438
Switch	S2	0.00438
Switch	S3	0.00438
Resistor	R1	0.00263
Lamp	L1	0.00876

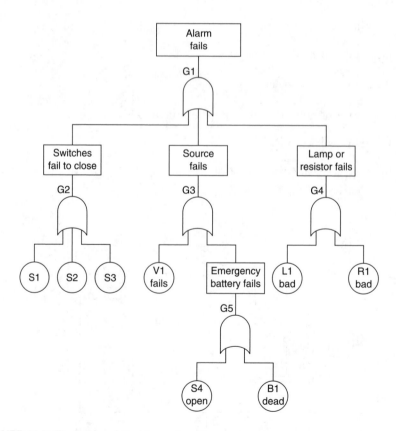

FIGURE 11-7 Fault tree of the alarm circuit

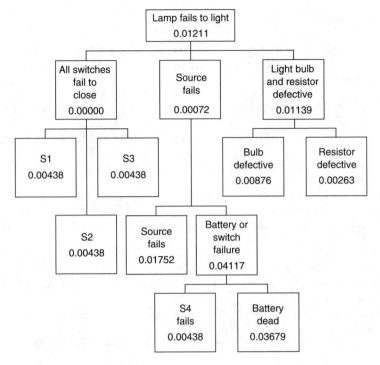

FIGURE 11-8 Probability tree

The lamp and resistor fail if:

    the bulb is defective
        or
    the resistor is defective

At the lowest level, the emergency battery is ineffective if:

    the switch fails to close
        or
    the battery is dead

Figure 11-7 shows the fault tree for the circuit.

    Once the fault tree is developed, the probabilities for each level can be entered in a probability tree and the probability of failure for the top event calculated, using the equations for the gates. Figure 11-8 shows the probability tree for the alarm circuit.

REFERENCES

AAMI/ISO 14971-1, *Medical Devices – Risk Management – Part 1: Application of Risk Analysis*, Association for the Advancement of Medical Instrumentation, Arlington, VA, 1998.

Anderson, F.A., Medical device risk assessment, in *The Medical Device Industry – Science, Technology, and Regulation in a Competitive Environment*, Marcel Dekker, Inc., New York, 1990.

Banta, H.D., The regulation of medical devices, *Preventive Medicine*, 19(6), November, 1990.

Boehm, B.W., *Software Risk Management*, IEEE Computer Society Press, Washington, DC, 1989.

Brooks, F., *The Mythical Man-Month*, Addison-Wesley Publishers, Reading, MA, 1975.

Fairley, R., Risk management for software projects, *IEEE Software*, 11(3), May, 1994.

Fries, R.C., *Reliability Assurance for Medical Devices, Equipment and Software*, Interpharm Press Inc., Buffalo Grove, IL, 1991.

Fries, R.C., *Reliable Design of Medical Devices*, Marcel-Dekker, Inc., New York, 1997.

Fries, R.C., *Handbook of Medical Device Design*, Marcel-Dekker, Inc., New York, 2001.

King, P.H. and Fries, R.C., *Design of Biomedical Devices and Systems*, Marcel Dekker, Inc., New York, 2002.

Levenson, N.G., Software safety: why, what and how, *Computing Surveys*, 18(2), June, 1986.

Levenson, N.G., *Safeware*, Addison-Wesley Publishers, Reading, MA, 1995.

12 Liability

CONTENTS

12.1 Negligence 178
12.2 Strict liability 179
12.3 Breach of warranty... 179
    12.3.1 Implied warranties...................................... 179
    12.3.2 Exclusion of warranties................................ 180
12.4 Defects... 180
12.5 Failure to warn of dangers 182
12.6 Plaintiff's conduct 182
12.7 Defendant's conduct 183
12.8 Defendant-related issues....................................... 183
12.9 Manufacturer's and physician's responsibilities.................. 183
12.10 Conclusion.. 184
References.. 185

Law can be defined as the collection of rules and regulations by which society is governed. The law regulates social conduct in a formal binding way while it reflects society's needs, attitudes, and principles. Law is a dynamic concept that lives, grows, and changes. It can be described as a composite of court decisions, regulations and sanctioned procedures, by which laws are applied and disputes adjudicated.

The three most common theories of liability for which a manufacturer may be held liable for personal injury caused by its product are negligence, strict liability, and breach of warranty. These are referred to as common-law causes of action, which are distinct from causes of action based on federal or state statutory law. Although within the last decade federal legislative action that would create a uniform federal product liability law has been proposed and debated, no such law exists today. Thus, such litigation is governed by the laws of each state.

These three doctrines are called "theories of recovery" because an injured person cannot recover damages against a defendant unless he alleges and proves, through use of one or more of these theories, that the defendant owed him a legal duty and that the defendant breached that duty, thereby causing the plaintiff's injuries. Although each is conceptually distinct, similarities exist between them. Indeed, two or more theories are asserted in many product defect suits.

12.1 NEGLIGENCE

Since much of medical malpractice litigation relies on negligence theory, it is important to clearly establish the elements of that cause of action. Negligence may be defined as conduct which falls below the standard established by law for the protection of others against unreasonable risk of harm. There are four major elements of the negligence action:

- That a person or business owes a duty of care to another
- That the applicable standard for carrying out the duty be breached
- That as proximate cause of the breach of duty a compensable injury results
- That there be compensable damages or injury to the plaintiff

The burden is on the plaintiff to establish each and every element of the negligence action.

The basic idea of negligence law is that one should have to pay for injuries that he or she causes when acting below the standard of care of a reasonable, prudent person participating in the activity in question. This standard of conduct relates to a belief that centers on potential victims: that people have a right to be protected from unreasonable risks of harm. A fundamental aspect of the negligence standard of care resides in the concept of foreseeability.

A plaintiff in a product liability action grounded in negligence, then, must establish a breach of the manufacturer's or seller's duty to exercise reasonable care in the manufacture and preparation of a product. The manufacturer in particular must be certain that the product is free of any potentially dangerous defect that might become dangerous upon the happening of a reasonably anticipated emergency. The obligation to exercise reasonable care has been expanded to include reasonable care in the inspection or testing of the product, the design of the product, or the giving of warnings concerning the use of the product.

A manufacturer must exercise reasonable care even though he is but a link in the production chain that results in a finished product. For example, a manufacturer of a product which is designed to be a component part of another manufactured product is bound by the standard of reasonable care. Similarly, a manufacturer of a finished product which incorporates component parts fabricated elsewhere has the same legal obligation.

A seller of a product, on the other hand, is normally held to a less stringent standard of care than a manufacturer. The lesser standard is also applied to distributors, wholesalers, or other middlemen in the marketing chain. This rule pertains because a seller or middleman is viewed as simply a channel through which the product reaches the consumer.

In general, the duty owed at any particular time varies with the degree of risk involved in a product. The concept of reasonable care is not static, but changes with the circumstances of the individual case. The care must be commensurate with the risk of harm involved. Thus, manufacturers or sellers of certain hazardous products must exercise a greater degree of care in their operations than manufacturers or sellers of other less dangerous products.

12.2 STRICT LIABILITY

Unlike the negligence suit, in which the focus is on the defendant's conduct, in a strict liability suit, the focus is on the product itself. The formulation of strict liability states that one who sells any product in a defective condition unreasonably dangerous to the user or consumer or to his property is subject to liability for physical harm thereby caused to the ultimate user or consumer or to his property if the seller is engaged in the business of selling such a product, and it is expected to and does reach the user or consumer without substantial change to the condition in which it is sold. Therefore, the critical focus in a strict liability case is on whether the product is defective and unreasonably dangerous. A common standard applied in medical device cases to reach that determination is the risk/benefit analysis – that is, whether the benefits of the device outweigh the risks attendant with its use.

The result of strict liability is that manufacturers, distributors, and retailers are liable for the injuries caused by defects in their products, even though the defect may not be shown to be the result of any negligence in the design or manufacture of the product. Moreover, under strict liability, the manufacturer cannot assert any of the various defenses available to him in a warranty action.

Strict liability means that a manufacturer may be held liable even though he has exercised all possible care in the preparation and sale of this product. The sole necessity for manufacturer liability is the existence of a defect in the product and a causal connection between this defect and the injury which resulted from the use of the product.

12.3 BREACH OF WARRANTY

A warranty action is contractual rather than tortious in nature. Its basis lies in the representations, either express or implied, which a manufacturer or a seller makes about its product.

A third cause of action that may be asserted by a plaintiff is breach of warranty. There are three types of breaches of warranty that may be alleged:

1. Breach of the implied warranty of merchantability
2. Breach of the implied warranty of fitness for a particular purpose
3. Breach of an express warranty

12.3.1 IMPLIED WARRANTIES

Some warranties accompany the sale of an article without any express conduct on the part of the seller. These implied warranties are labeled the warranties of merchantability and of fitness for a particular purpose.

A warranty that goods shall be merchantable is implied in a contract for their sale, if the seller is a merchant who commonly deals with such goods. At a minimum, merchantable goods must:

- Pass without objection in the trade under the contract description
- Be fit for the ordinary purposes for which they are used
- Be within the variations permitted by the sales agreement, of even kind, quality, and quantity within each unit and among all units involved
- Be adequately contained, packaged, and labeled as the sales agreement may require
- Conform to the promises or affirmations of fact made on the container or label

The implied warranty of fitness for a particular purpose arises when a buyer makes known to the seller the particular purpose for which the goods are to be used, and the buyer, relying on the seller's skill or judgement, receives goods which are warranted to be sufficient for that purpose.

12.3.2 EXCLUSION OF WARRANTIES

The law has always recognized that sellers may explicitly limit their liability upon a contract of sale by including disclaimers of any warranties under the contract. The Uniform Commercial Code embodies this principle and provides that any disclaimer, exclusion, or modification is permissible under certain guidelines. However, a disclaimer is not valid if it deceives the buyer.

These warranty causes of action do not offer any advantages for the injured plaintiff that cannot be obtained by resort to negligence and strict liability claims and, in fact, pose greater hurdles to recovery. Thus, although a breach of warranty claim is often pled in the plaintiff's complaint, it is seldom relied on at trial as the basis for recovery.

12.4 DEFECTS

The term "defect" is used to describe generically the kinds and definitions of things that courts find to be actionable wrong with products when they leave the seller's hands. In the decisions, however, the courts sometimes distinguish between defectiveness and unreasonable danger. Other considerations in determining defectiveness are:

- Consumer expectations
- Presumed seller knowledge
- Risk–benefit balancing
- State of the art
- Unavoidably unsafe products

A common and perhaps the prevailing definition of product unsatisfactoriness is that of "unreasonable danger." This has been defined as the article sold must be dangerous to an extent beyond that which would be contemplated by the ordinary consumer who purchases it, with the ordinary knowledge common to the community as to its characteristics.

Another test of defectiveness sometimes used is that of presumed seller knowledge: would the seller be negligent in placing a product on the market if he had knowledge of its harmful or dangerous condition? This definition contains a standard of strict liability, as well as one of defectiveness, since it assumes the seller's knowledge of a product's condition even though there may be no such knowledge or reason to know.

Sometimes a risk–benefit analysis is used to determine defectiveness, particularly in design cases. The issue is phrased in terms of whether the cost of making a safer product is greater or less than the risk or danger from the product in its present condition. If the cost of making the change is greater than the risk created by not making the change, then the benefit or utility of keeping the product as is outweighs the risk and the product is not defective. If, on the other hand, the cost is less than the risk then the benefit or utility of not making the change is outweighed by the risk and the product in its unchanged condition is defective.

Risk–benefit or risk–burden balancing involves questions concerning state of the art, since the burden of eliminating a danger may be greater than the risk of that danger if the danger cannot be eliminated. State of the art is similar to the unavoidably unsafe defense where absence of the knowledge or ability to eliminate a danger is assumed for purposes of determining if a product is unavoidably unsafe. "State of the art" is defined as the state of scientific and technological knowledge available to the manufacturer at the time the product was placed in the market.

Determining defectiveness is one of the more difficult problems in product liability, particularly in design litigation. There are three types of product defects:

1. Manufacturing or production defects
2. Design defects
3. Defective warnings or instructions

The issue implicates questions of the proper scope of the strict liability doctrine, and the overlapping definitions of physical and conceptual views of defectiveness.

Manufacturing defects can rarely be established on the basis of direct evidence. Rather, a plaintiff who alleges the existence of a manufacturing defect in the product must usually resort to the use of circumstantial evidence in order to prove that the product was defective. Such evidence may take the form of occurrence of other similar injuries resulting from use of the product, complaints received about the performance of the product, defectiveness of other units of the product, faulty methods of production, testing, or analysis of the product, elimination of other causes of the accident, and comparison with similar products.

A manufacturer has a duty to design his product so as to prevent any foreseeable risk of harm to the user or patient. A product which is defectively designed can be distinguished from a product containing a manufacturing defect. While the latter involves some aberration or negligence in the manufacturing process, the former encompasses improper planning in connection with the preparation of the product. Failure to exercise reasonable care in the design of a product is negligence. A product which is designed in a way which makes it unreasonably dangerous will subject the manufacturer to strict liability. A design defect, in contrast to a manufacturing defect, is the result of the manufacturer's conscious decision to design the product in a certain manner.

Product liability cases alleging unsafe design may be divided into three basic categories:

- Cases involving concealed dangers
- Cases involving a failure to provide appropriate safety features
- Cases involving construction materials of inadequate strength

A product has a concealed danger when its design fails to disclose a danger inherent in the product which is not obvious to the ordinary user.

Some writers treat warning defects as a type of design defect. One reason for doing this is that a warning inadequacy, like a design inadequacy, is usually a characteristic of a whole line of products, while a production or manufacturing flaw is usually random and atypical of the product.

12.5   FAILURE TO WARN OF DANGERS

An increasingly large portion of product liability litigation concerns the manufacturer's or seller's duty to warn of actual or potential dangers involved in the use of the product. Although the duty to warn may arise under all three theories of product liability, as mentioned above, most warning cases rely on negligence principles as the basis for the decision. The general rule is that a manufacturer or seller who has knowledge of the dangerous character of the product has a duty to warn users of this danger. Thus, failure to warn where a reasonable man would do so is negligence.

12.6   PLAINTIFF'S CONDUCT

A manufacturer or seller may defend a product liability action by demonstrating that the plaintiff either engaged in negligent conduct that was a contributing factor to his injury, or used a product when it was obvious that a danger existed and thereby assumed the risk of his injury. Another type of misconduct which may defeat recovery is when the plaintiff misuses the product by utilizing it in a manner not anticipated by the manufacturer. The applicability of these defenses in any given product suit is dependent upon the theory or theories of recovery which are asserted by the plaintiff.

12.7 DEFENDANT'S CONDUCT

Compliance with certain standards by a manufacturer may provide that party with a complete defense if the product leaves the manufacturer's or seller's possession or control and when it is a substantial or proximate cause of the plaintiff's injury. Exceptions to this rule include alterations or modifications made with the manufacturer's or seller's consent, or according to manufacturer's/seller's instructions.

12.8 DEFENDANT-RELATED ISSUES

When a medical device proves to be defective, potential liability is created for many parties who may have been associated with the device. Of all the parties involved, the injured patient is least able to bear the financial consequences. To place the financial obligation upon the proper parties, the courts must consider the entire history of the product involved, often from the time the design concept was spawned until the instant the injury occurred. The first parties encountered in this process are the designers, manufacturers, distributors, and sellers of the product.

Physicians and hospitals are subject to liability through medical malpractice actions for their negligence, whether or not a defective product is involved. Where such a product is involved, the doctor or hospital may be liable for:

- Negligent misuse of the product
- Negligent selection of the product
- Failure to inspect or test the product
- Using the product with knowledge of its defect

12.9 MANUFACTURER'S AND PHYSICIAN'S RESPONSIBILITIES

Manufacturers of medical devices have a duty with regard to manufacture, design, warnings, and labeling. A manufacturer is required to exercise that degree of care which a reasonable, prudent manufacturer would use under the same or similar conditions. A manufacturer's failure to comply with the standard in the industry, including failing to warn or give adequate instructions, may result in a finding of liability against the manufacturer.

With regard to medical devices, a manufacturer must take reasonable steps to warn physicians of dangers of which it is aware or reasonably should be aware, where the danger would not be obvious to the ordinary competent physician dispensing a particular device. The responsibility for the prudent use of the medical device is with a physician. A surgeon who undertakes to perform a surgical procedure has the responsibility to act reasonably.

It is therefore required of the manufacturer to make a full disclosure of all known side effects and problems with a particular medical device by use of appropriate warnings given to physicians. The physician is to act as the learned intermediary between the manufacturer and the patient and transmit appropriate information to the patient. The manufacturer, however, must provide the physician with the information in order that he can pass it on to the patient.

In addition, the manufacturer's warnings must indicate the scope of potential danger from the use of a medical device and the risks of its use. This is particularly important where there is "off label use" (the practice of using a product approved for one application in a different application) by a physician.

The manufacturer's warnings must detail the scope of potential danger from the use of a medical device, including the risks of misuse. The warnings must alert a reasonably competent physician to the dangers of not using a product as instructed. It would seem then that the manufacturer may be held liable for failing to disclose the range of possible consequences of the use of a medical device if it has knowledge that the particular device is being used "off label."

The duty of a manufacturer and physician for use of a medical device will be based upon the state of knowledge at the time of the use. The physician therefore has a responsibility to be aware of the manufacturer's warnings as he considers the patient's condition. This dual responsibility is especially relevant in deciding what particular medical device to use. Physician judgement and an analysis of the standard of care in the community should predominate the court's analysis in determining liability for possible misuses of the device.

A concern arises if the surgeon has received instruction as to the specific device from a manufacturer outside an investigative device exemption (IDE) clinical trail approved by the FDA. In such circumstances, plaintiffs will maintain that the manufacturer and physician conspired to promote a product that is unsafe for "off label use."

12.10 CONCLUSION

Products liability will undoubtedly continue to be a controversial field of law, because it cuts across so many fundamental issues of our society. It will also remain a stimulating field of study and practice, since it combines a healthy mixture of the practical and theoretical. The subject will certainly continue to change, both by statutory and by common law modification.

Products liability implicates many of the basic values of our society. It is a test of the ability of private industry to accommodate competitiveness and safety. It tests the fairness and the workability of the tort system of recovery, and of the jury system as a method of resolving disputes.

REFERENCES

Boardman, T.A. and Dipasquale, T., Product liability implications of regulatory compliance or non-compliance, in *The Medical Device Industry – Science, Technology, and Regulation in a Competitive Environment*, Marcel-Dekker, Inc., New York, 1990.

Boumil, M.M. and Elias, C.E., *The Law of Medical Liability in a Nutshell*, West Publishing Co., St. Paul, MN, 1995.

Buchholz, S.D., Defending pedicle screw litigation, in *For the Defense*, 38(3), March, 1996.

Fries, R.C., *Reliable Design of Medical Devices*, Marcel-Dekker, Inc., New York, 1997.

Fries, R.C., *Handbook of Medical Device Design*, Marcel-Dekker, Inc., New York, 2001.

Gingerich, D., *Medical Product Liability: A Comprehensive Guide and Sourcebook*, F & S Press, New York, 1981.

Kanoti, G.A., Ethics, medicine, and the law, in *Legal Aspects of Medicine*, Springer-Verlag, New York, 1989.

King, P.H. and Fries, R.C., *Design of Biomedical Devices and Systems*, Marcel-Dekker, Inc., New York, 2002.

Phillips, J.J., *Products Liability in a Nutshell*, 4th edition, West Publishing Co., St. Paul, MN, 1993.

Shapo, M.S., *Products Liability and the Search for Justice*, Carolina Academic Press, Durham, NC, 1993.

13 Intellectual property

CONTENTS

13.1	Patents		188
	13.1.1	What qualifies as a patent	188
		13.1.1.1 Patentable subject matter	189
		13.1.1.2 Usefulness	189
		13.1.1.3 Novelty	189
		13.1.1.4 Non-obviousness	189
		13.1.1.5 Improvement of an existing invention	190
		13.1.1.6 A design	190
	13.1.2	The patent process	191
	13.1.3	Patent claims	192
	13.1.4	Protecting your rights as an inventor	192
	13.1.5	Patent infringement	193
13.2	Copyrights		194
	13.2.1	What can be copyrighted?	195
	13.2.2	The copyright process	196
		13.2.2.1 Copyright notice	196
		13.2.2.2 Copyright registration	197
	13.2.3	Copyright duration	197
	13.2.4	Protecting your copyright rights	198
	13.2.5	Infringement	198
13.3	Trademarks		198
	13.3.1	Selecting a trademark	199
		13.3.1.1 What is a distinctive trademark?	200
	13.3.2	The trademark process	201
	13.3.3	Intent to use registration	201
	13.3.4	Protecting your trademark rights	202
13.4	Trade secrets		202
	13.4.1	What qualifies for trade secrecy	203
	13.4.2	Trade secrecy authorship	203
	13.4.3	How trade secrets are lost	203
	13.4.4	Duration of trade secrets	204
	13.4.5	Protecting your trade secret rights	204
	13.4.6	A trade secrecy program	204

13.4.7   Use of trade secrecy with copyrights and patents......... 205
          13.4.7.1   Trade secrets and patents 205
          13.4.7.2   Trade secrets and copyrights 205
References.. 205

Intellectual property is a generic term used to describe the products of the human intellect that have economic value. Intellectual property is "property" because a body of laws has been created over the last 200 years that gives owners of such works legal rights, similar in some respects to those given to owners of real estate or tangible personal property. Intellectual property may be owned, bought, and sold the same as other types of property.

There are four separate bodies of law that may be used to protect intellectual property. These are patent law, copyright law, trademark law, and trade secret law. Each of these bodies of law may be used to protect different aspects of intellectual property, although there is a great deal of overlap among them.

13.1   PATENTS

A patent is an official document, issued by the U.S. government or another government, that describes an invention and confers on the inventors a monopoly over the use of the invention. The monopoly allows the patent owner to go to court to stop others from making, selling, or using the invention without the patent owner's permission.

Generally, an invention is any device or process that is based on an original idea conceived by one or more inventors and is useful in getting something done or solving a problem. An invention may also be a non-functional unique design or a plant. But when the word "invention" is used out in the real world, it almost always means a device or process. Many inventions, while extremely clever, do not qualify for patents, primarily because they are not considered to be sufficiently innovative in light of previous developments. The fact that an invention is not patentable does not mean necessarily that it has no value for its owner.

There are three types of patents that can be created: utility, design, and plant patents. Table 13-1 compares the three type of patents and the monopoly each type grants to the author.

13.1.1   WHAT QUALIFIES AS A PATENT

An invention must meet several basic legal tests in order to qualify as a patent. These include:

• Patentable subject matter
• Usefulness
• Novelty

TABLE 13-1
Patent monopolies

Type of patent	Length of monopoly (years)
Utility	20
Design	14
Plant	20

- Non-obviousness
- An improvement over an existing invention
- A design

13.1.1.1   Patentable subject matter

The most fundamental qualification for a patent is that the invention consists of patentable subject matter. The patent laws define patentable subject matter as inventions that are one of the following:

- A process or method
- A machine or apparatus
- An article of manufacture
- A composition of matter
- An improvement of an invention in any of these classes

13.1.1.2   Usefulness

Almost always, an invention must be useful in some way to qualify for a patent. Fortunately, this is almost never a problem, since virtually everything can be used for something.

13.1.1.3   Novelty

As a general rule, no invention will receive a patent unless it is different in some important way from previous inventions and developments in the field, both patented and unpatented. To use legal jargon, the invention must be novel over the prior art. As part of deciding whether an invention is novel, the U.S. patent law system focuses on two issues: when the patent application is filed, and when the invention was first conceived.

13.1.1.4   Non-obviousness

In addition to being novel, an invention must have a quality that is referred to as "non-obviousness." This means that the invention would have been surprising or unexpected to someone who is familiar with the field of the invention. And, in deciding whether an invention is non-obvious, the U.S. Patent and Trademark Office (PTO) may consider all previous developments (prior art) that existed when the invention was conceived. Obviousness is a quality that is difficult to define, but supposedly a patent examiner knows when they see it.

As a general rule, an invention is considered non-obvious when it does one of the following:

- Solves a problem that people in the field have been trying to solve for some time
- Does something significantly quicker that was previously possible
- Performs a function that could not be performed before

13.1.1.5 Improvement of an existing invention

Earlier we noted that, to qualify for a patent, an invention must fit into at least one of the statutory classes of matter entitled to a patent – a process, a machine, a manufacture, a composition of matter, or an improvement of any of these. As a practical matter, this statutory class is not very important since even an improvement on an invention in one of the other statutory classes will also qualify as an actual invention in that class. In other words, an invention will be considered as patentable subject matter as long as it fits within at least one of the other four statutory classes – whether or not it is viewed as an improvement or an original invention.

13.1.1.6 A design

Design patents are granted to new, original and ornamental designs that are a part of articles of manufacture. Articles of manufacture are in turn defined as anything made by the hands of humans. In the past, design patents have been granted to items such as truck fenders, chairs, fabric, athletic shoes, toys, tools, and artificial hip joints.

The key to understanding this type of patent is the fact that a patentable design is required to be primarily ornamental and an integral part of an item made by humans.

A design patent provides a 14-year monopoly to industrial designs that have no functional use. That is, contrary to the usefulness rule discussed above, designs covered by design patents must be purely ornamental. The further anomaly of design patents is that while the design itself must be primarily ornamental, as opposed to primarily functional, it must at the same time be embodied in something people-made. Design patents are easy to apply for, as they do not require much written description. They require drawings for the design, a short description of each figure or drawing, and one claim that says little more than the inventor claims the ornamental design depicted on the attached drawings. In addition, the design patent is less expensive to apply for than a utility patent, lasts for 14 rather than 20 years, and requires no maintenance fees.

13.1.2 THE PATENT PROCESS

The patent process consists of the following steps:

- Note all problems caused by equipment, supplies, or non-existing devices when performing a task
- Focus on the problem every time you perform the task or use the item
- Concentrate on solutions
- Keep a detailed, dated diary of problems and solutions; include drawings and sketches
- Record the benefits and usefulness of your idea
- Evaluate the marketability of your idea. It if does not have a wide application, it may be more advantageous to abandon the idea and focus on another
- Do not discuss your idea with anyone except one person you trust who will maintain confidentially
- Prepare an application with a patent attorney
- Have a search done; first a computer search, then a hand search

Purchase a composition book with bound pages for keeping your notes. Start each entry with the date, and include all details of problem identification and solutions. Use drawings or sketches of your idea. Never remove any pages. If you do not like an entry or have made a mistake, simply make an X through the entry or write "error." Sign all entries and have a witness sign and date them as frequently as possible. Your witness should be someone you trust who understands your idea and will maintain confidentiality.

The patent document contains:

- A title for the invention and the names and addresses of the inventors
- Details of the patent search made by the PTO
- An abstract that concisely describes the key aspects of the invention
- Drawings or flowcharts of the invention
- Very precise definitions of the invention covered by the patent (called the patent claims)
- A brief summary of the invention

Taken together, the various parts of the patent document provide a complete disclosure of every important aspect of the covered invention. When a U.S. patent is issued, all the information in the patent is readily accessible to the public in the PTO and in patent libraries across the U.S. and through on-line patent database services.

U.S. patents are obtained by submitting to the PTO a patent application and an application fee. Once the application is received, the PTO assigns it to an examiner who is supposed to be knowledgeable in the technology underlying the invention. The patent examiner is responsible for deciding whether the invention qualifies for a patent and, assuming it does, what the scope of the patent should be. Usually, back and forth communications – called patent prosecution – occur between the applicant and the examiner regarding these issues. Clearly the most serious and hard-to-fix issue is whether the invention qualifies for a patent.

Eventually, if all of the examiner's objections are overcome by the applicant, the invention is approved for a patent. A patent issue fee is paid and the applicant receives an official copy of the patent deed. Three additional fees must be paid over the life of the patent to keep it in effect.

13.1.3 PATENT CLAIMS

Patent claims are the part of the patent application that precisely delimits the scope of the invention – where it begins and where it ends. Perhaps it will help understand what patent claims do if you analogize them to real estate deeds. A deed typically includes a description of the parcel's parameters precise enough to map the exact boundaries of the plot of land in question which, in turn, can be used as the basis of a legal action to toss out any trespassers.

With patents, the idea is to similarly draw in the patent claims a clear line around the property of the inventor so that any infringer can be identified and dealt with. Patent claims have an additional purpose. Because of the precise way in which they are worded, claims also are used to decide whether, in light of previous developments, the invention is patentable in the first place.

Unfortunately, to accomplish these purposes, all patent claims are set forth in an odd, stylized format. But the format has a big benefit. It makes it possible to examine any patent application or patent granted by the PTO and get a pretty good idea about what the invention covered by the patent consists of. While the stylized patent claim language and format have the advantage of lending a degree of precision to a field that badly needs it, there is an obvious and substantial downside to the use of the arcane patent-speak. Mastering it amounts to climbing a fairly steep learning curve.

It is when you set out to understand a patent claim that the rest of the patent becomes crucially important. The patent's narrative description of the invention – set out in the patent specification – with all or many of the invention's possible uses, and the accompanying drawings or flowcharts, usually provide enough information in combination to understand any particular claim. And, of course, the more patent claims you examine, the more adept you will become in deciphering them.

13.1.4 PROTECTING YOUR RIGHTS AS AN INVENTOR

If two inventors apply for a patent around the same time, the patent will be awarded to the inventor who came up with the invention first. This may or may not be the inventor who was first to file a patent application. For this reason, it is vital that one carefully document the inventive activities. If two or more pending patent applications by different inventors claim the same invention, the PTO will ask the inventors to establish the date each of them first conceived the invention and the ways in which they then showed diligence in "reducing the invention to practice."

Inventors can reduce the invention to practice in two ways: (1) by making a working model – a prototype – which works as the idea of the invention dictates it should or (2) by constructively reducing it to practice – that is, by describing the invention in sufficient detail for someone else to build it – in a document that is then filed as a patent application with the PTO.

The inventor who conceived the invention first will be awarded the patent if he or she also showed diligence in either building the invention or filing a patent application. If the inventor who was second to conceive the invention was the first one to reduce it to practice – for instance by filing a patent application – that inventor may end up with the patent.

It is often the quality of the inventor's documentation (dated, written in a notebook, showing the conception of the invention and the steps that were taken to reduce the invention to practice) that determines which invention ends up with the patent.

You especially should be aware that you can unintentionally forfeit your right to obtain patent protection. This can happen if you disclose your invention to others, such as a company interested in the invention, and then do not file an application within 1 year from that disclosure date. The same 1-year period applies if you offer your invention, or a product made by your invention, for sale. You must file your patent application in the U.S. within 1 year from any offer of sale.

Even more confusing is the fact that most other countries do not allow this 1-year grace period. Any public disclosure before you file your first application will prevent you from obtaining patent protection in nearly every country other than the U.S.

13.1.5 PATENT INFRINGEMENT

Patent infringement occurs when someone makes, uses, or sells a patented invention without the patent owner's permission. Defining infringement is one thing, but knowing when it occurs in the real world is something else. Even with common technologies, it can be difficult for experienced patent attorneys to tell whether patents have been infringed.

There are multiple steps in deciding whether infringement of a patent has occurred:

- Identify the patent's independent apparatus and method claims
- Break these apparati and method claims into their elements
- Compare these elements with the alleged infringing device or process and decide whether the claim has all of the elements that constitute

the alleged infringing device or process. If so, the patent has probably been infringed. If not, proceed to the next step

- If the elements of the alleged infringing device or process are somewhat different than the elements of the patent claim, ask if they are the same in structure, function, and result. If yes, you probably have infringement. Note that for infringement to occur, only one claim in the patent needs to be infringed

A patent's independent claims are those upon which usually one or more claims immediately following depend. A patent's broadest claims are those with the fewest words and that therefore provide the broadest patent coverage. The patent's broadest claims are its independent claims. As a general rule, if you find infringement of one of the broadest claims, all the other patent's claims that depend on that claim are infringed. Conversely, if you don't find infringement by comparison with a broad claim, then you won't find infringement of claims which depend on it. Although an infringement is declared on a claim-by-claim basis, generally it will be declared that the patent itself is infringed.

In apparatus (machine) claims, the elements are usually conceptualized as the (a), (b), (c), etc., parts of the apparatus that are listed, interrelated, and described in detail following the word "comprising" at the end of the preamble of the claim. Elements in method (process) claims are the steps of the method and sub-parts of those steps.

If each and every element of the patent's broadest claims are in the infringing device, the patent is probably infringed. The reason you start by analyzing the broadest claim is that, by definition, that claim has the fewest elements and it is therefore easier to find infringements.

Even if infringement can't be found on the basis of the literal language in the claims, the courts may still find infringement if the alleged infringing device's elements are equivalent to the patent claims in structure, function, and result. Known as the Doctrine of Equivalents, this rule is difficult to apply in practice.

13.2   COPYRIGHTS

A copyright is a legal device that provides the creator of a work of authorship the right to control how the work is used. If someone wrongfully uses material covered by a copyright, the copyright owner can sue and obtain compensation for any losses suffered, as well as an injunction requiring the copyright infringer to stop the infringing activity.

A copyright is a type of tangible property. It belongs to its owner and the courts can be asked to intervene if anyone uses it without permission. Like other forms of property, a copyright may be sold by its owner, or otherwise exploited by the owner for economic benefit.

The Copyright Act of 1976 grants creators many intangible, exclusive rights over their work, including reproduction rights – the right to make copies of a protected work; distribution rights – the right to sell or otherwise distribute copies to the public; the right to create adaptations – the right to prepare new works based on the protected work; performance and display rights – the right to perform a protected work or display a work in public.

Copyright protects all varieties of original works of authorship, including:

- Literary works
- Motion pictures, videos, and other audiovisual works
- Photographs, sculpture, and graphic works
- Sound recordings
- Pantomimes and choreographic works
- Architectural works

13.2.1 WHAT CAN BE COPYRIGHTED?

Not every work of authorship receives copyright protection. A program or other work is protected only if it satisfies all three of the following requirements:

- Fixation
- Originality
- Minimal creativity

The work must be fixed in a tangible medium of expression. Any stable medium from which the work can be read back or heard, either directly or with the aid of a machine or device, is acceptable.

Copyright protection begins the instant you fix your work. There is no waiting period and it is not necessary to register the copyright. Copyright protects both completed and unfinished works, as well as works that are widely distributed to the public or never distributed at all.

A work is protected by copyright only if, and to the extent, it is original. But this does not mean that copyright protection is limited to works that are novel – that is new to the world. For copyright purposes, a work is "original" if at least a part of the work owes its origin to the author. A work's quality, ingenuity, aesthetic merit, or uniqueness is not considered.

A minimal amount of creativity over and above the independent creation requirement is necessary for copyright protection. Works completely lacking creativity are denied copyright protection even if they have been independently created. However, the amount of creativity required is very slight.

In the past, some courts held that copyright protected works that may have lacked originality and/or creativity if a substantial amount of work was involved in their creation. Recent court cases have outlawed this "sweat of the brow" theory. It is now clear that the amount of work put in to create a work of authorship has absolutely no bearing on the degree of copyright protection it will receive. Copyright only protects fixed, original, minimally creative expressions, not hard work.

Perhaps the greatest difficulty with copyrights is determining just what aspects of any given work are protected. All works of authorship contain elements that are protected by copyright and elements that are not protected. Unfortunately, there is no system available to precisely identify which aspects of a given work are protected. The only time we ever obtain a definitive answer as to how much any particular work is protected is when it becomes the subject of a copyright infringement lawsuit. However, there are two tenets which may help in determining what is protected and what is not. The first tenet states that a copyright only protects "expressions," not ideas, systems, or processes. Tenet two states the scope of copyright protection is proportional to the range of expression available. Let us look at both in detail.

Copyright only protects the tangible expression of an idea, system, or process – not the idea, system, or process itself. Copyright law does not protect ideas, procedures, processes, systems, mathematical principles, formulas, algorithms, methods of operation, concepts, facts, or discoveries. Remember, copyright is designed to aid the advancement of knowledge. If the copyright law gave a person a legal monopoly over ideas, the progress of knowledge would be impeded rather than helped.

The scope of copyright protection is proportional to the range of expression available. The copyright law only protects original works of authorship. Part of the essence of original authorship is the making of choices. Any work of authorship is the end result of a whole series of choices made by its creator. For example, the author of a novel expressing the idea of love must choose the novel's plot, characters, locale, and the actual words used to express the story. The author of such a novel has a nearly limitless array of choices available. However, the choices available to the creators of many works of authorship are severely limited. In these cases, the idea or ideas underlying the work and the way they are expressed by the author are deemed to "merge." The result is that the author's expression is either treated as if it were in the public domain or protected only against virtually verbatim or "slavish" copying.

13.2.2 THE COPYRIGHT PROCESS

13.2.2.1 Copyright notice

Before 1989, all published works had to contain a copyright notice, (the "©" symbol followed by the publication date and copyright owner's name) to be protected by copyright. This is no longer necessary. Use of copyright notices is now optional in the U.S. Even so, it is always a good idea to include a copyright notice on all work distributed to the public so that potential infringers will be informed of the underlying claim to copyright ownership.

In addition, copyright protection is not available in some 20 foreign countries unless a work contains a copyright notice.

There are strict technical requirements as to what a copyright notice must contain. A valid copyright must contain three elements:

- The copyright symbol – use the familiar "©" symbol, i.e., the lower case letter "c" completely surrounded by a circle. The word "Copyright" or the abbreviation "Copr." are also acceptable in the U.S., but not in many foreign countries. So if your work might be distributed outside the U.S., always use the "©" symbol
- The year in which the work was published – you only need to include the year the work was first published
- The name of the copyright owner – the owner is (1) the author or authors of the work, (2) the legal owner of a work made for hire, or (3) the person or entity to whom all the author's exclusive copyright rights have been transferred

Although the three elements of a copyright notice need not appear in a particular order, it is common to list the copyright symbol, followed by the date and owners.

According to Copyright Office regulations, the copyright notice must be placed so as not to be concealed from an ordinary user's view upon reasonable examination. A proper copyright notice should be included on all manuals and promotional materials. Notices on written works are usually placed on the title page or the page immediately following the title page.

13.2.2.2   Copyright registration

Copyright registration is a legal formality by which a copyright owner makes a public record in the U.S. Copyright Office in Washington, DC, of some basic information about a protected work, such as the title of the work, who wrote it and when, and who owns the copyright. It is not necessary to register to create or establish a copyright.

Copyright registration is a relatively easy process. You must fill out the appropriate pre-printed application form, pay an application fee, and mail the application and fee to the Copyright Office in Washington, DC, along with two copies of the work being registered.

13.2.3   Copyright duration

One of the advantages of copyright protection is that it lasts a very long time. The copyright in a protectable work created after 1977 by an individual creator lasts for the life of the creator plus an additional 50 years. If there is more than one creator, the life plus 50 term is measured from the date the last creator dies. The copyright in works created by employees for their employers last for 75 years from the date of publication, or 100 years from the date of creation, whichever occurs first.

13.2.4 PROTECTING YOUR COPYRIGHT RIGHTS

The exclusive rights granted by the Copyright Act initially belong to a work's author. There are four ways to become an author:

- An individual may independently author a work
- An employer may pay an employee to create the work, in which case, the employer is the author under the work made for hire rule
- A person or business entity may specially commission an independent contractor to create the work under a written work made for hire contract, in which case the commissioning party becomes the author
- Two or more individuals or entities may collaborate to become joint authors

The initial copyright owner of a work is free to transfer some or all copyright rights to other people or businesses, who will then be entitled to exercise the rights transferred.

13.2.5 INFRINGEMENT

Copyright infringement occurs when a person other than the copyright owner exploits one or more of the copyright owner's exclusive rights without the owner's permission. A copyright owner who wins an infringement suit may stop any further infringement, obtain damages from the infringer and recover other monetary losses. This means, in effect, that a copyright owner can make a copyright infringer restore the author to the same economic position they would have been in had the infringement never occurred.

Copyright infringement is usually proven by showing that the alleged infringer had access to the copyright owner's work and that the protected expression in the two works is substantially similar. In recent years, the courts have held that the person who claims his work was infringed upon must subject his work to a rigorous filtering process to find out which elements of the work are and are not protected by copyright. In other words, the plaintiff must filter out from his work ideas, elements dictated by efficiency or external factors, or taken from the public domain. After this filtration process is completed, there may or may not be any protectable expression left.

13.3 TRADEMARKS

A trademark is a work, name, symbol, or a combination used by a manufacturer to identify its goods and distinguish them from others. Trademark rights continue indefinitely as long as the mark is not abandoned and it is properly used.

A federal trademark registration is maintained by filing a declaration of use during the sixth year after its registration and by renewal every 20 years, as long as the mark is still in use. The federal law provides that non-use of a mark for two consecutive years is ordinarily considered abandonment, and the first subsequent user of the mark can claim exclusive trademark rights. Trademarks, therefore, must be protected or they will be lost. They must be distinguished in print form from other words and must appear in a distinctive manner.

Trademarks should be followed by a notice of their status. If it has been registered in the U.S. Patent Office, the registration notice "®" or "Reg. U.S. Pat OFF," should be used. Neither should be used however, if the trademark has not been registered, but the superscripted letter "TM" should follow the mark, or an asterisk can be used to refer to a footnote starting "a trademark of xxx." The label compliance manager should remember that trademarks are proper adjectives and must be accompanied by the generic name for the product they identify. Trademarks are not to be used as possessives, nor in the plural form.

A trademark is any visual mark that accompanies a particular tangible product, or line of goods, and serves to identify and distinguish it from products sold by others and it indicates its source. A trademark may consist of letters, words, names, phrases, slogans, numbers, colors, symbols, designs, or shapes. As a general rule, to be protected from unauthorized use by others, a trademark must be distinctive in some way.

The word "trademark" is also a generic term used to describe the entire broad para of state and federal law that covers how businesses distinguish their products and services from the competition. Each state has its own set of laws establishing when and how trademarks can be protected. There is also a federal trademark law, called the Lanham Act, which applies in all 50 states. Generally, state trademark laws are relied upon for marks used only within one particular state, while the Lanham Act is used to protect marks for products that are sold in more than one state or across territorial or national borders.

13.3.1 SELECTING A TRADEMARK

Not all trademarks are treated equally by the law. The best trademarks are "distinctive" – that is, they stand out in a customer's mind because they are inherently memorable. The more distinctive the trademark is, the stronger it will be and the more legal protection it will receive. Less distinctive marks are "weak" and may be entitled to little or no legal protection.

Generally, selecting a mark begins with brainstorming for general ideas. After several possible marks have been selected, the next step is often to use formal or informal market research techniques to see how the potential marks will be accepted by customers. Next, a "trademark search" is conducted. This means that an attempt is made to discover whether the same or similar marks are already in use.

13.3.1.1   What is a distinctive trademark?

A trademark should be created that is distinctive rather than descriptive. A trademark is "distinctive" if it is capable of distinguishing the product to which it is attached from competing products. Certain types of marks are deemed to be inherently distinctive and are automatically entitled to maximum protection. Others are viewed as not inherently distinctive and can be protected only if they acquire "secondary meaning" through use.

Arbitrary, fanciful, or coined marks are deemed to be inherently distinctive and are therefore very strong marks. These are words and/or symbols that have absolutely no meaning in the particular trade or industry prior to their adoption by a particular manufacturer for use with its goods or services. After use and promotion, these marks are instantly identified with a particular company and product, and the exclusive right to use the mark is easily asserted against potential infringers.

Fanciful or arbitrary marks consist of common words used in an unexpected or arbitrary way so that their normal meaning has nothing to do with the nature of the product or service they identify. Some examples would be APPLE COMPUTER and PEACHTREE SOFTWARE.

Coined words are words made up solely to serve as trademarks, such as ZEOS or INTEL.

Suggestive marks are also inherently distinctive. A suggestive mark indirectly describes the product it identifies but stays away from literal descriptiveness. That is, the consumer must engage in a mental process to associate the mark with the product it identifies. For example, WORDPERFECT and VISICALC are suggestive marks.

Descriptive marks are not considered to be inherently distinctive. They are generally viewed by the courts as weak and thus not deserving of much, if any, judicial protection unless they acquire a "secondary meaning" – that is, become associated with a product in the public's mind through long and continuous use. There are three types of descriptive marks: (1) marks that directly describe the nature or characteristics of the product they identify (for example, QUICK MAIL), (2) marks that describe the geographic location from which the product emanates (for example, OREGON SOFTWARE), (3) marks consisting primarily of a person's last name (for example, NORTON'S UTILITIES. A mark that is in continuous and exclusive use by its owner for a 5-year period is presumed to have acquired secondary meaning and qualifies for registration as a distinctive mark.

A generic mark is a word(s) or symbol that is commonly used to describe an entire category or class of products or services, rather than to distinguish one product or service from another. Generic marks are in the public domain and cannot be registered or enforced under the trademark laws. Some examples of generic marks include "computer," "mouse," and "RAM." A term formerly protestable as a trademark may lose such protection if it becomes generic. This often occurs when a mark is assimilated into common use to such an extent that it becomes the general term describing an entire product category. Examples would be ESCALATOR and XEROX.

13.3.2 THE TRADEMARK PROCESS

A trademark is registered by filing an application with the PTO in Washington, DC. Registration is not mandatory. Under both federal and state law, a company may obtain trademark rights in the states in which the mark is actually used. However, federal registration provides many important benefits including:

- The mark's owner is presumed to have the exclusive right to use the mark nationwide
- Everyone in the country is presumed to know that the mark is already taken
- The trademark owner obtains the right to put an "®" after the mark
- Anyone who begins using a confusingly similar mark after the mark has been registered will be deemed a willful infringer
- The trademark owner obtains the right to make the mark "incontestable" by keeping it in continuous use for 5 years

To qualify for federal trademark registration, a mark must meet several requirements. The mark must:

- Actually be used in commerce
- Be sufficiently distinctive to reasonably operate as a product identifier
- Not be confusingly similar to an existing, federally registered trademark

A mark you think will be good for your product could already be in use by someone else. If your mark is confusingly similar to one already in use, its owner may be able to sue you for trademark infringement and get you to change it and even pay damages. Obviously, you do not want to spend time and money marketing and advertising a new mark only to discover that it infringes on another preexisting mark and must be changed. To avoid this, state and federal trademark searches should be conducted to attempt to discover if there are any existing similar marks. You can conduct a trademark search yourself, either manually or with the aid of computer databases. You may also pay a professional search firm to do so.

13.3.3 INTENT TO USE REGISTRATION

If you seriously intend to use a trademark on a product in the near future, you can reserve the right to use the mark by filing an intent to use registration. If the mark is approved, you have 6 months to actually use the mark on a product sold to the public. If necessary, this period may be increased by 6-month intervals up to 24 months if you have a good explanation for the delay. No one else may use the mark during this interim period. You should promptly file an intent to use registration as soon as you have definitely selected a trademark for a forthcoming product.

13.3.4 PROTECTING YOUR TRADEMARK RIGHTS

The owner of a valid trademark has the exclusive right to use the mark on its products. Depending on the strength of the mark and whether and where it has been registered, the trademark owner may be able to bring a court action to prevent others from using the same or similar marks on competing or related products.

Trademark infringement occurs when an alleged infringer uses a mark that is likely to cause consumers to confuse the infringer's products with the trademark owner's products. A mark need not be identical to one already in use to infringe upon the owner's rights. If the proposed mark is similar enough to the earlier mark to risk confusing the average consumer, its use will constitute infringement.

Determining whether an average consumer might be confused is the key to deciding whether infringement exists. The determination depends primarily on whether the products or services involved are related, and, if so, whether the marks are sufficiently similar to create a likelihood of consumer confusion.

If a trademark owner is able to convince a court that infringement has occurred, she may be able to get the court to order the infringer to stop using the infringing mark and to pay monetary damages. Depending on whether the mark was registered, such damages may consist of the amount of the trademark owner's losses caused by the infringement or the infringer's profits. In cases of willful infringement, the courts may double or triple the damages award.

A trademark owner must be assertive in enforcing its exclusive rights. Each time a mark is infringed upon, it loses strength and distinctiveness and may eventually die by becoming generic.

13.4 TRADE SECRETS

Trade secrecy is basically a do-it-yourself form of intellectual property protection. It is based on the simple idea that by keeping valuable information secret, one can prevent competitors from learning about and using it. Trade secrecy is by far the oldest form of intellectual property, dating back at least to ancient Rome. It is as useful now as it was then.

A trade secret is any formula, pattern, physical device, idea, process, compilation of information, or other information that (1) is not generally known by a company's competitors, (2) provides a business with a competitive advantage, and (3) is treated in a way that can reasonably be expected to prevent the public or competitors from learning about it, absent improper acquisition, or theft.

Trade secrets may be used to:

- Protect ideas that offer a business a competitive advantage
- Keep competitors from knowing that a program is under development and from learning its functional attributes
- Protect source code, software development tools, design definitions and specifications, manuals, and other documentation
- Protect valuable business information such as marketing plans, cost and price information, and customer lists

Unlike copyrights and patents, whose existence is provided and governed by federal law that applies in all 50 states, trade secrecy is not codified in any federal statute. Instead, it is made up of individual state laws. Nevertheless, the protection afforded to trade secrets is much the same in every state. This is partly because some 26 states have based their trade secrecy laws on the Uniform Trade Secrecy Act, a model trade secrecy law designed by legal scholars.

13.4.1 WHAT QUALIFIES FOR TRADE SECRECY

Information that is public knowledge or generally known cannot be trade secret. Things that everybody knows cannot provide anyone with a competitive advantage. However, information comprising a trade secret need not be novel or unique. All that is required is that the information not be generally known by people who could profit from its disclosure and use.

13.4.2 TRADE SECRECY AUTHORSHIP

Only the person that owns a trade secret has the right to seek relief in court if someone else improperly acquires or discloses the trade secret. Only the trade secret owner may grant others a license to use the secret.

As a general rule, any trade secrets developed by an employee in the course of employment belong to the employer. However, trade secrets developed by an employee on their own time and with their own equipment can sometimes belong to the employee. To avoid possible disputes, it is a very good idea for employers to have all the employees who may develop new technology sign an employee agreement that assigns in advance all trade secrets developed by the employee during their employment to the company.

13.4.3 HOW TRADE SECRETS ARE LOST

A trade secret is lost if either the product in which it is embodied is made widely available to the public through sales and displays on an unrestricted basis, or the secret can be discovered by reverse engineering or inspection.

13.4.4 DURATION OF TRADE SECRETS

Trade secrets have no definite term. A trade secret continues to exist as long as the requirements for trade secret protection remain in effect. In other words, as long as secrecy is maintained, the secret does not become generally known in the industry, and the secret continues to provide a competitive advantage, it will be protected.

13.4.5 PROTECTING YOUR TRADE SECRET RIGHTS

A trade secret owner has the legal right to prevent the following two groups of people from using and benefitting from its trade secrets or disclosing them to others without the owner's permission:

- People who are bound by a duty of confidentiality not to disclose or use the information
- People who steal or otherwise acquire the trade secret through improper means

A trade secret owner's rights are limited to the two restricted groups of people discussed above. In this respect, a trade secret owner's rights are much more limited than those of a copyright owner or patent holder.

A trade secret owner may enforce their rights by bringing a trade secret infringement action in court. Such suits may be used to:

- Prevent another person or business from using the trade secret without proper authorization
- Collect damages for the economic injury suffered as a result of the trade secret's improper acquisition and use

All persons responsible for the improper acquisition and all those who benefitted from the acquisition are typically named as defendants in trade secret infringement actions. To prevail in a trade secret infringement suit, the plaintiff must show that the information alleged to be secret is actually a trade secret. In addition, the plaintiff must show that the information was either improperly acquired by the defendant or improperly disclosed, or likely to be so, by the defendant.

There are two important limits on trade secret protection. It does not prevent others from discovering a trade secret through reverse engineering, nor does it apply to persons who independently create or discover the same information.

13.4.6 A TRADE SECRECY PROGRAM

The first step in any trade secret protection program is to identify exactly what information and material is a company trade secret. It makes no difference in what form a trade secret is embodied. Trade secrets may be stored on computer hard disks or floppies, written down, or exist only in employees' memories.

Once a trade secret has been established, the protection program should include the following steps:

- Maintain physical security
- Enforce computer security
- Mark confidential documents "Confidential"
- Use non-disclosure agreements

13.4.7 USE OF TRADE SECRECY WITH COPYRIGHTS AND PATENTS

Trade secrecy is a vitally important protection for any medical device, but because of its limitations listed above, it should be used in conjunction with copyright and, in some cases, patent protection.

13.4.7.1 Trade secrets and patents

The federal patent laws provide the owner of a patentable invention with far greater protection than that available under trade secrecy laws. Trade secret protection is not lost when a patent is applied for. The Patent Office keeps patent applications secret unless or until a patent is granted. However, once a patent is granted and an issue fee paid, the patent becomes public record. Then all the information disclosed in the patent application is no longer a trade secret. This is so even if the patent is later challenged in court and invalidated.

If, for example, a software program is patented, the software patent applies only to certain isolated elements of the program. The remainder need not be disclosed in the patent and can remain a trade secret.

13.4.7.2 Trade secrets and copyrights

Trade secrecy and copyright are not incompatible. To the contrary, they are typically used in tandem to provide the maximum legal protection available.

REFERENCES

American Intellectual Property Law Association, *How to Protect and Benefit From Your Ideas*, American Intellectual Property Law Association Inc., Arlington, VA, 1988.

Banner and Allegretti, *An Overview of Changes to U.S. Patent and Trademark Office Rules and Procedures Effective June 8, 1995*, Banner & Allegretti, Ltd., Chicago, IL, 1995.

Fishman, S., *Software Development – A Legal Guide*, Nolo Press, Berkeley, CA, 1994.

Fries, R.C., *Reliable Design of Medical Devices*, Marcel-Dekker, Inc., New York, 1997.

Fries, R.C., *Handbook of Medical Device Design*, Marcel-Dekker, Inc., New York, 2001.

King, P.H. and Fries, R.C., *Design of Biomedical Devices and Systems*, Marcel-Dekker, Inc., New York, 2002.

Noonan, W.D., Patenting medical technology, *The Journal of Legal Medicine*, 11(3), September, 1990.

Rebar, L.A., The nurse as inventor – obtain a patent and benefit from your ideas, *AORN Journal*, 53(2), February, 1991.

Sherman, M., Developing a labeling compliance program, in *The Medical Device Industry*, Marcel-Dekker, Inc., New York, 1990.

U.S. Department of Commerce, *General Information Concerning Patents*, U.S. Government Printing Office, Washington, DC, 1993.

Section 4

Designing the product

14 Six Sigma and product design

CONTENTS

14.1 Design for Six Sigma 210
14.2 Methodologies 210
14.3 Structure 212
14.4 Design for Six Sigma tools 213
    14.4.1 Robust design 213
        14.4.1.1 Why use the robust design methodology? 213
        14.4.1.2 Typical problems addressed by
                robust design 214
        14.4.1.3 Robustness strategy 214
                14.4.1.3.1 P-diagram 216
        14.4.1.4 Quality measurement 216
        14.4.1.5 Signal to noise (S/N) ratios 216
                14.4.1.5.1 Static vs. dynamic
                          S/N ratios 217
                14.4.1.5.2 Steps in robust parameter
                          design 217
    14.4.2 Quality function deployment 218
    14.4.3 Robust design failure mode and effects analysis 218
        14.4.3.1 Benefits of a robust DFMEA 219
        14.4.3.2 The parameter diagram 219
        14.4.3.3 Performing a robust DFMEA.................. 221
        14.4.3.4 Conclusion 225
    14.4.4 Axiomatic design 226
        14.4.4.1 What is axiomatic design? 226
        14.4.4.2 Mapping of axiomatic design 227
References 229

Six Sigma is a revolutionary business process geared toward dramatically reducing organizational inefficiencies that translate into bottom-line profitably. It started in the 1980s at Motorola and spread to such organizations as Allied Signal, Seagate, and General Electric. The process consists of five steps known as DMAIC:

- Define
- Measure
- Analyze
- Improve
- Control

By systematically applying these steps, with the appropriate tools, practitioners of this approach have been able to save substantial dollars.

The basis of Six Sigma is measuring a process in terms of defects. The statistical concept of Six Sigma means your processes are working nearly perfectly, delivering only 3.4 defects per million opportunities (DPMO). Most organizations in the U.S. are operating at a 3–4 sigma quality level. This means they could be losing up to 25% of their total revenue due to processes that deliver too many defects, defects that take up time and effort to repair, as well as making customers unhappy.

The central idea of Six Sigma management is that if you can measure the defects in a process, you can systematically figure out ways to eliminate them, thus approaching a quality level of zero defects. The goal is to get the maximum return on your Six Sigma investment by spreading it throughout your company, continuing to train employees in the Six Sigma methodology and tools to lead process improvement teams, and sustaining the exponential gains you achieve by continuing to improve. One area the methodology of Six Sigma can be extended to is product design.

14.1   DESIGN FOR SIX SIGMA

Design for Six Sigma (DFSS) is an approach to designing or re-designing product and/or services to meet or exceed customer requirements and expectations. Like its parent Six Sigma initiative, Design for Six Sigma uses a disciplined methodology and set of tools to bring high quality to product development. It begins by conducting a gap analysis of your entire product development system This analysis finds the gaps in your processes that are negatively affecting new product performance. It also addresses a highly significant factor, the Voice of the Customer (VOC). Every new product decision must be driven by the Voice of the Customer. Otherwise, what basis is there for introducing it? By learning how to identify that voice and respond to it, the designer is in a far better position to deliver a new product or service that the customer actually wants.

14.2   METHODOLOGIES

Once the gap analysis is completed and the Voice of the Customer defined, Design for Six Sigma applies its own version of the Six Sigma DMAIC methodology. The steps in the Design for Six Sigma methodology, known as DMADV, include:

- Define
- Measure
- Analyze
- Design
- Verify

The Define step determines the project goals and the requirements of both internal and external customers. The Measure step assesses customer needs and specifications. The Analyze step examines process options to meet customer requirements. The Design step develops the process to meet the customer requirements. The Verify step checks the design to ensure that it meets customer requirements.

There are other methodologies for Design for Six Sigma that have been used, including:

- DMADOV
- IDEAS
- IDOV
- DMEDI
- DCCDI

DMADOV is a slight modification of the DMADV methodology mentioned above. The addition to DMADV is the Optimize step, where the design is optimized.

IDEAS is a methodology with the following steps:

- Identify
- Design
- Evaluate
- Affirm
- Scale up

IDOV is a well-known design methodology, especially in the manufacturing world. The Identify step identifies the customer and the critical-to-quality specifications. The Design step translates the customer specifications into functional requirements and into solution alternatives. A selection process brings the list of solutions down to the "best" solution. The Optimize step uses advanced statistical tools and modeling to predict and optimize the design and performance. The Validate step ensures the design that was developed will meet the customer specifications.

DMEDI is a methodology with the following steps:

- Define
- Measure

- Explore
- Develop
- Implement

DCCDI is a methodology that is fairly new. The Define step defines the project goals. The Customer step ensures the analysis of the potential customer and their requirements is complete. The Concept step is where ideas are developed, reviewed, and selected. The Design step is performed to meet the customer and business specifications. The Implementation step is completed to develop and commercialize the product or service.

14.3   STRUCTURE

The Design for Six Sigma approach can utilize any of the many possible methodologies. The fact is that all of these methodologies use the same advanced design tools, such as Quality Function Deployment, Failure Modes and Effects Analysis, benchmarking, Design of Experiments, simulation, Robust Design, etc. Each methodology primarily differs in the name of each phase and the number of phases.

Design for Six Sigma packages methods and tools in a framework that promotes cultural change under a recognized brand name that helps overcome an initial resistance to change. It is most useful if it generates permanent behavior changes that outlast its own life as a brand. Given the Design for Six Sigma toolset is not substantially new, the rationale for Design for Six Sigma should not focus on tools. Over time, Design for Six Sigma should emerge as a scientific approach to product development that leverages the Six Sigma culture. It will become a means to reinstill rigorous deductive and inductive reasoning in product development processes. It requires:

- Identifying customer desires
- Developing validated transfer functions that describe product performance through objective measures
- Correlating these objective measures to customer desires
- Effectively assessing the capability to meet those desires well before product launch
- Applying transfer function knowledge to optimize designs to satisfy customer desires and avoid failure modes

Six Sigma culture aids implementation of these steps by providing:

- A cross company common language for problem resolution and prevention
- A mind-set that demands the use of valid data in decision making
- An expectation across the organization that results should be measurable

- A disciplined project management system to help achieve timely results

None of the elements of this approach is revolutionary, but together they provide a template for success.

14.4 DESIGN FOR SIX SIGMA TOOLS

The use of Six Sigma tools and techniques should be introduced in a well-thought-out manner at various phases of the project. Tools that should be considered during a product development process include:

- Robust design
- Quality function deployment
- Design failure modes and effects analysis
- Axiomatic design

14.4.1 ROBUST DESIGN

The robust design method, also called the Taguchi Method, pioneered by Dr. Genichi Taguchi, greatly improves engineering productivity. By consciously considering the noise factors (environmental variation during the product's usage, manufacturing variation, and component deterioration) and the cost of failure in the field the robust design method helps ensure customer satisfaction. Robust design focuses on improving the fundamental function of the product or process, thus facilitating flexible designs and concurrent engineering. Indeed, it is the most powerful method available to reduce product cost, improve quality, and simultaneously reduce development interval.

14.4.1.1 Why use the robust design methodology?

Over the last 5 years many leading companies have invested heavily in the Six Sigma approach aimed at reducing waste during manufacturing and operations. These efforts have had great impact on the cost structure and hence on the bottom line of those companies. Many of them have reached the maximum potential of the traditional Six Sigma approach. What would be the engine for the next wave of productivity improvement?

Brenda Reichelderfer of ITT Industries reported on their benchmarking survey of many leading companies, "design directly influences more than 70% of the product life cycle cost; companies with high product development effectiveness have earnings three times the average earnings; and companies with high product development effectiveness have revenue growth two times the average revenue growth." She also observed, "40% of product development costs are wasted!"

These and similar observations by other leading companies are compelling them to adopt improved product development processes under the banner Design for Six Sigma. The Design for Six Sigma approach is focused on (1) increasing engineering productivity so that new products can be developed rapidly and at low cost, and (2) value-based management.

The robust design method is central to improving engineering productivity. Pioneered by Dr. Genichi Taguchi after the end of the Second World War, the method has evolved over the last five decades. Many companies around the world have saved hundreds of millions of dollars by using the method in diverse industries: automobiles, xerography, telecommunications, electronics, software, etc.

14.4.1.2 Typical problems addressed by robust design

A team of engineers was working on the design of a radio receiver for ground to aircraft communication requiring high reliability, i.e., low bit error rate, for data transmission. On the one hand, building series of prototypes to sequentially eliminate problems would be forbiddingly expensive. On the other hand, computer simulation effort for evaluating a single design was also time consuming and expensive. Then, how can one speed up development and yet assure reliability?

In another project, a manufacturer had introduced a high-speed copy machine to the field only to find that the paper feeder jammed almost ten times more frequently than what was planned. The traditional method for evaluating the reliability of a single new design idea used to take several weeks. How can the company conduct the needed research in a short time and come up with a design that would not embarrass the company again in the field? The robust design method has helped reduce the development time and cost by a factor of two or better in many such problems.

In general, engineering decisions involved in product/system development can be classified into two categories:

- Error-free implementation of the past collective knowledge and experience
- Generation of new design information, often for improving product quality/reliability, performance, and cost

While CAD/CAE tools are effective for implementing past knowledge, robust design method greatly improves productivity in the generation of new knowledge by acting as an amplifier of engineering skills. With robust design, a company can rapidly achieve the full technological potential of their design ideas and achieve higher profits.

14.4.1.3 Robustness strategy

Variation reduction is universally recognized as a key to reliability and productivity improvement. There are many approaches to reducing the variability, each one having its place in the product development cycle.

By addressing variation reduction at a particular stage in a product's life cycle, one can prevent failures in the downstream stages. The Six Sigma approach has made tremendous gains in cost reduction by finding problems that occur in manufacturing or white-collar operations and fixing the immediate causes. The robustness strategy is to prevent problems through optimizing product designs and manufacturing process designs.

The manufacturer of a differential op-amplifier used in coin telephones faced the problem of excessive offset voltage due to manufacturing variability. High offset voltage caused poor voice quality, especially for phones further away from the central office. So, how to minimize field problems and associated cost? There are many approaches:

- Compensate the customers for their losses
- Screen out circuits having large offset voltage at the end of the production line
- Institute tighter tolerances through process control on the manufacturing line
- Change the nominal values of critical circuit parameters such that the circuit's function becomes insensitive to the cause, namely, manufacturing variation

The approach is the robustness strategy. As one moves from approach 1 to 4, one progressively moves upstream in the product delivery cycle and also becomes more efficient in cost control. Hence it is preferable to address the problem as upstream as possible. The robustness strategy provides the crucial methodology for systematically arriving at solutions that make designs less sensitive to various causes of variation. It can be used for optimizing product design as well as for manufacturing process design.

The robustness strategy uses five primary tools:

1. P-diagram is used to classify the variables associated with the product into noise, control, signal (input), and response (output) factors
2. Ideal function is used to mathematically specify the ideal form of the signal–response relationship as embodied by the design concept for making the higher-level system work perfectly
3. Quadratic loss function (also known as quality loss function) is used to quantify the loss incurred by the user due to deviation from target performance
4. Signal-to-noise ratio is used for predicting the field quality through laboratory experiments
5. Orthogonal arrays are used for gathering dependable information about control factors (design parameters) with a small number of experiments

14.4.1.3.1 P-diagram

P-diagram is a must for every development project. It is a way of succinctly defining the development scope. It is discussed in detail in Section 14.4.3.2.

14.4.1.4   Quality measurement

In quality improvement and design optimization the metric plays a crucial role. Unfortunately, a single metric does not serve all stages of product delivery. It is common to use the fraction of products outside the specified limits as the measure of quality. Though it is a good measure of the loss due to scrap, it miserably fails as a predictor of customer satisfaction. The quality loss function serves that purpose very well.

Let us define the following variables:
m: target value for a critical product characteristic
$+/- \Delta_0$: allowed deviation from the target
A_0: loss due to a defective product

Then the quality loss, L, suffered by an average customer due to a product with y as the value of the characteristic is given by the following equation:

$$L = k * (y - m)^2$$

where

$$k = (A_0 / \Delta_0^2)$$

If the output of the factory has distribution of the critical characteristic with mean μ and variance σ^2, then the average quality loss per unit of the product is given by:

$$Q = k\{(\mu - m)^2 + s^2\}$$

14.4.1.5   Signal to noise (S/N) ratios

The product/process/system design phase involves deciding the best values/levels for the control factors. The signal to noise (S/N) ratio is an ideal metric for that purpose. The equation for average quality loss, Q, says that the customer's average quality loss depends on the deviation of the mean from the target and also on the variance. An important class of design optimization problem requires minimization of the variance while keeping the mean on target.

Between the mean and standard deviation, it is typically easy to adjust the mean on target, but reducing the variance is difficult. Therefore, the designer should minimize the variance first and then adjust the mean on target. Among the available control factors most of them should be used to reduce variance. Only one or two control factors are adequate for adjusting the mean on target.

The design optimization problem can be solved in two steps:

1. Maximize the S/N ratio, η, defined as

$$\eta = 10 \log_{10}(\eta^2/\sigma^2)$$

This is the step of variance reduction.

2. Adjust the mean on target using a control factor that has no effect on h. Such a factor is called a scaling factor. This is the step of adjusting the mean on target.

One typically looks for one scaling factor to adjust the mean on target during design and another for adjusting the mean to compensate for process variation during manufacturing.

14.4.1.5.1 Static vs. dynamic S/N ratios

In some engineering problems, the signal factor is absent or it takes a fixed value. These problems are called static problems and the corresponding S/N ratios are called static S/N ratios. The S/N ratio described in the preceding section is a static S/N ratio.

In other problems, the signal and response must follow a function called the ideal function. In the cooling system example described earlier, the response (room temperature) and signal (set point) must follow a linear relationship. Such problems are called dynamic problems and the corresponding S/N ratios are called dynamic S/N ratios. The dynamic S/N ratio will be illustrated in a later section using a turbine design example. Dynamic S/N ratios are very useful for technology development, which is the process of generating flexible solutions that can be used in many products.

14.4.1.5.2 Steps in robust parameter design

Robust parameter design has four main steps:

- Problem formulation: This step consists of identifying the main function, developing the P-diagram, defining the ideal function and S/N ratio, and planning the experiments. The experiments involve changing the control, noise, and signal factors systematically using orthogonal arrays.
- Data collection/simulation: The experiments may be conducted in hardware or through simulation. It is not necessary to have a

full-scale model of the product for the purpose of experimentation. It is sufficient and more desirable to have an essential model of the product that adequately captures the design concept. Thus, the experiments can be done more economically.

- Factor effects analysis: The effects of the control factors are calculated in this step and the results are analyzed to select optimum setting of the control factors.
- Prediction/confirmation: In order to validate the optimum conditions we predict the performance of the product design under baseline and optimum settings of the control factors. Then we perform confirmation experiments under these conditions and compare the results with the predictions. If the results of confirmation experiments agree with the predictions, then we implement the results. Otherwise, the above steps must be iterated.

14.4.2   QUALITY FUNCTION DEPLOYMENT

Quality function deployment is discussed in Chapter 9.

14.4.3   ROBUST DESIGN FAILURE MODE AND EFFECTS ANALYSIS

FMEA is a methodology that has been used in the medical industry for many years. It is usually developed early in the product development cycle, in conjunction with a risk analysis. Risk by definition is the probable rate of occurrence of a hazard causing harm. Risk can be associated with device failure and also can be present in a normally operating device. The FMEA is an enhancement to the risk analysis by analyzing the potential failure down to the component level. Robust design FMEA, the subject of this paper, is an enhancement to the normal FMEA by anticipating safety and reliability failure modes through use of parameter diagram (P-diagram).

Given the fact that product design responsibility starts at concept phase and ends when the product is obsolete, special emphases should be implemented to achieve design reliability and robustness. Robust design FMEA (DFMEA) fits very well into this methodology. It is an invaluable tool to shorten product development times.

Robust DFMEA fits very well into the concept of concurrent engineering. It necessitates a close and continuous working relationship between design, manufacturing, service, suppliers, and customers. Robust DFMEA is best generated for the system level and used to derive through analysis the system's key subsystems and key components. Robust DFMEA preparation should incorporate inputs from a cross-functional team with expertise in design, human factors, manufacturing, testing, service, quality, reliability, clinical, regulatory, supplier or other fields, as appropriate.

The robust DFMEA is an integral part of the robust design methodology (RDM) currently being used in Europe and is an essential tool of the Design for Six Sigma (DFSS) process. Robust DFMEA should be generated to analyze device design through a comprehensive and structured approach using the concept of a P-diagram. Robust DFMEA takes the failure mode analysis into a structural five dimensional failure-cause brainstorming approach, including:

- Total design and manufacturing variation: Design variability refers to the ability of the design to allow a misuse (i.e. design symmetry, can be installed upside down). Manufacturing variability refers to the special design characteristics that are sensitive to variation in manufacturing/assembly processes
- Changes over time: refers to changes over time in dimensions or strength such as wear out or degradation
- Customer usage: refers to customer misuse and abuse of the product
- External environment: refers to external environmental conditions
- System interaction: refers to the interaction of the various subsystems and components

14.4.3.1   Benefits of a robust DFMEA

There are many benefits when using the Robust DFMEA, including:

1. Improved design reliability through a detailed analysis of system, subsystems, and components
2. Traceability back to customer needs (Voice of the Customer) for validation
3. Ability to recognize and evaluate potential design failure modes and their effects
4. Ability to recognize and evaluate potential special design characteristics
5. Assure the implementation of proper mitigation, before the event action, to improve product reliability and robustness
6. Improve or modify design verification/validation planning
7. Analysis of interactions among various subsystems/components as well as interfaces to external systems
8. Analysis of all interfaces and interactions with the customer and environment
9. Definition of all stresses needed for testing

14.4.3.2   The parameter diagram

The parameter diagram (P-diagram) (Figure 14-1) is a block diagram used to facilitate the understanding of robust design as a concept. The P-diagram shows factors that affect a product. It models the product as a box affected

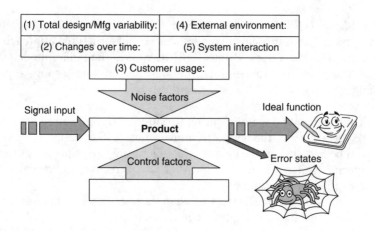

FIGURE 14-1 P-diagram

by three types of parameters or factors that affect the response of the product, i.e., how the product performs its intended function:

- Signal factors
- Noise factors
- Control factors

Two types of factors are controllable, whereas noise factors are uncontrollable in natural conditions of use.

- Signal factors: set by the user at a level that corresponds to the desired response
- Control factors: set by the designer

There are five elements to every P-diagram:

1. Inputs: any or all of the energy, material and information that the product requires to deliver the desirable or undesirable output
2. Ideal functions: also called desirable output, which is referred to as the physical and performance requirements of an item that are used as a basis for design. Those requirements are stated in engineering terms that are unambiguous, complete, verifiable, and not in conflict with one another.
3. Error states: error states are also called undesirable output or failure modes, which are referred to as the ways in which the product may fail to meet the ideal function. Error states occur in one or all of the four states listed below:
    1. No function
    2. Over/under/degraded function

    3. Intermittent function
    4. Unintended function
4. Noise Factors: noise factors are also called potential cause/ mechanism of failure. Noise factors are the source of variation that can cause the error states/failure modes to occur. Noise factors are categorized in five categories; any or all of the below-mentioned five categories may cause the error states/failure modes to occur:

Noise 1:   total design/manufacturing variability
- design variability refers to the ability of the design to allow a misuse (i.e. design symmetry, can be installed upside down).
- manufacturing variability refers to the key design character-istics that are sensitive to variation in manufacturing.

Noise 2:   changes over time
It is the changes over time in dimensions or strength such as wear out or degradation

Noise 3:   customer usage
It is customer misuse and abuse of the product

Noise 4:   external environment
It is external environmental conditions

Noise 5:   system interaction
It is the interaction of the various subsystems and components

5. Control factors: control factors are the design parameters used to optimize performance in the presence of noise factors

14.4.3.3   Performing a robust DFMEA

The DFMEA form is illustrated in Figure 14-2. The form contains the following sections:

- Number (No.): Enter ideal function number, start with ideal function number 1
- Item/Function: Enter the name of the product being analyzed. Use the nomenclature and show the design level as indicated on the engineering drawing/specification. Robust DFMEA is best gene-rated in the following order system, key subsystems then key components. Product under analysis in the P-diagram corresponds to item in item/function column. Enter, as concisely as possible, the function of the product being analyzed to meet the design intent. If the system has more than one function, list all the functions separately. Ideal functions in the P-diagram corresponds to function in item/function column
- Potential failure mode: List each potential failure mode for the particular product function. A recommended starting point is

No	Item/ function	Potential failure mode	Potential effect(s) of failure	S E V	Potential cause(s) mechanism(s) of failure	O C C	C L A S S	Current mitigations	Verification	D E T	Recommended actions	Action results			
												S E V	O C C	D E T	C L A S S
1	Ideal functions	Error states			Noise factors										
2															
3															

POTENTIAL FAILURE MODE AND EFFECTS ANALYSIS IN DESIGN (Robust DESIGN FMEA) Baxter confidential

Project Number: Product Number: FMEA Number: Page   of

Project Name: Product Name: Rev:

FIGURE 14-2 DFMEA form

a review of product quality history, complaint reports, and group brainstorming. Remember that a hierarchical relationship exists between the components, subsystems, and system levels

- Potential effect(s) of failure: Potential effects of failure are defined as the effects of the failure mode on the function, as perceived by the customer. Describe the effects of the failure in terms of what the customer might notice or experience, remembering that the customer may be an internal customer as well as the ultimate end user. State clearly if the function could impact safety or non-compliance to regulations. Remember that a hierarchical relationship exists between the components, subsystems, and system levels

- Severity (S): Severity is an assessment of the seriousness of the effect of the potential failure mode to customer if it occurs. Severity is rated and recorded for the worst-case scenario potential effect. To ensure continuity, the robust DFMEA team should use a consistent severity ranking system

- Potential cause(s)/mechanism(s) of failure: Causes are the source of variation that causes the failure modes/error states to occur. Noise factors in the P-diagram correspond to potential cause(s)/mechanism of failure column

- Occurrence (O): Occurrence is the likelihood that a specific cause/ noise factor will occur and cause the potential failure during the design life. The likelihood of occurrence ranking number has a meaning rather than a value; below are some guidelines for defining an occurrence value:
  - What is the field experience with similar components, subsystems, or system?

- Is it carryover or similar to a previous level component, subsystem, or system?
- How significant are the changes from a previous level component, subsystem, or system?
- Is it radically different from a previous level design?
- Is it completely new?
- Has its application/use changed?
- What are the environmental changes?
- Has any analysis (e.g., simulation) been used to estimate the expected comparable occurrence rate?
- Has prevention mitigation been put in place? To ensure continuity, the robust DFMEA team should use a consistent occurrence ranking system
- Classification: This column may be used to classify any special product characteristics (safety and key design characteristics) for components, subsystems, and system that require mitigations. This column may also be used to highlight high-priority failure modes for assessment. The classification codes are illustrated in Figure 14-3
- Current mitigations: Current mitigations are the activities that will assure the design adequacy for the failure mode and/or cause under consideration. Those activities will prevent the cause/mechanism or failure mode/effect from occurring, or reduce the rate of occurrence, such as:
  - Proven modeling/simulation (e.g., finite element analysis)
  - Tolerance stack up study (e.g., geometric dimensional tolerance)
  - Material compatibility study (e.g., thermal expansion, corrosion)
  - Subjective design and manufacturing reviews
  - Redundancy
  - Labeling
  - Design of experiments studies
  - Parameter design studies
  - Tolerance design studies
- Verification: Verify the design adequacy against cause/mechanism of failure or verify the design adequacy against failure mode, either by analytical or physical methods, such as:
  - Tests on pre-production samples or prototype samples
  - Analytical tests
  - Design verification plan tests

Manufacturing tests or inspections conducted as part of the manufacturing and/or assembly process are not acceptable verification in design phase

- Detection (D): Detection is the ability (detection likelihood) of the current mitigations/verification to detect a potential

Classification		
Code	To indicate	Criteria
SC	Potential safety characteristics	Severity = 5 and Occurrence = 2 to 5
KC	Potential key design characteristics	Severity = 4 and Occurrence = 3 to 5 Severity = 3 and Occurrence = 3 to 5 Severity = 2 and Occurrence = 4 to 5
AO	Action is optional	Not SC nor KC

		Severity				
		None	Low	Moderate	High	Very high
Occurrence	Sev. / Occ.	1	2	3	4	5
Remote: Failure is unlikely, improbable	1	AO	AO	AO	AO	AO
Low: Relatively few failures	2	AO	AO	AO	AO	SC
Moderate: Occasional failures	3	AO	AO	KC	KC	SC
High: Repeated/frequent failures	4	AO	KC	KC	KC	SC
Very high: Failure is almost inevitable, frequent, persistent failures	5	AO	KC	KC	KC	SC

FIGURE 14-3 Classification codes for DFMEA

cause/mechanism or failure mode and lead to corrective actions. Timeliness of current mitigations and verification application, such as early in design concept stage or just prior to released for production, plays a major role in ranking the detection level. To ensure continuity, the robust DFMEA team should use a consistent detection ranking system

• Recommended actions: Recommended actions intent is to reduce any one or all of the severity, occurrence, and detection rankings. Only a design revision/technology change can bring a reduction in the severity ranking. Occurrence reduction can be achieved by removing or controlling the cause/mechanism of the failure mode, where detection reduction can be achieved by increasing the design validation/verification actions. Additional mitigations and/or recommended actions shall be implemented, as illustrated in Figure 14-4. If no actions are recommended for a specific cause,

Code	To indicate	Criteria	Additional mitigation and/or recommended actions
SC	Potential safety characteristics	Severity = 5 and Occurrence = 2 to 5	Risk must be mitigated and all current mitigations must be traced back to requirement. All recommended actions must be tracked via issues tracking system until Occurrence brought to less or equal to 1 and Detection brought to less or equal to 2.
KC	Potential key design characteristics	Severity = 4 and Occurrence = 3 to 5	All current mitigations must be traced back to requirement. All recommended actions must be tracked via issues tracking system until Occurrence brought to less or equal to 2 and Detection brought to less or equal to 3.
		Severity = 3 and Occurrence = 3 to 5	All current mitigations must be traced back to requirement. All recommended actions must be tracked via issues tracking system until Occurrence brought to less or equal to 2 and Detection brought to less or equal to 3.
		Severity = 2 and Occurrence = 4 to 5	All current mitigations must be traced back to requirement. All recommended actions must be tracked via issues tracking system until Occurrence brought to less or equal to 3 and Detection brought to less or equal to 3.
AO	Action optional	Not SC nor KC	Project team decides actions required.

FIGURE 14-4 Recommended actions for DFMEA

indicate this by entering a "NONE" or "None at this time" in this column
- Action Results: Estimate and record the resulting severity, occurrence, and detection rankings and also assess classification. If no actions result, indicate this by entering a "NR" in the severity, occurrence, and detection columns

14.4.3.4 Conclusion

As a result of performing the step-by-step robust DFMEA one should be able to define the special design characteristics (safety and reliability product characteristics) that contribute directly to a failure mode/error state of the medical device under analysis.

Special design characteristics (safety and reliability product characteristics) defined for the product under analysis are dependent on the robust DFMEA scope and boundary, when performed on a system, a subsystem, or a component. For example, in a system-level robust DFMEA, system-level characteristics are defined, in a subsystem-level Robust DFMEA, subsystem-level characteristics are defined, and in a component-level Robust DFMEA, component-level characteristics are defined.

In many cases a system contains purchased subsystems and/or components, robust DFMEA is capable of defining all appropriate safety and reliability product characteristics that need to be reached to an agreement with the purchased subsystems and/or components suppliers.

Adding to all that, all safety and reliability product characteristics that are sensitive to the manufacturing process defined in the robust DFMEA (designed in-house or purchased subsystems and components) need to derive the process FMEAs and control plans in order to achieve product reliability and robustness.

14.4.4 AXIOMATIC DESIGN

Axiomatic design, a theory and methodology developed at Massachusetts Institute of Technology (MIT; Cambridge, MA) 20 years ago, helps designers focus on the problems in bad designs. Says the theory's creator, Professor Nam Suh, "The goal of axiomatic design is to make human designers more creative, reduce the random search process, minimize the iterative trial-and-error process, and determine the best design among those proposed." And this applies to designing all sorts of things: software, business processes, manufacturing systems, work flows, etc. What's more, it can be used for diagnosing and improving existing designs.

14.4.4.1 What is axiomatic design?

While "MIT" and "axiomatic" might suggest some lofty academic theory, axiomatic design is well grounded in reality. It is a systematic, scientific approach to design. It guides designers through the process of first breaking up customer needs into functional requirements (FRs), then breaking up these requirements into design parameters (DPs), and then finally figuring out a process to produce those design parameters. In MIT-speak, axiomatic design is a decomposition process going from customer needs to FRs, to DPs, and then to process variables (PVs), thereby crossing the four domains of the design world: customer, functional, physical, and process.

The fun begins in decomposing the design. A designer first "explodes" higher-level FRs into lower-level FRs, proceeding through a hierarchy of levels until a design can be implemented. At the same time, the designer "zigzags" between pairs of design domains, such as between the functional and physical domains. Ultimately, zigzagging between "what" and "how" domains reduces the design to a set of FR, DP, and PV hierarchies.

Along the way, there are these two axioms: the independence axiom and the information axiom. (From these two axioms come a bunch of theorems that tell designers "some very simple things," says Suh. "If designers remember these, then they can make enormous progress in the quality of their product design.") The first axiom says that the functional requirements within a good design are independent of each other. This is the goal of the whole exercise: Identifying DPs so that "each FR can be satisfied without affecting the other FRs," says Suh.

The second axiom says that when two or more alternative designs satisfy the first axiom, the best design is the one with the least information. That is, when a design is good, information content is zero. (That's "information" as in the measure of one's freedom of choice, the measure of uncertainty, which is the basis of information theory.) "Designs that satisfy the independence axiom are called uncoupled or decoupled," explains Robert Powers, President of Axiomatic Design Software, Inc. (Boston, MA), developers of Acclaro, a software application that prompts designers through the axiomatic design process. "The difference is that in an uncoupled design, the DPs are totally independent; while in a decoupled design, at least one DP affects two or more FRs. As a result, the order of adjusting the DPs in a decoupled design is important."

The approach for design is to spend time upfront understanding customer expectations and delights (customer attributes) together with corporate and regulatory requirements. Then the following mappings are necessary:

- Perform QFD by mapping critical to satisfaction (CTS) to functional requirements
- Perform mapping of axiomatic design between the functional requirements (FRs) and design parameters (DPs)
- Perform mapping of axiomatic design between the design parameters (DPs) and the process variables (PVs)

The design process involves three mappings between four domains as shown in Figure 14-5. The first mapping involves the mapping from critical-to-satisfaction (CTSs) metrics to the functional requirements (FRs) and then to design parameters. The last mapping occurs between design parameters and the process variables.

14.4.4.2 Mapping of axiomatic design

The axiomatic design method provides the process as the means to define physical and process structures. The design is first identified in terms of its FRs and then progressively detailed in terms of its lower-level functional

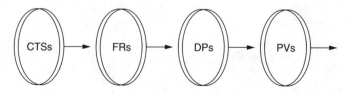

FIGURE 14-5 Axiomatic design process mapping

requirements and design parameters. Hierarchy is built by the decomposing design into a number of functional requirements and design parameters. The principles that are used as guidance are:

- Principle of independence – maintain the independence of the functional requirements
- Principle of information – minimize the information content in a design: reduce complexity

The principle of independence states that the optimal design maintains the independence of the functional requirements. An acceptable design will have the FRs and DPs related in such a way that a specific DP can be adjusted to satisfy a corresponding FR without affecting other FRs.

There are three possible mappings – uncoupled (optimal), decoupled (semi-optimal), and coupled. These mappings can be explained by use of matrices as follows:

$$\{FRs\} = [A]\{DPs\}$$

The elements of the design matrix, A, indicate the effects of changes of DPs on the FRs; as an example, consider the design equation shown below:

$$\begin{Bmatrix} FR_1 \\ FR_2 \\ FR_3 \end{Bmatrix} = \begin{bmatrix} a_{11} & 0 & a_{13} \\ a_{21} & a_{22} & 0 \\ a_{31} & 0 & a_{33} \end{bmatrix} \begin{bmatrix} DP_1 \\ DP_2 \\ DP_3 \end{bmatrix}$$

Uncoupled design is represented as follows showing the independence of functional requirements

$$\begin{Bmatrix} FR_1 \\ FR_2 \\ FR_3 \end{Bmatrix} = \begin{bmatrix} a_{11} & 0 & 0 \\ 0 & a_{22} & 0 \\ 0 & 0 & a_{33} \end{bmatrix} \begin{bmatrix} DP_1 \\ DP_2 \\ DP_3 \end{bmatrix}$$

Functional requirements are represented as:

$$FR_1 = a_{11} \times DP_1$$
$$FR_2 = a_{22} \times DP_2$$
$$FR_3 = a_{33} \times DP_3.$$

Decoupled design is represented as follows showing the semi-independence of functional requirements:

$$\begin{Bmatrix} FR_1 \\ FR_2 \\ FR_3 \end{Bmatrix} = \begin{bmatrix} a_{11} & 0 & 0 \\ a_{21} & a_{22} & 0 \\ a_{31} & a_{32} & a_{33} \end{bmatrix} \begin{bmatrix} DP_1 \\ DP_2 \\ DP_3 \end{bmatrix}$$

Functional requirements are represented as:

$$FR_1 = a_{11} \times DP_1 + 0 \times DP_2 + 0 \times DP_3$$

$$= a_{11} \times DP_1$$

$$FR_2 = a_{21} \times DP_1 + a_{22} \times DP_2 + 0 \times DP_3$$

$$= a_{21} \times DP_1 + a_{22} \times DP_2$$

$$FR_3 = a_{31} \times DP_1 + a_{32} \times DP_2 + a_{33} \times DP_3.$$

Coupled design is represented as follows showing the interdependencies of functional requirements:

$$\begin{Bmatrix} FR_1 \\ FR_2 \\ FR_3 \end{Bmatrix} = \begin{bmatrix} a_{11} & 0 & a_{13} \\ a_{21} & a_{22} & 0 \\ a_{31} & 0 & a_{33} \end{bmatrix} \begin{bmatrix} DP_1 \\ DP_2 \\ DP_3 \end{bmatrix}$$

The functional requiremements are highly inter-dependent that lead to a mediocre design.

$$FR_1 = a_{11} \times DP_1 + 0 \times DP_2 + a_{13} \times DP_3$$

$$= a_{11} \times DP_1 + a_{13} \times DP_3$$

$$FR_2 = a_{21} \times DP_1 + a_{22} \times DP_2 + 0 \times DP_3$$

$$= a_{21} \times DP_1 + a_{22} \times DP_2$$

$$FR_3 = a_{31} \times DP_1 + a_{32} \times DP_2 + a_{33} \times DP_3$$

This concept is valid during mapping between DPs and PVs. In each stage, during mapping between FRs and DPs, and mapping between DPs and PVs the principles of axiomatic design should be followed.

REFERENCES

AIAG (Automotive Industry Action Group), *Potential Failure Mode and Effects Analysis*, Reference Manual, Third Edition.

ANSI/AAMI/ISO-14971-2000, *Medical Devices – Application of Risk Management to Medical Devices*.

Brue, G. and Launsby, R.G., *Design for Six Sigma*, McGraw-Hill, New York, 2003.

EURobust Partnership, *Use and Knowledge of Robust Design Methodology*, Chalmers University, Sweden, 2003.

Fries, R.C., *Reliable Design of Medical Devices*, Marcel-Dekker, Inc., New York, 1997.

Fries, R.C., *Handbook of Medical Device Design*, Marcel-Dekker, Inc., New York, 2001.

Gaydos, W., *Dynamic Parameter Design for an FM Data Demodulator*, ITT Industries Annual Taguchi Symposium, October, 1994.

Huber, C., et al., Straight talk on DFSS, *Six Sigma Forum Magazine*, 1(4), August, 2002.

IEC-60812 1985, *Analysis Techniques for System Reliability – Procedure for Failure Mode and Effects Analysis (FMEA)*.

Phadke, M.S., *Quality Engineering Using Robust Design*, Englewood Cliff, NJ, Prentice Hall.

Taguchi, G., *System of Experimental Design*, Clausing, D. (ed.) UNIPUB/ Krass International Publications, New York, Volumes 1 & 2, 1987.

15 Hardware design

CONTENTS

15.1 Block diagram 232
15.2 Redundancy 232
    15.2.1 Active redundancy..................................... 233
    15.2.2 Standby redundancy................................... 234
15.3 Component selection 235
    15.3.1 Component fitness for use............................. 236
    15.3.2 Component reliability 236
    15.3.3 Component history.................................... 237
    15.3.4 Component safety..................................... 238
15.4 Component derating 238
15.5 Safety margin 239
15.6 Load protection... 240
15.7 Environmental protection 240
15.8 Product misuse.. 240
15.9 Initial reliability prediction 241
    15.9.1 Parts count prediction 242
    15.9.2 Parts count prediction example 244
    15.9.3 Summary of reliability prediction 248
15.10 Design for variation.. 248
15.11 Design of experiments... 249
    15.11.1 The Taguchi method 249
15.12 Design changes.. 249
15.13 Design reviews 250
References.. 252

Design input provides the foundation for product development. The objective of the design input process is to establish and document the design input requirements for the device. The design input document is as comprehensive and precise as possible. It contains the information necessary to direct the remainder of the design process. It includes design constraints, but does not impose design solutions.

Once the documentation describing the design and the organized approach to the design is complete, the actual design work begins. As the design activity proceeds, there are several failure-free or failure-tolerant principles that must

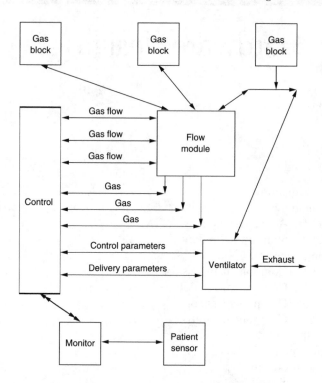

FIGURE 15-1 Block diagram

be considered to make the design more reliable. Each is important and has its own place in the design process.

15.1 BLOCK DIAGRAM

The first step in an organized design is the development of a block diagram of the device (see Figure 15-1). The block diagram is basically a flow chart of the signal movement within the device and is an aid to organizing the design. Individual blocks within the block diagram can be approached for component design, making the task more organized and less tedious. Once all blocks have been designed, their connections are all that remain.

15.2 REDUNDANCY

One method of addressing the high failure rate of certain components is the use of redundancy, that is, the use of more than one component for the same purpose in the circuit. The philosophy behind redundancy is if one component fails another will take its place and the operation will continue. An example would be the inclusion of two reed switches in parallel, where, if one fails because the reeds have stuck together, the other is available to continue the operation.

Redundancy may be of two types:

- Active
- Standby

15.2.1 ACTIVE REDUNDANCY

Active redundancy occurs when two or more components are placed in parallel, with all components being operational. Satisfactory operation occurs if at least one of the components functions. If one component fails, the remaining parts will function to sustain the operation. Active redundancy is important in improving the reliability of a device. Placing components redundantly increases the MTBF of the circuit, thus improving reliability. Consider the following example.

Figure 15-2 shows a circuit for an amplifier. Let's use the component U1 as our candidate for redundancy. Determining the failure rate for the component in MIL-HDBK-215 gives a value for our intended use of 0.320 failures/million hours. The failure rate assumption is that the component was in its useful life period. Therefore, the reciprocal of the failure rate is the mean time between failure (MTBF). When calculating the MTBF, the failure rate must be specified in failures per hour. Therefore, the failure rate, as listed in the handbook or in vendor literature, must be divided by one million.

$$\text{MTBF} = 1/\lambda$$
$$= 1/0.00000032$$
$$= 3\,125\,000 \text{ hours}$$

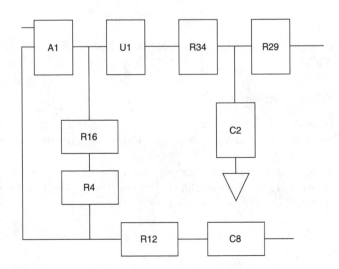

FIGURE 15-2 Circuit example

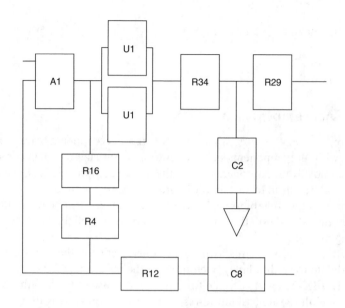

FIGURE 15-3 Active redundancy

Let's assume, for our particular application, this MTBF value is not acceptable. Therefore, we decide to put two components in parallel (Figure 15-3). Again, we assume the useful life period of the component. For this case:

$$MTBF = 3/2\lambda$$
$$= 3/2(0.00000032)$$
$$= 3/0.00000064$$
$$= 4\,687\,500 \text{ hours}$$

By putting two components in active redundancy, the MTBF of the circuit has increased by 50%.

15.2.2 STANDBY REDUNDANCY

Standby redundancy occurs when two or more components are placed in parallel, but only one component is active. The remaining components are in standby mode.

Returning to our previous example, we have decided to use standby redundancy to increase our reliability (Figure 15-4). Again assuming the useful life period and ignoring the failure rate of the switch,

$$MTBF = 2/\lambda$$
$$= 2/0.00000032$$
$$= 6\,250\,000 \text{ hours}$$

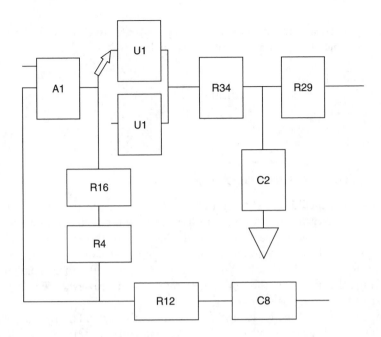

FIGURE 15-4 Standby redundancy

By using standby redundancy, the MTBF has increased by 100% over the use of the single component and by 33% over active redundancy.

Obviously, the use of redundancy is dependent upon the circuit and the failure rates of the individual components in the circuit. However, the use of redundancy definitely increases the reliability of the circuit. What type of redundancy is used again depends on the individual circuit and its intended application.

15.3 COMPONENT SELECTION

As certain portions of the design become firm, the job of selecting the proper components becomes a primary concern, especially where there are long lead times for orders. How are the vendors for these components chosen? If one is honest in looking back at previous design developments and honest in listing the three main criteria for choosing a component vendor, they would be:

- Lowest cost
- Lowest cost
- Lowest cost

The only other parameter which may play a part in choosing a vendor is loyalty to a particular vendor, no matter what his incoming quality may be.

Obviously, these are not the most desirable parameters to consider if the design is to be reliable. The parameters of choice include:

- Fitness for use
- Criticality versus non-criticality
- Reliability
- History
- Safety

15.3.1 COMPONENT FITNESS FOR USE

Fitness for use includes analyzing a component for the purpose to which it is designed. Many vendors list common applications for their components and tolerances for those applications. Where the desired application is different than that listed, the component must be analyzed and verified in that application. This includes specifying parameters particular to its intended use, specifying tolerances, inclusion of a safety margin and a review of the history of that part in other applications.

For components being used for the first time in a particular application and for which no history or vendor data are available, testing in the desired application should be conducted. More is said about this in Chapter 21.

15.3.2 COMPONENT RELIABILITY

The process of assuring the reliability of a component is a multi-step procedure, including:

- Initial vendor assessment
- Vendor audit
- Vendor evaluation
- Vendor qualification

The initial vendor assessment should be a review of any past history of parts delivery, including on-time deliveries, incoming rejection rate, willingness of the vendor to work with the company and handling of rejected components. The vendor should also be questioned as to the nature of his acceptance criteria, what type of reliability tests were performed and what the results of the tests were. It is also important to determine whether the nature of the test performed was similar to the environment the component will experience in your device.

Once the initial vendor assessment is satisfactorily completed, an audit of the vendor's facility is in order. The vendor's processes should be reviewed, the production capabilities assessed, rejection rates and failure analysis discussed. Sometimes the appearance of the facility provides a clue as to what type of vendor you are dealing with. A facility that is unorganized or dirty may tell you about the quality of the work performed.

Once components are shipped, you want to ensure that the quality of the incoming product is what you expect. A typical approach to the evaluation would be to do 100% inspection on the first several lots to check for consistent quality. Once you have an idea of the incoming quality and you are satisfied with it, components can be randomly inspected or inspected on a skip-lot basis.

Many companies have established a system of qualified vendors to determine what components will be used and the extent of incoming inspection. Some vendors qualify through a rigorous testing scheme that determines the incoming components meet the specification. Other companies have based qualification on a certain number of deliveries with no failures at incoming. Only components from qualified vendors should be used in any medical device. This is especially important when dealing with critical components.

15.3.3 COMPONENT HISTORY

Component history is an important tool in deciding what components to use in a design. It is important to review the use of the component in previous products, whether similar or not. When looking at previous products, the incoming rejection history, performance of the component in field use and failure rate history need to be analyzed.

A helpful tool in looking at component history is the use of available data banks of component information. One such data bank is MIL-HDBK-217. This military standard lists component failure rates based upon the environment in which they are used. The information has been accumulated from the use of military hardware. Some environments are similar to that seen by medical devices and the data is applicable. MIL-HDBK-217 is discussed in greater detail later in this chapter.

Another component data bank is a government program named GIDEP. The only cost for joining this group is a report listing failure rates of components in your applications. You receive reports listing summaries of other reports the group has received. It is a good way to get a history on components you intend to use. More information may be obtained by writing to:

GIDEP Operations Center
P.O. Box 8000
Corona, CA 92878-8000
http://www.gidep.org

A good source for both mechanical and electrical component failure rates is the books produced by the Reliability Analysis Center. They may be contacted at:

Reliability Analysis Center
201 Mills Street
Rome, NY 13440-6916
Telephone: +1+888+RAC-USER
http://rac.alionscience.com

15.3.4 COMPONENT SAFETY

The safety of each component in your application must be analyzed. Do this by performing a fault tree analysis, where possible failures are traced back to the components causing them. This is discussed later in this chapter.

A failure mode analysis can be performed that looks at the results of single point failures of components. Unlike the fault tree, which works from the failure back to the component, failure mode analysis works from the component to the resultant failure. This is also discussed in more detail later in the chapter.

15.4 COMPONENT DERATING

Component failure in a given application is determined by the interaction between the strength and the stress level. When the operational stress levels of a component exceed the rated strength of the component, the failure rate increases. When the operational stress level falls below the rated strength, the failure rate decreases.

With the various ways for improving the reliability of products, derating of components is an often-used method to guarantee the good performance as well as the extended life of a product. Derating is the practice of limiting the stresses which may be applied to a component to levels below the specified maximum.

Derating enhances reliability by:

- Reducing the likelihood that marginal components will fail during the life of the system
- Reducing the effects of parameter variations
- Reducing the long-term drift in parameter values
- Providing allowance for uncertainty in stress calculations
- Providing some protection against transient stresses, such as voltage spikes

An example of component derating is the use of a 2-watt resistor in a 1-watt application. It has been shown that derating a component to 50% of its operating value generally decreases its failure rate by a factor greater than 30%. As the failure rate is decreased, the reliability is increased.

Components are derated with respect to those stresses to which the component is most sensitive. These stresses fall into two categories, operational stresses and application stresses. Operational stresses include:

- Temperature
- Humidity
- Atmospheric pressure

Application stresses include:

- Voltage
- Current

- Friction
- Vibration

These latter stresses are particularly applicable to mechanical components.

Electrical-stress usage rating values are expressed as ratios of maximum applied stress to the component's stress rating. The equation for table guidelines is:

usage ratio = maximum applied stress/component stress rating

For most electronic components, the usage ratio varies between 0.5 and 0.9.

Thermal derating is expressed as a maximum temperature value allowed or as a ratio of "actual junction temperature" to "maximum allowed junction temperature" of the device. The standard expression for temperature measurement is the Celsius scale.

Derating guidelines should be considered to minimize the degradation effect on reliability. In examining the results from a derating analysis, one often finds that a design needs less than 25 components aggressively derated to greatly improve its reliability. And, depending on the design of the product, these components often relate to an increase in capacitance voltage rating, a change of propagation speed, an increase in the wattage capacity of a selected few power resistors, etc.

15.5 SAFETY MARGIN

Components or assemblies will fail when the applied load exceeds the strength at the time of application. The consideration of the load should take into account combined loads, such as voltage and temperature or humidity and friction. Combined loads can have effects which are out of proportion to their separate contributions, both in terms of instantaneous effects and strength degradation effects.

Tolerancing is an essential element of assuring adequate safety margins. Tolerancing, with appropriate controls on manufacturing, provides control over the resulting strength distributions. Analysis should be based on worst-case strength or distributional analysis, rather than on an anticipated strength distribution. Safety margin is calculated as follows:

$$\text{Safety margin} = (\text{mean safety factor}) - 1$$

$$= (\text{mean strength/mean stress}) - 1$$

An example illustrates the concept.

A structure is required to withstand a pressure of 20 000 psi. A safety margin of 0.5 is to be designed into the device. What is the strength that must be designed in?

$$\text{Safety margin} = (\text{strength}/\text{stress}) - 1$$
$$0.5 = (\text{strength}/20\,000) - 1$$
$$1.5 = \text{strength}/20\,000$$
$$(20\,000 \times 1.5) = \text{strength}$$
$$30\,000 \text{ psi} = \text{strength}$$

Most handbooks list a safety margin of 2.0 as the minimum required for high-reliability devices. In some cases, this may result in an over-design. The safety margin must be evaluated according to device function, the importance of its application and the safety requirements. For most medical applications, a minimum safety margin of 0.5 is adequate.

15.6　LOAD PROTECTION

Protection against extreme loads should be considered whenever practicable. In many cases, extreme loading situations can occur and must be protected against. When overload protection is provided, the reliability analysis should be performed on the basis of the maximum load which can be anticipated, bearing in mind the tolerances of the protection system.

15.7　ENVIRONMENTAL PROTECTION

Medical devices should be designed to withstand the worst-case environmental conditions in the product specification, with a safety margin included. Some typical environmental ranges which the device may experience include:

Operating temperature	0° to +55° centigrade
Storage temperature	−40° to +65° centigrade
Humidity	95% RH at 40° centigrade
Mechanical vibration	5 to 300 Hz at 2 Gs
Mechanical shock	24" to 48" drop
Mechanical impact	10 Gs at a 50 msec pulse width
Electrostatic discharge	Up to 50 000 volts

Electromagnetic compatibility becomes an issue in an environment, like an operating room. Each medical device should be protected from interference from other equipment, such as electrocautery and should be designed to eliminate radiation to other equipment.

15.8　PRODUCT MISUSE

An area of design concern that was briefly addressed earlier in this chapter is the subject of product misuse. Whether through failure to properly read the operation manual or through improper training, medical devices are going to be misused and even abused. There are many stories of product misuse, such as the hand-held monitor that was dropped into the toilet bowl, the user who used a hammer to pound a 9-volt battery into a monitor backwards or the user who spilled a can of soda on and into a device. Practically, it is impossible to make a device completely misuse-proof. But it is highly desirable to design around the ones that can be anticipated.

Some common examples of product misuse include:

- Excess application of cleaning solutions
- Physical abuse
- Spills
- Excess weight applied to certain parts
- Excess torque applied to controls or screws
- Improper voltages, frequencies, or pressures
- Improper or interchangeable electrical or pneumatic connections

Product misuse should be discussed with Marketing to define as many possible misuse situations as can be anticipated. The designer must then design around these situations, including a safety margin, which will serve to increase the reliability of the device. Where design restrictions limit the degree of protection against misuse and abuse, the device should alarm or should malfunction in a manner that is obvious to the user.

15.9   INITIAL RELIABILITY PREDICTION

Once the design has proceeded to the point where parts have been defined and a parts list developed, an initial prediction based on the parts used may be performed to produce an initial MTBF value. This value may then be compared to the original reliability goal to determine if the design will meet the intended reliability. The initial prediction is also used to highlight certain areas of the design that have a high failure rate, such as a particular component or an assembly, such as a PC board or a pneumatic circuit. The prediction is also used to form the basis for future analysis, reliability growth, and change.

Certain limitations exist with the prediction method. The first deals with the ability to accumulate data of known validity for the new application. The design may contain many new components, some of which are new to the marketplace and are not included in MIL-HDBK-217. Also, a component may be used in an application for which failure rate data have not been accumulated. In these cases, you may have to rely on vendor data or on the history of similar components in similar products.

A second limitation is the complexity of the predicting technique. It takes a long time to list each component, look up each failure rate and then calculate the MTBF for each assembly and then the device. As the complexity of the product increases, the length of time increases. Several companies have advertised computer programs that perform the prediction. The program takes the individual components and their quantity and determines the failure rates from tables residing in the computer, which are periodically updated. No matter the effort it takes to complete, the prediction must be done to get the basis for future activities.

MIL-HDBK-217 contains two methods of doing a prediction, a parts stress analysis and a part count analysis. The parts stress analysis requires a greater amount of detail to complete and thus is applicable at a later stage in development, when hardware testing has been completed. The parts count analysis requires a minimum of information, including the parts, quantities, quality levels, and application environment. Because it does not require operational stress levels, it can be performed early in the design phase as soon as a parts list is developed. Only the parts count method will be discussed here. Details of the parts stress analysis may be found in MIL-HDBK-217.

15.9.1 PARTS COUNT PREDICTION

There are four items necessary to begin a parts count prediction:

- A schematic
- A parts list
- MIL-HDBK-217
- Marketing parameters

The marketing parameters include (1) the use rate, i.e., the number of hours the device is in operation per day, the number of days per week and the number of weeks per year, (2) the desired MTBF goal, (3) the desired life of the device, and (4) the desired warranty cost as a percentage of sales. These parameters are used for final calculations after the MTBF has been calculated.

The first step in completing a part count prediction is to choose the environment in which the product will be used from among the many listed in the handbook. The three most commonly experienced by medical devices, in order of increasing severity, are:

- GF (ground fixed)   Conditions less than ideal, such as installation in permanent racks, with adequate cooling air and possible installations in unheated buildings. An example would be a wall-mounted gas pressure alarm
- GB (ground benign)   Non-mobile, laboratory environment, readily accessible to maintenance. An example would be a CAT scan residing in one location or a monitor permanently set on a table or desk
- GM (ground mobile)   Equipment installed on wheeled or tracked vehicles. An example would be an evoked potential system that can be rolled from the operating room into a patient's room or a laboratory

INITIAL RELIABILITY PREDICTION

Device _____

Subsystem _____   Date _____

Component	Style	Quantity	Individual failure rate	Total failure rate

Total failure rate _____

MTBF _____

FIGURE 15-5 Parts count prediction sheet

Where a question exists as to which of two environments should be chosen, select the more severe of the two.

Once the environment is chosen, all parts in one particular assembly, such as a PC board or a pneumatic circuit, are listed on a form, such as that shown in Figure 15-5. The form lists the type of component, the style of part, where applicable, the quantity of that component in the assembly, the failure rate for that component, and the total failure rate for the quantity of that component.

When all parts are listed on the sheet, start the process of determining the individual failure rates. The individual components are found in the appropriate tables within the parts count analysis portion of MIL-HDBK-217. The base failure rate is listed as well as the quality factor and other parameters, where necessary. The component failure rate is found by multiplying the base failure rate and the quality factor and other listed factors. This number is then listed in the individual component failure rate. This number is multiplied by the quantity included in the assembly and the total failure rate is determined. This process continues for the remainder of the items in the assembly. When all components are determined, the total failure rates are summed to determine the failure rate for the assembly. This failure rate is listed as failure per million hours. To calculate the MTBF for the assembly, the total failure rate is divided by one million and the reciprocal taken. This will be the MTBF in hours.

The above process is repeated for each assembly. When completed, the total failure rates for each assembly are summed, yielding the total failure rate for the device. The MTBF for the device is calculated as it was above, for the assembly. An example will help illustrate the method.

15.9.2 PARTS COUNT PREDICTION EXAMPLE

A company is developing the model 3322 Monitor. The device consists of several PC boards and a display. Reliability engineering has the task of determining the MTBF of the device, based on the hardware components used, for comparison to the reliability goal.

The device will be stationary during use. Thus the environment "GB" is chosen from MIL-HDBK-217. The parts for each PC board are listed on separate worksheets and the failure rates calculated. Figure 15-6 shows a sample worksheet for the ADC board.

The PC board is listed in the Generic Failure Rate for Inductive and Electromechanical Parts Table of MIL-HDBK-217F (Figure 15-7) under the term "PCBs." Read across the line until the column GB is found. The value

INITIAL RELIABILITY PREDICTION

Device __3322 Monitor__

Subsystem___ADC board___   Date _____5/3/95_____

Component	Style	Quantity	Individual failure rate	Total failure rate
PC board		1		
Resistors	RN	30		
Capacitors	CK	5		
Capacitors	CM	10		
Diodes	Zener	18		
Transistors	Si NPN	8		
54LS164		2		
8259		1		
54LS240		3		
54LS00		5		

Total failure rate _____

MTBF_____

FIGURE 15-6 Worksheet for the ADC board

Part type	GB
SWITCHES	
Toggles & pushbutton	0.001
Sensitive	0.15
Thumbwheel	0.56
CIRCUIT BREAKERS	
Magnetic	0.06
CONNECTORS	
Cir/rack/panel	0.011
Coaxial	0.012
PCBs	0.0054
IC SOCKETS	0.0019
INTERCONNECT ASSY	0.053

FIGURE 15-7 Sample of generic failure rate for Inductive and Electromechanical Parts Table

Part type	Quality MIL-SPEC	Level NON-MIL
Inductive devices	1	10
Quartz crystals	1	2.1
Relays, solid states	1	4
Relays, time delay	1	4
Relays, mechanical	3	9
Switches, toggle & sensitive	1	20
Switches, thumbwheel	1	10
Switches, rotary wafer	1	50
Circuit breakers, thermal	1	8.4
Connectors	1	2
Interconnection assemblies	1	2

FIGURE 15-8 Sample of π_Q factor for use with Section 11-22 Devices Table

there is 0.0054. The quality factor for the interconnects is found in the π_Q Factor for Use with Section 11-22 Devices Table (Figure 15-8). Since this board is a MIL-SPEC board, the quality factor is 1. The total failure rate for the board is then the product of the initial failure rate and the quality factor.

Total failure rate = component failure rate (quality factor)

Part type	GB
Composition	0.00050
Film, insulated	0.0012
Film, RN (R, C, or N)	0.0014
Film, power	0.012
Film, network	0.0023
Wirewound, accurate	0.0085
Wirewound, power	0.014

FIGURE 15-9 Sample of generic failure rate for resistors table

Established reliability styles	Quality factor
S	0.030
R	0.10
P	0.30
M	1.0
MIL-SPEC	3.0
Lower	10

FIGURE 15-10 Sample of quality factors for resistors table

Therefore, the failure rate for the PC board is 0.0054 failures per million hours. The total failure rate for the assembly is the failure rate multiplied by the number of PC boards, in this case one. The total failure rate is 0.0054 failures per million hours.

The resistors are type "RN." The data for resistors are found in the Generic Failure Rate for Resistors Table (Figure 15-9). Find style "RN" and column GB. The value is 0.0014. The quality value for resistors of two letter types found in this table (Figure 15-10) is 10. Therefore the failure rate for the resistors is 0.014 failures per million hours. The total failure rate for the assembly is the failure rate multiplied by the number of resistors, in this case 30. The total failure rate for the resistors is 0.042 failures per million hours.

Other parts have their failure rates calculated in the same manner, using the appropriate MIL-HDBK-217 tables. They are then summed to give the total failure rate for the board. The failure rate is then divided by one million to yield the failure rate per hour. The reciprocal of this number yields the MTBF in hours.

The total failure rate for the device is calculated by summing the individual failure rates for the subassemblies and other components. The parts previously calculated are included along with other parts whose failure rate may be obtained from the vendor or component testing. The MTBF of the monitor is then calculated.

This value may then be compared to the reliability goal to determine if the values are comparable. It is also important to look at the individual subassemblies to determine which have the highest failure rates. The designer should then determine how the subassembly may be changed to reduce the failure rate. This may include using a component with a higher reliability or by using redundant components.

The prediction value may also be used to calculate the warranty cost for the device. To do this, several parameters for the device are necessary, including:

Operating time per year	2500 hours
Number of units sold per year	200 units
Selling price	$ 58,000
Average charge for a service call	$ 850

The following calculations can then be made:

$$\text{Total sales per year} = 200 \text{ units (\$ 58\,000 per unit)}$$
$$= \$ 11\,600\,000$$

Assuming the device has an MTBF of 39 626 hours, the reliability of the device based on 2500 hours operating time per year is:

$$\text{Reliability} = \exp{-\text{usetime}/\text{MTBF})}$$
$$= \exp(-2500/39\,626)$$
$$= \exp(-0.0631)$$
$$= 0.94$$

This means 94% of the 200 units will survive the first year of operation without a failure, while 5%, or 12 units, will fail. Therefore, the total service charges are:

$$\text{Service charge} = 12 \text{ units (\$850 per service call)}$$
$$= \$10\,200$$

The warranty cost as a percentage of sales is thus:

$$\text{Warranty cost} = (\text{service charges}/\text{total sales})/100$$
$$= (\$10\,200/\$11\,600\,000)/100$$
$$= 0.09\% \text{ of sales}$$

This value should be compared to the company standard for warranty cost.

15.9.3 SUMMARY OF RELIABILITY PREDICTION

There are computer programs which will calculate a reliability prediction. The programs usually come with a database of components and failure rates. When such a program is purchased, it is essential to get periodic updates to the component database to assure the program is using the latest failure rate values.

Experience comparing initial predictions with actual field data has shown that the parts count value is approximately 10% to 20% below the actual value calculated from field data. However, the prediction values are good indicators of trends with regard to warranty costs, serve to highlight parts of the device with high failure rates, and provide valuable information for the Service Department in planning the inventory of replacement parts. Predictions can be updated after reliability testing is completed to establish a greater confidence in the calculated value.

In addition to the parts count prediction, MIL-HDBK-217 provides a second type of prediction, based on more detail of how the component operates. This second type of prediction requires information such as component current, component voltage, ambient temperature, etc. This prediction provides a more detailed calculation for the reliability but would occur later in the development process because of the details required. The choice of the type of prediction will depend on the type of information desired and how early in the development process it is desired.

15.10 DESIGN FOR VARIATION

During design, one may need to deal with the problem of assessing the combined effects of multiple variables on a measurable output or other characteristic of a product, by means of experiments. This is not a problem that is important in all designs, particularly when there are fairly large margins between capability and required performance, or for design involving negligible risk or uncertainty, or when only one or a few items are to be manufactured. However, when designs have to be optimized in relation to variations in parameter values, processes, and environmental conditions, particularly if these variations can have combined effects, it is necessary to use methods that can evaluate the effects of the simultaneous variations.

Statistical methods of experimentation have been developed which enable the effects of variation to be evaluated in these types of situation. They are applicable whenever the effects cannot be theoretically evaluated, particularly when there is a large component of random variation or interactions between variables. For multivariable problems, the methods are much more economical than traditional experiments, in which the effect of one variable is evaluated at a time. The traditional approach also does not enable interactions to be analyzed, when these are not known empirically.

15.11   DESIGN OF EXPERIMENTS

The statistical approach to design of experiments is a very elegant, economical, and powerful method for determining the significant effects and interactions in multivariable situations.

15.11.1   THE TAGUCHI METHOD

Genichi Taguchi developed a framework for statistical design of experiments adapted to the particular requirements of engineering design. Taguchi suggested that the design process consists of three phases: system design, parameter design, and tolerance design. In the system design phase, the basic concept is decided, using theoretical knowledge and experience to calculate the basic parameter values to provide the performance required. Parameter design involves refining the values so that the performance is optimized in relation to factors and variation which are not under the effective control of the designer, so that the design is robust in relation to these. Tolerance design is the final stage, in which the effects of random variation of manufacturing processes and environments are evaluated, to determine whether the design of the product and the production processes can be further optimized, particularly in relation to cost of the product and the production processes.

Taguchi separates variables into two types. Control factors are those variables which can be practically and economically controlled, such as a controllable dimensional or electrical parameter. Noise factors are the variables which are difficult or expensive to control in practice, though they can be controlled in an experiment, e.g., ambient temperature, or parameter variation with a tolerance range. The objective is then to determine the combination of control factor settings (design and process variables) which will make the product have the maximum robustness to the expected variation in the noise factors.

15.12   DESIGN CHANGES

Design changes occur throughout the design process. Often, assessing the impact of changes of all aspects of the project can be very difficult. This is particularly true for large projects involving multifunctional design teams. It is important to have the design under revision control, so that the history of changes may be tracked. To accomplish this, a design change methodology should be employed. Each change to the design should be reviewed, documented and approved before it is implemented. A simple change form, such as that indicated in Figure 15-11, can be used. This type of form limits the number of reviewers, but assures the appropriate personnel on the development team are informed of the change.

The basic question for design change is "When is a design put under revision control?" For example, the product specification changes frequently in the beginning of the process, as will other documentation. To institute a change

DESIGN REVISION CONTROL SHEET

Revision control number: _____

Subsystem:		Old revision:	
Origination date:		New revision:	
Origination site:			

Summary (additional information may be attached):

Change description:
Reason for the change:

Functional review:

Function	Signature
Project leader	
System coordinator	
Validation coordinator	

Non-approval (additional information may be attached):

Reason for non-approval:

Document information:

Effectivity date:	
Originator signature:	

FIGURE 15-11 Sample design change form

process too early will cause an excessive amount of documentation to become part of the project file. It is far better for all design activity that revision control be instituted after the initial flurry of changes has occurred. The activity, whether a specification, drawing, program, etc., should be fairly stable and have been reviewed at least once. This will allow for an orderly control of the design without excessive documentation.

15.13 DESIGN REVIEWS

Despite discipline, training, and care, it is inevitable that occasional oversights or errors will occur in new designs. Design reviews are held to highlight critical aspects of the design and to focus attention on possible shortfalls. Design reviews are held to:

- Review the progress of a design
- Monitor reliability growth
- Assure all specifications are being addressed
- Peer review the design approach

The primary purpose of the design review is to make a choice among alternative design approaches. The output of the review should include an understanding of the weak areas in the design and the areas of the design in need of special attention. Topics to be covered in a design review include:

- Redundancy versus derating
- Redesign of weak areas versus high-reliability parts
- Review of failure mode and effects analysis
- Review of potential product misuse
- Review overstressed areas

The design review should follow a structured order and be well documented with topics discussed, decisions reached, and resulting action items.

There are three overall types of design reviews:

- Informal design reviews: To address detailed technical design and performance issues, usually for an isolated part of the product
- Formal design review: To address technical performance issues for the entire product and correlate activities with the project objectives and the product specifications
- Program review: To examine the project relative to budget and schedule performance, technical discoveries or limitations. Program reviews, also known as progress (or project) reviews, are generally conducted by senior managers and do not concern themselves with technical reviews of design

Formal design reviews are generally held according to the project plan and are convened to support major project milestones. Plenty of time should be allowed for the review meeting. People should be invited who will challenge the design, including experts. The purpose is to review theory, technical design specs, implementation, and performance to specification. The design review should be held to challenge the design, not familiarize people with it. If familiarization is needed, a separate session should be held prior to the actual review. People should be allowed to talk freely. Criticism should be expected and accepted. A dedicated person not expected to participate in the review should be asked to take the minutes.

Informal design reviews are generally not scheduled per the project plan and are convened when the need arises to address specific concerns. Informal design reviews are generally not scheduled per the project plan and are convened when the need arises to address specific concerns. Generally, only local reviewers are invited. The informal reviews are used to brainstorm a particularly tough problem or to analyze alternate design approaches. These reviews are generally extremely detailed and focus on a particular sub-system, module, or component. Informal review results are usually documented in lab notebooks or supporting memos.

For all design reviews, it is optimal to assure the design review personnel have not taken part in the actual design activity. This gives a fresh and unbiased look at the design. Some of the guidelines for design reviewers include:

- Design reviewers have a serious responsibility to comment on the potential outcome of the project
- When notice of review meetings is announced, reviewers should plan ahead and take time to prepare for the reviews
- The reviewers should assure they understand project objectives and the product specification
- Reviewers should attend all formally planned learning sessions
- If possible, reviewers should submit concerns and questions to the review chair in advance of the design review meeting. The issues and concerns can be discussed in depth at the meeting
- Reviewers should help the design review leader during the meeting by questioning the design's performance relative to the product specification, design specification, project objectives, safety, effectiveness, and reliability of the product's functioning. At this stage, being harshly, constructively, critical is being helpful

REFERENCES

Fries, R.C., *Reliability Assurance for Medical Devices, Equipment and Software*, Interpharm Press, Inc., Buffalo Grove, IL, 1991.

Fries, R.C., *Reliable Design of Medical Devices*, Marcel-Dekker, Inc., New York, 1997.

Fries, R.C., *Handbook of Medical Device Design*, Marcel-Dekker, Inc., New York, 2001.

Government – Industry Data Exchange Program, *Program Summary*, June, 1979.

Jensen, F. and Peterson, N.E., *Burn-In*, John Wiley and Sons, New York, 1982.

King, P.H. and Fries, R.C., *Design of Biomedical Devices and Systems*, Marcel-Dekker, Inc., New York, 2002.

Lloyd, D.K., and Lipow, M., *Reliability Management, Methods and Management*, 2nd edition, American Society for Quality Control, Milwaukee, WI, 1984.

Logothetis, N. and Wynn, H.P., *Quality Through Design*, Oxford University Press, London, UK, 1990.

Mason, R.L., Hunter, W.G., and Hunter, J.S., *Statistical Design and Analysis of Experiments*, John Wiley & Sons, New York, 1989.

MIL-STD-202, *Test Methods for Electronic and Electrical Component Parts*, Department of Defense, Washington, DC, 1980.

MIL-HDBK-217F, *Reliability Prediction of Electronic Equipment*, Department of Defense, Washington, DC, 1991.

MIL-STD-750, *Test Methods for Semiconductor Devices*, Department of Defense, Washington, DC, 1983

MIL-STD-781, *Reliability Design Qualification and Production Acceptance Tests: Exponential Distribution*, Department of Defense, Washington, DC, 1977.

MIL-STD-883, *Test Methods and Procedures for Microelectronics*, Department of Defense, Washington, DC, 1983.

Montgomery, D.C., *Design and Analysis of Experiments*, 2nd edition, John Wiley & Sons, New York, 1984.

O'Connor, P.D.T., *Practical Reliability Engineering*, 3rd edition, John Wiley & Sons, Chichester, UK, 1991.

Reliability Analysis Center, *Nonelectronic Parts Reliability Data: 1995*, Reliability Analysis Center, Rome, NY, 1994.

Ross, P.J., *Taguchi Techniques for Quality Engineering*, McGraw-Hill, New York, 1988.

Taguchi, G., *Systems of Experimental Design*, Unipub/Asian Productivity Association, 1978.

Taguchi, G., *Introduction to Quality Engineering*, Unipub/Asian Productivity Association, 1986.

16 Software design

CONTENTS

16.1   Software design levels 256
    16.1.1   Top-level design 256
    16.1.2   Detailed design 256
16.2   Design alternatives and tradeoffs 256
16.3   Software architecture 257
16.4   Choosing a methodology 259
16.5   Structured analysis 260
16.6   Object-oriented design 260
16.7   Choosing a language 261
16.8   Software risk analysis 263
16.9   The requirements traceability matrix 265
16.10   Software review 266
16.11   Design techniques 269
16.12   Performance predictability and design simulation 269
16.13   Module specifications 270
16.14   Coding 270
16.15   Design support tools 270
16.16   Design as the basis for verification and validation activity 271
16.17   Conclusion 272
References 272

Software design and implementation is a multi-staged process in which system and software requirements are translated into a functional program that addresses each requirement. Good software designs are based on a combination of creativity and discipline. Creativity provides resolution to new technical hurdles and the challenges of new market and user needs. Discipline provides quality and reliability to the final product.

Software design begins with the Software Requirements Specification. The design itself is the system architecture, which addresses each of the requirements of the specification and any appropriate software standards or regulations.

The top-level design begins with the analysis of software design alternatives and their tradeoffs. The overall software architecture is then established along with the design methodology to be used and the programming language to be implemented. A risk analysis is performed and then refined to ensure that malfunction of any software component will not cause harm to the patient,

255

the user, or the system. Metrics are established to check for program effectiveness and reliability. The Requirements Traceability Matrix is reviewed to assure all requirements have been addressed. The software design is reviewed by peers for completeness.

The detailed design begins with modularizing the software architecture, assigning specific functionality to each component and assuring both internal and external interfaces are well defined. Coding style and techniques are chosen based on their proven value and the intended function and environment of the system. Peer reviews assure the completeness and effectiveness of the design. The detailed design also establishes the basis for subsequent verification and validation activity. The use of automated tools throughout the development program is an effective method for streamlining the design and development process and assists in developing the necessary documentation.

16.1   SOFTWARE DESIGN LEVELS

Software design may be divided into two distinct stages.

16.1.1   TOP-LEVEL DESIGN

- Design alternatives and tradeoffs
- Software architecture
- Choosing a methodology
- Structural analysis
- Object-oriented design
- Choosing a language
- Software risk analysis
- The Software Requirements Traceability Matrix
- Software review

16.1.2   DETAILED DESIGN

- Design techniques
- Performance predictability and design simulation
- Module specification
- Coding
- Design support tools
- Design as a basis for verification and validation testing

16.2   DESIGN ALTERNATIVES AND TRADEOFFS

The determination of the design and the allocation of requirements is a very iterative process. Alternative designs are postulated that are candidates to satisfy the requirements. The determination of these designs is a fundamentally creative activity, a "cut and try" determination of what might work. The specific techniques used are numerous and call upon a broad range of skills.

They include control theory, optimization, consideration of the man–machine interface, use of modern control test equipment, queuing theory, communication and computer engineering, statistics, and other disciplines. These techniques are applied to factors such as performance, reliability, schedule, cost, maintainability, power consumption, weight, and life expectancy.

Some of the alternative designs will be quickly discarded, while others will require more careful analysis. The capabilities and quality of each design alternative are assessed using a set of design factors specific to each application and the methods of representing the system design.

Certain design alternatives will be superior in some aspects, while others will be superior in different aspects. These alternatives are "traded off," one against the other, in terms of the factors important for the system being designed. The design ensues from a series of technology decisions, which are documented with architecture diagrams that combine aspects of data and control flow. As an iterative component of making technology decisions, the functionality expressed by the data flow and control flow diagrams from system requirements analysis is allocated to the various components of the system. Although the methods for selection of specific technology components are not a part of the methodology, the consequences of the decisions are documented in internal performance requirements and timing diagrams.

Finally, all factors are taken into account, including customer desires and political issues to establish the complete system design. The product of the system design is called an architecture model. The architecture includes the components of the system, allocation of requirements, and topics such as maintenance, reliability, redundancy, and self-test.

16.3   SOFTWARE ARCHITECTURE

Software architecture is the high-level part of software design, the frame that holds the more detailed parts of the design. Typically, the architecture is described in a single document referred to as the architecture specification. The architecture must be a prerequisite to the detailed design, because the quality of the architecture determines the conceptual integrity of the system. This in turn determines the ultimate quality of the system.

A system architecture first needs an overview that describes the system in broad terms. It should also contain evidence that alternatives to the final organization have been considered and the reasons the organization used was chosen over the alternatives. The architecture should also contain:

- Definition of the major modules in a program. What each module does should be well defined, as well as the interface of each module
- Description of the major files, tables, and data structures to be used. It should describe alternatives that were considered and justify the choices that were made
- Description of specific algorithms or reference to them

- Description of alternative algorithms that were considered and indicate the reasons that certain algorithms were chosen
- In an object-oriented system, specification of the major objects to be implemented. It should identify the responsibilities of each major object and how the object interacts with other objects. It should include descriptions of the class hierarchies, of state transitions, and of object persistence. It should also describe other objects that were considered and give reasons for preferring the organization that was chosen
- Description of a strategy for handling changes clearly. It should show that possible enhancements have been considered and that the enhancements most likely are also easiest to implement
- Estimation of the amount of memory used for nominal and extreme cases

Software architecture alludes to two important characteristics of a computer program: (1) the hierarchical structure of procedural components (modules) and (2) the structure of data. Software architecture is derived through a partitioning process that relates elements of a software solution to parts of a real world problem implicitly defined during requirements analysis. The evolution of a software structure begins with a problem definition. The solution occurs when each part of the problem is solved by one or more software elements.

An architectural template may be developed that gives a general layout for all the architectural model diagrams to follow. This template indicates the physical perspectives that had not existed in the system requirements. Areas that may be included in the template are:

- User interface processing
- Maintenance, self test, and redundancy requirements
- Input processing
- Output processing

User interface processing is the system-to-user interface, requiring some technology-based enhancements that were omitted in the requirements model. These enhancements are based on use of available technology and on various cost, operational environment, and other criteria. The architecture should be flexible so that a new user interface can be substituted without affecting the processing and output parts of the program.

Maintenance, self test, and redundancy processing requirements are also technology dependent. These requirements cannot be identified until an implementation technology has been selected that meets the system's reliability and performance criteria.

Input/output is another area that deserves attention in the architecture. Input processing refers to the communications across the system's boundary that were not addressed in the system requirements and are not part of the user interface or a maintenance interface. Additional processing is added depending on technology decisions. Output processing involves the same considerations as input processing. Output processing takes the system's logical output and converts it to a physical form. The architecture should specify a look-ahead, look-behind, or just-in-time reading scheme and it should describe the level at which I/O errors are detected.

The detailed architecture may be expressed in various forms. Examples include:

- Architecture context diagram: the top-level diagram for the architecture model. It contains the system's place in its environment and, in addition, the actual physical interface to the environment
- Architecture flow diagram: the network representation of the system's physical configuration

16.4   CHOOSING A METHODOLOGY

It seems there are about as many design methodologies as there are engineers to implement them. Typically, the methodology selection entails a prescription for the requirements analysis and design processes. Of the many popular methods, each has its own merit based on the application to which the methods are applied. The toolset and methodology selection should run hand-in-hand. Tools should be procured to support established or tentative design methodology and implementation plans. In some cases, tools are purchased to support a methodology already in place. In other cases the methodology is dictated by an available toolset. Ideally, the two are selected at the same time following a thorough evaluation of need.

Selecting the right toolset and design methodology should not be based on a flashy advertisement or suggestion from an authoritative methodology guru. It is important to understand the environment in which it will be employed and the product to which it will be applied. Among other criteria, the decision should be based on the size of the project (number of requirements), type of requirements (hard or soft real-time), complexity of the end-product, number of engineers, experience and skill level of the engineers, project schedules, project budget, reliability requirements, and future enhancements to the product (maintenance concerns). Weight factors should be applied to the evaluation criteria. One way or another, whether the evaluation is done in a formal or informal way, involving one or more than one person, it should be done to assure a proper fit for the organization and product.

Regardless of the approach used, the most important factor to be considered for the successful implementation of a design methodology is software development team buy-in. The software development team must possess the confidence that the approach is appropriate for the application and be willing and "excited" to tackle the project. The implementation of a design methodology takes relentless discipline. Many projects have been unsuccessful as a result of lack of commitment and faith.

The two most popular formal approaches applied to the design of medical products are the object-oriented analysis/design and, the more traditional, (top-down) structured analysis/design. There are advantages and disadvantages to each. Either approach, if done in a disciplined and systematic manner, along with the electrical system design, can provide for a safe and effective product.

16.5 STRUCTURED ANALYSIS

Structured analysis is the process of examining the software requirements for the purposes of generating a structural model of the requirements. This activity focuses on data flowing through the system. In particular, data transformations are identified which occur in the process of delivering the required outputs from given inputs. A thorough structured analysis of the system will provide a complete and well-understood set of software requirements which is highly conducive to the ensuing structured design process.

Structured design entails an abstraction of the analysis results into a top-down, functional decomposition of the requirements. Structured design focuses on the decomposition of the operations to be performed on the data. At the onset a series of high-level functional blocks are identified which, in collection, address all processing expectations of the system. In a systematic manner, a hierarchy of ever-smaller processing units are evolved from the high-level blocks. This iterative partitioning produces a series of small, procedural components which, when integrated together, form a system capable of satisfying all functional requirements.

Structured design is the most common approach to software design today. Designing systems from the functional decomposition perspective has been around for decades and its approach is the most well understood and mature. Its weaknesses, however, lie in the emphasis on sequential thinking and the generation of solutions based on procedural connection among functional blocks. Most software developers will agree that this is not a natural representation of real-world objects and the relationships between them.

Although normally manageable in small- to medium-scale software systems, it is inherent that most product requirements changes result in significant design changes unless they were anticipated from the start. Certain types of changes can be very expensive to make because of their disturbance of some of the predefined high-level procedural flows. Unforeseen changes can also lead to reduced product confidence and reliability. Increased complexity often results when trying to retain harmony among existing components in the presence of new and sometimes foggy relationships.

16.6 OBJECT-ORIENTED DESIGN

The object-oriented design paradigm seeks to mimic the way that people form models of the real world. In contrast to procedural design methods, it de-emphasizes the underlying computer representation. Its major modeling concept is that of the object, which is used to symbolize real-world entities and their interactions. Objects are entities which have state and behavior. They can be implemented in computer systems as data and a set of operations defined over those data.

Although at its lowest level of design, object-oriented design resembles structured design and traditional code development, during the analysis and high-level design phases a different mind set surrounds the attack of the problem. Object-oriented design hinges on approaching design solutions in terms of the identification of objects, associated object attributes, and operations performed on and among the objects. This approach generates designs which map very well to "real-world" items and operations, thus leading to designs which can be easier to understand and maintain.

Object-oriented designs have been found to be a very successful approach to the design of some large, more complex systems. This has garnished the attention of software developers around the world. There are, however, two generally recognized blemishes currently associated with the approach. Developers often have difficulty agreeing on the definitions of objects and object classes. This has resulted in system designs which are not as easy to understand as expectations would have. Also, an additional processing overhead is associated with the implementation of object-oriented programming languages. This inefficiency has deterred many from using the approach on embedded real-time medical systems because of the increased hardware cost incurred to deliver acceptable system performance. Still, as the price of processing power for the dollar decreases it can be expected that object-oriented programming will increase in popularity as a viable approach to the development of high-performance, competitively priced medical products.

16.7 CHOOSING A LANGUAGE

Programming languages are the notational mechanisms used to implement software products. Features available in the implementation language exert a strong influence on the architectural structure and algorithmic details of the software. Choice of language has also been shown to have an influence on programmer productivity. Industry data have shown that programmers are more productive using a familiar language than an unfamiliar one. Programmers working with high-level languages achieve better productivity than those working with lower-level languages. Developers working in interpreted languages tend to be more productive than those working in compiled languages. In languages that are available in both interpreted and compiled forms, programs can be productively developed in the interpreted form and then released in the better-performing compiled form.

Computer languages are the malleable tools for program design and implementation alike. From one perspective, they offer representations of computer procedures that can consolidate the understanding gained from a prototyping process and then link these key requirements to machine capabilities. From another perspective, they can impose structure and clarity on the logical flow of a system with an eye toward operational efficiency and reliability. In principle, these two perspectives should converge. In actual practice, they often conflict. The problem of how to move from an initial design through the necessary revisions to implementation is the underlying issue in the choice and use of language in medical systems.

Modern programming languages provide a variety of features to support development and maintenance of software products. These features include:

- Strong type checking
- Separate compilation
- User-defined data types
- Data encapsulation
- Data abstraction

The major issue in type checking is flexibility versus security. Strongly typed languages provide maximum security, while automatic type coercion provides maximum flexibility. The modern trend is to augment strong type checking with features that increase flexibility while maintaining the security of strong type checking.

Separate compilation allows retention of program modules in a library. The modules are linked into the software system, as appropriate, by the linking loader. The distinction between independent compilation and separate compilation is that type checking across compilation–unit interfaces is performed by a separate compilation facility, but not by an independent compilation facility.

User-defined data types, in conjunction with strong type checking, allow the programmer to model and segregate entities from the problem domain using a different data type for each type of problem entity.

Data encapsulation defines composite data objects in terms of the operations that can be performed on them, and the details of data representation and data manipulation are suppressed by the mechanisms. Data encapsulation differs from abstract data types in that encapsulation provides only one instance of an entity.

Data abstraction provides a powerful mechanism for writing well-structured, easily modified programs. The internal details of data representation and data manipulation can be changed at will and, provided the interfaces of the manipulation procedures remain the same, other components of the program will be unaffected by the change, except perhaps for changes in performance characteristics and capacity limits. Using a data abstraction facility, data entities can be defined in terms of predefined types, user-defined types, and other data abstractions, thus permitting systematic development of hierarchical abstractions.

One of the most striking things about computer languages is that there are so many of them. All have struggled to keep up with the increasing

TABLE 16-1
Language suitability for programming situtations

Kind of programs	More effective languages	Less effective languages
Structured data	Ada, C/C++, Pascal	Assembler, Basic
Quick and dirty project	Basic	Ada, Assembler, Pascal
Fast execution	Assembler, C	Interpreted languages
Mathematical calculations	Fortran	Pascal
Easy to maintain	Ada, Pascal	C, Fortran
Dynamic memory usage	C, Pascal	Basic
Limited memory environments	Assembler, Basic, C	Ada, Fortran
Real time program	Ada, Assembler, C	Basic, Fortran
String manipulation	Basic, Pascal	C

individuality and complexity of modern computer systems. To be successful, a language must mediate between (1) the capabilities and limitations of the machine on which the applications run, (2) the properties of the information domain that is to be addressed, (3) the characteristics of the user and (4) the exchange of information between machines. Ideally, every language should be a proper reflection of these four perspectives.

When choosing a language, careful evaluation is necessary for a particular program. Table 16-1 lists some languages and their suitability for various purposes. The classifications are broad, so care must be taken in their use.

Among the many languages available, each has its pros and cons, depending on its specific application. Table 16-2 lists some of the pros and cons for individual languages. In addition to the pros and cons, the following language characteristics should be analyzed in making a choice:

- Clarity, simplicity, and unity of language concept
- Clarity of program syntax
- Naturalness of application
- Support for abstraction
- Ease of verification
- Programming environment
- Portability of programs
- Cost of use

16.8 SOFTWARE RISK ANALYSIS

Software risk analysis techniques identify software hazards and safety-critical single and multiple failure sequences, determine software safety requirements, including timing requirements, and analyze and measure software for safety. While functional requirements often focus on what the system shall do, risk requirements must also include what the system shall not do – including

TABLE 16-2
Pros and cons of software languages

Language	Pros	Cons
Ada	Some software engineering techniques are embedded in the language. Portable, broad range of language constructs. Built in microprocessing	Large, overkill for many applications. Development systems are expensive to purchase. Life cycle costs are up front
Assembler	Very fast, low-level programming when other languages are unsuitable	High maintenance cost due to level or readability. High portability of errors, not portable, old, low-level language
Basic	Good beginner language. Straight-forward commands	Slow, unstructured, difficult to maintain
C	Wide usage, portable, fast, powerful. Recently became an ANSI standard language	Too powerful for the inexperienced programmer
Cobol	Good for large amounts of data, simple calculations, business record processing	Bad for scientific applications, poor support of complex calculations, slow
Fortran	Well suited for scientific and engineering applications	Old technology
Modula-2	Pascal-like, yet modular	Not widely used, no language standard, several dialects
Pascal	Flexible data typing, structured, good beginner language	Monolithic, confining

means of eliminating and controlling system hazards and of limiting damage in case of a mishap. An important part of the risk requirements is the specification of the ways in which the software and the system can fail safely and to what extent failure is tolerable.

Several techniques have been proposed and used for doing risk analysis, including:

- Software hazard analysis
- Software fault tree analysis
- Real time logic

Software hazard analysis, like hardware hazard analysis, is the process whereby hazards are identified and categorized with respect to criticality and probability. Potential hazards that need to be considered include normal operating modes, maintenance modes, system failure or unusual incidents in the environment, and errors in human performance. Once hazards are identified, they are assigned a severity and probability. Severity involves a qualitative measure of the worst credible mishap that could result from the hazard. Probability refers to the frequency with which the hazard occurs. Once the probability and severity are determined, a control mode is established, that is, a means of reducing the probability and/or severity of the associated potential hazard. Finally, a control method or methods are selected to achieve the associated Control Mode. Hazard and risk analysis were discussed in detail in Chapter 11.

Fault tree analysis is an analytical technique used in the risk analysis of electromechanical systems. An undesired system state is specified, and the system is analyzed in the context of its environment and operation to find credible sequences of events that can lead to the undesired state. The fault tree is a graphic model of various parallel and sequential combinations of faults or system states that will result in the occurrence of the predefined undesired event. It thus depicts the logical interrelationships of basic events that lead to the hazardous event. Fault tree analysis was discussed in Chapter 11.

Real time logic is a process wherein the system designer first specifies a model of the system in terms of events and actions. The event–action model describes the data dependency and temporal ordering of the computational actions that must be taken in response to events in a real-time application. The model can be translated into real time logic formulas. The formulas are transformed into predicates of Presburger arithmetic with uninterpreted integer functions. Decision procedures are then used to determine whether a given risk assertion is a theorem derivable from the system specification. If so, the system is safe with respect to the timing behavior denoted by that assertion, as long as the implementation satisfies the requirements specification. If the risk assertion is unsatisfiable with respect to the specification, then the system is inherently unsafe because successful implementation of the requirements will cause the risk assertion to be violated. Finally, if the negation of the risk assertion is satisfiable under certain conditions, then additional constraints must be imposed on the system to assure its safety.

16.9 THE REQUIREMENTS TRACEABILITY MATRIX

It is becoming more and more apparent how important thorough requirements traceability is during the design and development stages of a software product, especially in large projects with requirements numbering in the thousands or tens of thousands. Regardless of the design and implementation methodology, it is important to assure the design is meeting its requirements during all phases of design.

To ensure the product is designed and developed in accordance with its requirements throughout the development cycle, individual requirements should be assigned to design components. Each software requirement, as might appear in a Software Requirements Specification for example, should be uniquely identifiable. Requirements resulting from design decisions (i.e., implementation requirements) should be uniquely identified and tracked along with product functional requirements.

This process not only assures that all functional and safety features are built into the product as specified, but also drastically reduces the possibility of requirements "slipping through the cracks." Overlooked features can be

Requirement	Design	Code	Unit test	Integration test
Accept only valid input	check_input	check_num.c check_char.c check_mixed.c	num_only.tc char_only.tc mixed.tc	whole_valid.tc whole_invalid.tc
Requirement 2				

FIGURE 16-1 Requirements traceability matrix

much more expensive when they become design modifications at the tail end of development.

The requirements traceability matrix (RTM) is generally a tabular format with requirements identifiers as rows and design entities as column headings. Individual matrix cells are marked with file names or design model identifiers to denote a requirement is satisfied within a design entity.

A requirements traceability matrix assures completeness and consistency with the software specification. This can be accomplished by forming a table that lists the requirements from the specification versus how each is met in each phase of the software development process. Figure 16-1 is an example of a requirements traceability matrix.

16.10   SOFTWARE REVIEW

An integral part of all design processes includes timely and well-defined reviews. Each level of design should produce design review deliverables. Software project development plans should include a list of the design phases, the expected deliverables for each phase, and a sound definition of the deliverables to be audited at each review.

Reviews of all design material have several benefits. First and foremost, knowing that their work is being reviewed, authors are more compelled to elevate the quality of their work. Secondly, reviews often uncover design blind spots and alternative design approaches. Finally, the documentation generated by the reviews is used to acquire agency approvals for process and product.

Software reviews may take several different forms:

- Inspections of design and code
- Code walk-throughs
- Code reading
- Dog-and-pony shows

An inspection is a specific kind of review that has been shown to be extremely effective in detecting defects and to be relatively economical compared to testing. Inspections differ from the usual reviews in several ways:

- Checklists focus the reviewer's attention on areas that have been problems in the past

- The emphasis is on defect detection, not correction
- Reviewers prepare for the inspection meeting beforehand and arrive with a list of the problems they've discovered
- Data are collected at each inspection and are fed into future inspections to improve them

An inspection consists of several distinct stages:

- *Planning*: the moderator, after receiving the documentation, decides who will review the material and when and where the review will take place
- *Overview*: the author describes the technical environment within which the design or code has been created
- *Preparation*: each reviewer works alone to become familiar with the documents
- *Inspection meeting*: the moderator chooses someone, usually the author, to paraphrase the design or read the code. The scribe records errors as they are detected, but discussion of an error stops as soon as it is recognized as an error
- *Inspection report*: the moderator produces an inspection report that lists each defect, including its type and severity
- *Rework*: the moderator assigns defects to someone, usually the author, for repair. The assignee(s) resolve each defect on the list
- *Follow-up*: the moderator is responsible for seeing that all rework assigned during the inspection is carried out

The general experience with inspections has been that the combination of design and code inspections usually removes 60 to 90% of the defects in a product. Inspections identify error-prone routines early and reports indicate they result in 30% fewer defects per 1000 lines of code than walkthroughs do. The inspection process is systematic because of its standard checklists and standard roles. It is also self-optimizing because it uses a formal feedback loop to improve the checklists and to monitor preparation and inspection rates.

A walkthrough usually involves two or more people discussing a design or code. It might be as informal as an impromptu bull session around a whiteboard; it might be as formal as a scheduled meeting with overhead transparencies and a formal report sent to management. Some of the characteristics of a walkthrough include:

- The walkthrough is usually hosted and moderated by the author of the design or code under review
- The purpose of the walkthrough is to improve the technical quality of a program rather that to assess it
- All participants prepare for the walkthrough by reading design or code documents and looking for areas of concern

TABLE 16-3
Comparison of inspections and walkthroughs

Properties	Inspection	Walkthroughs
Formal moderator training	Yes	No
Distinct participant roles	Yes	No
Who "drives" the inspection or walkthrough	Moderator	Author
Checklists for finding errors	Yes	No
Focused review effort – looks for the most frequently found kinds of errors	Yes	No
Formal follow-up to reduce bad fixes	Yes	No
Fewer future errors because of detailed error feedback to individual programmers	Yes	Incidental
Improved inspection efficiency from analysis of results	Yes	No
Analysis of data leading to detection of problems in the process, which in turn leads to improvements in the process	Yes	No

- The emphasis is on error detection, not correction
- The walkthrough concept is flexible and can be adapted to the specific needs of the organization using it

Used intelligently, a walkthrough can produce results similar to those of an inspection – that is, it can typically find between 30 and 70% of the errors in a program. Walkthroughs have been shown to be marginally less effective than inspections but, in some circumstances, can be preferable. Table 16-3 is a comparison of inspections and walkthroughs.

Code reading is an alternative to inspections and walkthroughs. In code reading, you read source code and look for errors. You also comment on qualitative aspects of the code, such as its design, style, readability, maintainability, and efficiency.

A code reading usually involves two or more people reading code independently and then meeting with the author of the code to discuss it. To prepare for a meeting, the author hands out source listings to the code readers. Two or more people read the code independently. When the reviewers have finished reading the code, the code-reading meeting is hosted by the author of the code and focuses on problems discovered by the reviewers. Finally, the author of the code fixes the problems identified by the reviewers.

The difference between code reading on the one hand and inspections and walkthroughs on the other is that code reading focuses more on individual review of the code than on the meeting. The result is that each reviewer's time is focused on finding problems in the code. Less time is spent in meetings.

Dog-and-pony shows are reviews in which a software product is demonstrated to a customer. The purpose of the review is to demonstrate to the customer that the project is proceeding, so it's a management review rather than a technical review. They should not be relied on to improve the technical quality of a program. Technical improvement comes from inspections, walk-throughs and code reading.

The software development process now moves into the detailed design stage.

16.11   DESIGN TECHNIQUES

Good software design practice is more than a matter of applying one of the latest design methodologies. Thorough requirement generation, requirements tracking, requirements analysis, performance predictability, system simulation, and uniform design reviewing are all activities which contribute to the development of safe and effective software designs.

16.12   PERFORMANCE PREDICTABILITY AND DESIGN   SIMULATION

A key activity of design often overlooked by some software developers is the effort to predict the real-time performance of a system. During the integration phase, software designers often spend countless hours trying to finely tune a system which had bottlenecks "designed in." Execution estimates for the system interfaces, response times for external devices, algorithm execution times, operating system context switch time, and I/O device access times in the forefront of the design process provide essential input into software design specifications.

For single processor designs, mathematical modeling techniques such as Rate Monotonic Analysis (RMA) should be applied to assure all required operations of that processing unit can be performed in the expected time period. System designers often fall into the trap of selecting processors before the software design has been considered, only to experience major disappoint-ment and "finger pointing" when the product is released. It is imperative to a successful project that the processor selection comes after a processor loading study is complete.

In a multi-processor application, up-front system performance analysis is equally important. System anomalies can be very difficult to diagnose and resolve in multi-processor systems with heavy inter-processor communications and functional expectations. Performance shortcomings which appear to be the fault of one processor are often the result of a landslide of smaller inadequacies from one or more of the other processors or subsystems. Person-years of integration phase defect resolution can be eliminated by front-end system design analysis and/or design simulation. Commercial tools are readily available to help perform network and multi-processor communica-tions analysis and execution simulation. Considering the pyramid of effort needed in software design, defect correction in the forefront of design yields enormous cost savings and increased reliability in the end.

16.13   MODULE SPECIFICATIONS

The lowest level of software design is typically referred to as module specifications or "mspecs." A complete set of mspecs details the actual definitions for the routine names, interfaces (inputs and outputs) of the routines, resident data structures, and "pseudocode" for each routine. The pseudocode for each routine should explicitly detail the flow of logic through the routine, including the lowest level algorithms, decision branches, and usage of data structures. Module specifications are generated for both structured designs and object-oriented designs and usually become part of the documentation associated with the source code as routine header information. Accurate mspecs are an essential part of all software design, regardless of toolset and methodology selection. This is especially true when the mspec designer and the coder are not the same person.

16.14   CODING

For many years the term "software development" was synonymous with coding. Today, for many software development groups, coding is now one of the shortest phases of software development. In fact, in some cases, although very rare in a world of real-time embedded software development, coding is actually done automatically from higher level design (mspecs) documentation by automated tools called "code generators."

With or without automatic code generators, the effectiveness of the coding stage is dependent on the quality and completeness of the design documentation generated in the immediately preceding software development phase. The coding process should be a simple transition from the module specifications, and, in particular, the pseudocode. Complete mspecs and properly developed pseudocode leaves little to interpretation for the coding phase, thus reducing the chance of error.

The importance of coding style (how it looks) is not as great as the rules which facilitate comprehension of the logical flow (how it relates). In the same light, in-line code documentation (comments) should most often address "why" rather than "how" functionality is implemented. These two focuses help the code reader understand the context in which a given segment of code is used. With precious few exceptions (e.g., high-performance device drivers) quality source code should be recognized by its readability, and not by its raw size (number of lines) or its ability to take advantage of processor features.

16.15   DESIGN SUPPORT TOOLS

Software development is very labor intensive and is, therefore, prone to human error. In recent years, commercial software development support packages have become increasingly more powerful, less expensive, and readily available to reduce the time spent doing things that computers do better than people. Although selection of the right tools can mean up-front dedication of some of the most talented resources in a development team, it can bring about significant long-term increase in group productivity.

Good software development houses have taken advantage of CASE tools, which reduce the time spent generating clear and thorough design documentation. There are many advantages of automated software design packages. Formal documentation can be used as proof of product development procedure conformance for agency approvals. Clear and up-to-date design documents facilitate improved communications between engineers, leading to more effective and reliable designs. Standard documentation formats reduce learning curves associated with unique design depictions among software designers, leading to better and more timely design formulation. Total software life-cycle costs are reduced, especially during maintenance, due to reduced ramp-up time and more efficient and reliable modifications. Finally, electronic forms of documentation can be easily backed-up and stored off-site eliminating a crisis in the event of an environmental disaster. In summary, the adaptation of CASE tools has an associated up-front cost which is recovered by significant improvements in software quality and development time predictability.

16.16 DESIGN AS THE BASIS FOR VERIFICATION AND VALIDATION ACTIVITY

Verification is the process of assuring all products of a given development phase satisfy given expectations. Prior to proceeding to the next/lower level or phase of design, the product (or outputs) of the current phase should be verified against the inputs of the previous stage. A design process cannot be a "good" process without the verification process ingrained. That is, they naturally go hand-in-hand.

Software project management plans (or software quality assurance plans) should specify all design reviews. Each level of design will generate documentation to be reviewed or deliverables to verify against the demands of the previous stage. For each type of review, the software management plans should describe the purpose, materials required, scheduling rules, scope of review, attendance expectations, review responsibilities, what the minutes should look like, follow-up activities, and any other requirements that relate to company expectations.

At the code level, code reviews should assure that the functionality implemented within a routine satisfy all expectations documented in the "mspecs." Code should also be inspected to satisfy all coding rules.

The output of good software designs also includes implementation requirements. At minimum, implementation requirements include the rules and expectations placed on the designers to assure design uniformity as well as constraints, controls and expectations placed on designs to ensure upper-level requirements are met. General examples of implementation requirements might include rules for accessing I/O ports, timing requirements for memory accesses, semaphore arbitration, inter-task communication schemes, memory addressing assignments, and sensor or device control rules. The software verification and validation process must address implementation requirements as well as the upper-level software requirements to ensure the product works according to its specifications.

16.17 CONCLUSION

Software, in and as a medical device, is subjected to a rigorous, multi-staged design process to assure it is safe, effective, and reliable for its intended use. After taking the requirements from the Software Requirements Specification, including reviewing current standards and regulations for appropriate requirements, the top-level design consists of:

- Establishing the software architecture
- Choosing a methodology and a language
- Estimating the potential risks the software might produce
- Defining appropriate metrics to evaluate the design
- Checking for design completeness by use of a requirements traceability matrix
- Conducting various types of software reviews at appropriate times throughout the process

The detailed design consists of:

- Predicting real-time performance
- Conducting design simulation
- Repairing module specifications
- Coding the design
- Using support tools where appropriate

If done properly, the design will form the basis for the next phase in the development process, verification and validation. In addition to producing a safe and effective program, this process will also help reduce coding time. In the final analysis, the patient, the user, and the developer will all benefit from implementation of this structured development process.

REFERENCES

Boehm, B.W., Industrial software metrics top 10 list, *IEEE Software*, 4(9), p. 84–85, September, 1987.

Boehm, B.W., A spiral medel of software development and enhancement, *Computer*, May, 1988.

Boehm, B.W., *Software Risk Management*, IEEE Computer Society Press, Washington, DC, 1989.

Evans, M.W. and Marciniak, J.J., *Software Quality Assurance & Management*, John Wiley & Sons, Inc., New York, 1987.

Fagan, M.E., Design and code inspections to reduce errors in program development, *IBM Systems Journal*, 15(3), p. 182–211.

Fairley, R.E., *Software Engineering Concepts*, McGraw-Hill Book Company, New York, 1985.

Fries, R.C., *Reliability Assurance for Medical Devices, Equipment and Software*, Interpharm Press, Inc., Buffalo Grove, 1991.

Fries, R.C., Pienkowski, P., and Jorgens III, J., Safe, effective, and reliable software design and development for medical devices, *Medical Instrumentation*, 30(2), March/April, 1996.

Fries, R.C., *Reliable Design of Medical Devices*, Marcel-Dekker, Inc., New York, 1997.

Fries, R.C., *Handbook of Medical Device Design*, Marcel-Dekker, Inc., New York, 2001.

Heathfield, H., Armstrong, J., and Kirkham, N., Object-oriented design and programming in medical decision support, *Computer Methods and Programs in Biomedicine*, 36(4), December, 1991.

IEEE, *IEEE Standards Collection – Software Engineering*, The Institute of Electrical and Electronic Engineers, Inc., New York, 1993.

Jahanian, F. and Mok, A.K., Safety analysis of timing properties in real time systems, *IEEE Transactions on Software Engineering*, SE-12(9), September, 1986.

Keller, M. and Shumate, K., *Software Specification and Design – A Disciplined Approach for Real-Time Systems*, John Wiley & Sons, Inc., New York, 1992.

King, P.H. and Fries, R.C., *Design of Biomedical Devices and Systems*, Marcel-Dekker, Inc., New York, 2002.

Leveson, N.G., Software safety: why, what, and how, *Computing Surveys*, 18(2), June, 1986.

Lincoln, T.L., Programming languages, *Clinics in Laboratory Medicine*, 11(1), March, 1991.

McCabe, T., A complexity measure, *IEEE Transactions of Software Engineering*, SE-2(4), December, 1976.

McConnell, S., *Code Complete*, Microsoft Press, Redmond, Washington, 1993.

Möller, K.H. and Paulish, D.J., *Software Metrics – A Practitioner's Guide to Improved Product Development*, Chapman & Hall Computing, London, 1993.

Myers, G.J., *The Art of Software Testing*, John Wiley and Sons, New York, 1979.

Pressman, R., *Software Engineering – A Practitioner's Approach*, McGraw-Hill Book Company, New York, 2005.

Yourdon, E., *Modern Structured Analysis*, Yourdon Press, Englewood Cliffs, New Jersey, 1989.

Yourdan, E., *Structured Walkthroughs*, Yourdon Press, New York, 1989.

17 Software coding

CONTENTS

17.1 Structured coding techniques 276
17.2 Single-entry, single-exit constructs 276
17.3 Good coding practices... 277
    17.3.1 Review every line of code............................. 277
    17.3.2 Require coding sign-offs............................... 278
    17.3.3 Route good code examples for review.................. 278
    17.3.4 Emphasize that code listings are public assets 278
    17.3.5 Reward good code..................................... 278
    17.3.6 One easy standard.................................... 279
17.4 The coding process... 279
    17.4.1 Start with a PDL...................................... 279
    17.4.2 Writing the routine declaration 279
    17.4.3 Turning the PDL into high level comments 279
    17.4.4 Fill in the code below each comment.................... 281
    17.4.5 Check the code informally 281
    17.4.6 Clean up the leftovers 281
    17.4.7 Check the code formally............................... 282
17.5 Implementation checklist 282
References 282

The implementation phase of software development is concerned with translating design specifications into source code. The primary goal of implementation is to write source code and internal documentation so that conformance of the code to its specification can be easily verified, and so that debugging, testing, and modifications are eased. This goal can be achieved by making the source code as clear and straightforward as possible. Simplicity, clarity, and elegance are the hallmark of good programs. Obscurity, cleverness, and complexity are indications of inadequate design and misdirected thinking.

Source code clarity is enhanced by structured coding techniques, by good coding style, by appropriate supporting documents, by good internal comments, and by the features provided in modern programming languages.

17.1   STRUCTURED CODING TECHNIQUES

The goal of structured coding is to linearize control flow through a computer program so that the execution sequence follows the sequence in which the code is written. The dynamic structure of a program as it executes then resembles the state structure of the written text. This enhances readability of code, which eases understanding, debugging, testing, documentation, and modification of programs. It also facilitates formal verification of programs. Linear flow of control can be achieved by restricting the set of allowed program constructs to single-entry, single-exit formats. However, strict adherence to nested, single-entry, single-exit constructs leads to questions concerning efficiency, questions about reasonable violations of single-entry, single-exit, and questions about the proper role of the GOTO statement in structured coding.

17.2   SINGLE-ENTRY, SINGLE-EXIT CONSTRUCTS

In 1966, Bohm and Jacopini published a paper in which they demonstrated that sequencing, selection among alternative actions, and iteration are a sufficient set of constructs for describing the control flow of every conceivable algorithm. They argued that every Turing machine program can be written in this manner. Because the Turing machine is the fundamental model of computation, it follows that every algorithm can be written using sequencing, selection, and iteration.

A modified version of the Bohm-Jacopini theorem can be stated as follows:

> Any single-entry, single-exit program segment that has all statements on some path from the entry to the exit can be using only sequencing, selection, and iteration.

A sufficient set of single-entry, single-exit constructs for specifying control flow in algorithms is:

- Sequencing: S1; S2; S3
- Selection: IF B THEN S1 ELSE S2
- Iteration: WHILE B DO S

The single-entry, single-exit nature of these constructs is illustrated in Figure 17-1.

The single-entry, single-exit property permits nesting of constructs within one another in any desired fashion. Each statement Si might be an assignment statement, a procedure call, an IF...THEN...ELSE, or a WHILE...DO. Statements of the latter forms may in turn contain nested statements. The most important aspect of the single-entry, single-exit property is that linearity of control flow is retained, even with arbitrarily deep nesting of constructs. The set of structured constructs selected for use in any particular application is primarily a matter of notational convenience. However,

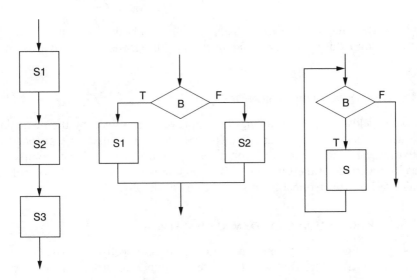

FIGURE 17-1 Single-entry, Single-exit constructs

the selected constructs should be conceptually simple and widely applicable in practice.

17.3 GOOD CODING PRACTICES

Since coding is the primary output of software construction, a key question in managing construction is "How does one encourage good coding practices?" In general, mandating a strict set of standards from the top is not a good idea. Programmers tend to view managers as being at a lower level of technical evolution and if there are going to be programming standards, programmers need to buy into them.

Standards should not be imposed at all, if they can be avoided. In contrast, flexible guidelines, a collection of suggestions rather than guidelines or a set of examples that embody the best practices may be an alternative to standards. The following are several techniques for achieving good coding practices, techniques that are not as heavy-handed as laying down rigid coding standards.

17.3.1 REVIEW EVERY LINE OF CODE

A code review typically involves the programmer and at least two reviewers. That means that at least three people read every line of code. Another name for peer review is "peer pressure." In addition to providing a safety net in case the original programmer leaves the project, reviews improve code quality because the programmer knows that the code will be read by others. Even if your shop hasn't created explicit coding standards, reviews provide a subtle way of moving toward a group coding standard – decisions are made by the group during reviews and over time the group will derive its own standards.

17.3.2 REQUIRE CODING SIGN-OFFS

In other fields, technical drawings are approved and signed by the managing engineer. The signature means that, to the best of the engineer's knowledge, the drawings are technically competent and error-free. Some companies treat software code the same way. Before code is considered to be complete, senior technical personnel must sign the code listing.

17.3.3 ROUTE GOOD CODE EXAMPLES FOR REVIEW

A big part of good management is communicating objectives clearly. One way to communicate objectives is to circulate good code to programmers or post it for public display. In doing so, you provide a clear example of the quality you're aiming for. Similarly, a coding standards manual can consist mainly of a set of "best code listings." Identifying certain listings as "best" sets an example for others to follow. Such a manual is easier to update than an English-language standards manual and effortlessly presents subtleties in coding style that are hard to capture point by point in prose descriptions.

17.3.4 EMPHASIZE THAT CODE LISTINGS ARE PUBLIC ASSETS

Programmers sometimes feel that the code they've written is "their code," as if it were private property. Although it is the result of their work, code is part of the project and should be freely available to anyone else on the project who needs it. It should be seen by others during reviews and maintenance, even if at no other time.

17.3.5 REWARD GOOD CODE

Use your organization's reward system to reinforce good coding practices. Keep these considerations in mind as you develop your reinforcement system:

- The reward should be something the programmer wants. Many programmers find "attaboy" rewards distasteful, especially when they come from non-technical managers
- Code that receives an award should be exceptionally good. If you give an award to a programmer everyone else knows does bad work, you look foolish. It doesn't matter that the programmer has a cooperative attitude or always comes to work on time. You lose credibility if your reward doesn't match the technical merits of the situation

17.3.6 ONE EASY STANDARD

If you are managing a programming project and you have a programming background, an easy and effective technique for eliciting good work is to say "I must be able to read and understand any code written for the project." This may discourage clever or tricky code.

17.4 THE CODING PROCESS

Once the problem has been defined, the requirements listed, the architecture and language selected, the program is ready to be implemented. Implementation (Figure 17-2) can be accomplished in a nearly standard order, although the steps may vary depending on the program to be written.

17.4.1 START WITH A PDL

Program Design Language (PDL) resembles English. However, it does not necessarily follow that any English-like description that collects one's thoughts will have roughly the same effect as any other. To use PDL effectively:

- Use English-like statements that precisely describe specific operations
- Avoid syntactic elements from the target programming language
- Write PDL at the level of intent
- Write PDL at a low enough level that generating code from it will be nearly automatic

Figure 17-3 is an example of Program Design Language.

17.4.2 WRITING THE ROUTINE DECLARATION

Write the routine interface statement. Turn the original header comment into a programming-language comment. Leave it in position above the PDL you've already written. This is a good time to make notes about any interface assumptions.

17.4.3 TURNING THE PDL INTO HIGH LEVEL
COMMENTS

Write the first and last statements. Then turn the PDL into comments. At this point, the character of the routine is evident. The design work is complete and one can sense how the routine works even without seeing any code. Converting the PDL into programming-language code should feel mechanical, natural, and easy. If not, continue designing in PDL until the design feels solid.

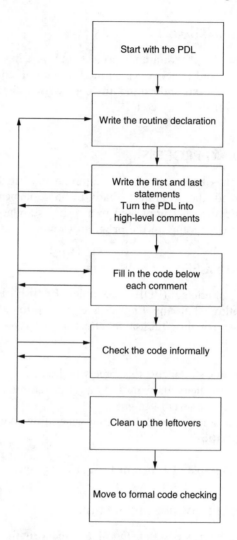

FIGURE 17-2 Coding implementation process

Keep track of current number of resources in use
If another resource is available
    Allocate a dialog box structure
    If a dialog box structure could be allocated
    Note that one more resource is in use
        Initialize the resource
        Store the resource number at the location provided by the caller
    Endif
Endif
Return TRUE if a new resource was created; else return FALSE

FIGURE 17-3 Sample program design language

17.4.4 FILL IN THE CODE BELOW EACH COMMENT

Fill in the code below each line of the PDL comment. This requires an outline, then a paragraph for each point in the outline. Each PDL comment describes a block or paragraph of code. Like the lengths of literary paragraphs, the lengths of code paragraphs vary according to the thought being expressed. The quality of the paragraphs depends on the vividness and focus of the thoughts in them. This is the start on the code.

Each comment has given rise to one or more lines of code. Each block of code forms a complete thought based on the comment. The comments have been retained to provide a higher-level explanation of the code. All the variables that have been used have been declared at the top of the routine.

17.4.5 CHECK THE CODE INFORMALLY

Mentally test each block of code as it is filled in below its comment. Think of what it would take to break that block, and then prove that it won't happen. Once the routine is implemented, check it for mistakes. Sometimes an important problem does not appear until the routine is implemented.

A problem might not appear until coding for several reasons. An error in the PDL might become more apparent in the detailed implementation logic. A design that looks elegant in PDL might become clumsy in the implementation language. Working with the detailed implementation might disclose an error in the architecture or the requirements analysis. Additionally, the code might have a coding error. For all these reasons, the code should be checked before moving to the next step.

17.4.6 CLEAN UP THE LEFTOVERS

When the code has been checked for problems, it should be checked for general characteristics including:

- Ensuring that all input and output data are accounted for
- Ensuring the routine does one thing and does it well, that it is loosely coupled to other routines, and is designed defensively
- Checking for inaccurate variable names, unused data, and undeclared data
- Checking for off-by-one errors, infinite loops, and improper nesting
- Ensuring white space has been used to clarify the logical structure of the routine, expressions, and parameter lists
- Ensuring the PDL that was translated into comments is still accurate. Check for algorithm descriptions, for documentation on interface assumptions and non-obvious dependencies, and for justification of unclear coding practices

17.4.7 CHECK THE CODE FORMALLY

After designing and implementing the routine, the next step is checking to be sure that what you've constructed is correct. Activity includes:

- Mentally checking the routine for errors
- Compiling the routine
- Using the computer to check the routine for errors
- Removal of errors from the routine

Remember, any errors that are missed at this stage will not be found until later testing. They are more expensive to find and correct then, so due diligence should be employed here.

17.5 IMPLEMENTATION CHECKLIST

After implementing the design, review these points to assure the implementation is robust and error resistant:

- Compare the implementation to the design. The design should be accurately implemented. Minor differences between the design and the implementation can cause problems
- Ensure no unnecessary assumptions have been made in the code. Check for any arbitrary aspect of the implementation
- Examine the expressions in the code for overflow or underflow. Variables should be checked as well
- Check for nested operators or other risky language idioms. Rewrite risky expressions using comparable, yet safer expressions
- Ensure the code does not contain arcane language that the average programmer would not understand
- Although each function may perform a single task, assure the task is implemented using a single code path. Avoid achieving a task using different code to implement various special codes
- Assure all memory that is referenced is memory that can be accessed
- Check to determine if the code restricts the references to pointers to inputs and outputs to only the memory required to hold those inputs and outputs
- Adding assertions and other debugging code to the implementations can reduce the time required to find any bugs hiding in the code.

REFERENCES

Bohm, C. and Jacopini, G., Flow diagrams, turing machines, and languages with only two formation rules, *Communications of the ACM*, 9(5), May, 1966.
Fairley, R.E., *Software Engineering Concepts*, McGraw-Hill Book Company, New York, 1985.

Fries, R.C., *Reliable Design of Medical Devices*, Marcel-Dekker, Inc., New York, 1997.

Fries, R.C., *Handbook of Medical Device Design*, Marcel-Dekker, Inc., New York, 2001.

King, P.H. and Fries, R.C., *Design of Biomedical Devices and Systems*, Marcel Dekker, Inc., New York, 2002.

Maguire, S.A., *Writing Solid Code: Microsoft's Techniques for Developing But-Free C Programs*, Microsoft Press, Redmond, WA, 1993.

McConnell, S.C., *Code Complete: A Practical Handbook of Software Construction*, Microsoft Press, Redmond, WA, 1993.

18 Establishing and using metrics

CONTENTS

18.1   Software metrics 286
18.2   Software complexity metrics..................................... 288
18.3   Objective and algorithmic measurements......................... 288
18.4   Process and product metrics.................................... 289
18.5   Meta-metrics... 289
18.6   Size metrics 290
      18.6.1   Lines of code... 290
      18.6.2   Token count 290
      18.6.3   Function count.. 291
18.7   McCabe's complexity.. 292
18.8   Halstead measures 293
      18.8.1   Vocabulary of the software 293
      18.8.2   Length of the program 294
      18.8.3   Volume of the software................................ 294
      18.8.4   The potential volume.................................. 294
      18.8.5   The program level..................................... 294
      18.8.6   Effort 294
18.9   Other metrics 295
18.10   Computer-aided metrics 295
18.11   Software metrics methodology................................... 295
      18.11.1   Establish software quality requirements............... 295
      18.11.2   Identify software quality metrics..................... 296
      18.11.3   Implement the software quality metrics 296
      18.11.4   Analyze the software quality metrics results.......... 296
      18.11.5   Validate the software quality metrics 296
18.12   Establish software quality requirements........................ 296
18.13   Identify a list of possible quality requirements 297
References 297

The field of software metrics is not a new phenomenon. Software metrics have been developed and used for some time. Many metrics and methods to measure software complexity have been proposed and explored. This activity has led to and been fueled by interest in software development models. Many of the proposed metrics can be measured objectively, but some can only be determined subjectively. Many models of the programming process have been constructed using various supposedly relevant factors that pertain to software size and complexity, programmer experience, and the program development procedure.

18.1   SOFTWARE METRICS

Software must be subjected to measurement in order to achieve a true indication of quality and reliability. Quality attributes must be related to specific product requirements and must be quantifiable. This is accomplished through the use of metrics.

Software quality metrics are defined as quantitative measures of an attribute that describes the quality of a software product or process. Using metrics for improving software quality, performance, and productivity begins with a documented software development process which will be incrementally improved over time. Goals are established with respect to the desired extent of quality and productivity improvements over a specified time period. These goals are derived from and are consistent with the strategic goals for the business enterprise.

Metrics must be selected that are useful to the specific objectives of the program, have been derived from the program requirements, and support the evaluation of the software consistent with the specified requirements. To develop accurate estimates, a historical baseline must be established consisting of data collected from previous software projects. The data collected should be reasonably accurate, collected from as many projects as possible, consistent, and representative of applications that are similar to work that is to be estimated. Once the data have been collected, metric computation is possible.

Metrics are then defined that can be used to measure periodic progress in achieving the improvement goals. The metric data collected can be used as an indicator of development process problem areas, and improvement actions identified. These actions can be compared and analyzed with respect to the best return-on-investment for the business. The measurement data provides information for investing wisely in tools for quality and productivity improvement.

There are six primary uses of metrics, including:

- Goal setting
- Improving quality
- Improving productivity
- Project planning
- Managing
- Improving customer confidence

Metric data are useful for establishing quantitative improvement objectives for company management, such as doubling the current development team productivity within 3 years. A metric can be used to measure the current productivity and then applied periodically to track progress until the goal is attained. If sufficient progress is not made and the goal is not achieved, additional actions and investments can be identified and implemented.

Metric data can be very useful when used in conjunction with a corporate quality improvement program. The goals of software quality improvement should be consistent with and supportive of the overall corporate quality improvement program. The software metrics should support the desired improvements for software quality.

Software metrics can also be applied to supporting a productivity improvement program in a manner similar to a quality improvement program. Direct goals and activities for improving productivity should be established.

The collection of metric data will improve over time the organization's skill in planning new projects. Metric data collected on prior projects will be available to project managers responsible for estimating complexity, schedule, required personnel resources, and budgets.

Software metrics are useful for managing and monitoring software projects. If metric data are made available to software project managers on a frequent basis, corrective actions can be made to the project plan to increase the probability of successful project completion.

A successful metrics program will ultimately result in higher-quality software system products which will in turn increase customer confidence. The metrics program is also useful for improving the confidence of internal customers, organizations within the business that depend on the output of another organization.

An initial small number of metrics should be selected to be consistent with the existing software development process and the organization/project objectives. The basic set of metrics should be of a limited number in order to maximize the visibility of each measurement. They should consist of objective and/or subjective measurements.

Objective metrics are easily quantified and measured. Examples include:

- Program size
- Effort
- Schedule
- Number of faults
- Quality costs

These basic metrics, after having been defined and implemented, can become the basis for a hierarchy of additional metrics, some of which can be calculated. One of the advantages of objective metrics is that they can often be collected more cost effectively using software tools.

Subjective metrics attempt to track less quantifiable data, such as quality attitudes. An example of a subjective metric would be the measurement of customer satisfaction. Data for subjective metrics would often be collected through interviews or surveys.

A feedback mechanism must be implemented so that the metrics data can provide guidance for identifying actions to improve the software development process. Continuous improvements to the software development process result in higher-quality products and increased development team productivity. The process improvement actions must be managed and controlled so as to achieve dynamic process improvement over time.

18.2   SOFTWARE COMPLEXITY METRICS

The term complexity appears so often and in so many different contexts in software engineering that it may be useful to discuss its various connotations. In theoretical circles, it is common to classify algorithms as to their computational complexity, which means the efficiency of the algorithm in its use of machine resources. On the other hand, the perceived complexity of software is often called psychological complexity because it is concerned with characteristics of the software that affect programmer performance in composing, comprehending, and modifying the software.

A definition of complexity would be:

> Complexity is a characteristic of the software interface which influences the resources another system will expend or commit while interacting with the software.

This definition implies that complexity is a function of both the software itself and its interactions with other systems. The word system in this context includes machines, people, and other software. This abstract definition of complexity can be made operational by defining and quantifying specific software metrics that are relevant to the phenomenon under study. When these operational metrics are further combined according to some hypothesis or theory, the result is a software complexity mode.

Specific types of complexity that have been considered include problem complexity, design complexity, as well as program or product complexity. For each of these complexity types, an appropriate metric accurately reflects the "difficulty" that a programmer or analyst encounters in performing such tasks as designing, coding, testing, or maintaining the software system.

18.3   OBJECTIVE AND ALGORITHMIC
MEASUREMENTS

An objective or algorithmic measurement is one that can be computed precisely according to an algorithm. Its value does not change due to changes in time, place, or observer. In theory, there should be no question of the replicability of an objective measurement. An algorithm should not change over time or among several observers. Any observer at any time should assign the same value to the same metric. Thus, software metrics that can be measured objectively should be comparable among several studies that allow the combination of data for research and analysis purposes. Furthermore, the algorithms for measurement may be included in software analyzers that compute objective metrics so that little human time is needed to obtain these values.

18.4   PROCESS AND PRODUCT METRICS

Process metrics quantify attributes of the development process and of the development environment. Process metrics include resource metrics, such as the experience of programmers, and the cost of development and maintenance. Examples of metrics for the levels of personnel experience are the number of years that a team has been using a programming language, the number of years that a programmer has been with the organization, the number of years that a programmer has been associated with a programming team, and the number of years of experience constructing similar software. Other factors related to development include such items as development techniques, programming aids, supervisory techniques, and resources. In many cases, the value of a particular technique could be either 0 or 1, representing the absence or presence of a particular technique or process.

Product metrics are measures of the software product. Note that they may reveal nothing about how the software has evolved into its current state. Product metrics include the size of the product, the logic structure complexity, the data structure complexity, the function, and combinations of these.

It may be difficult to classify certain metrics as either process- or product-related. For example, the number of defects discovered during formal testing depends both on the product and on the process used in the testing phase. In general, it is possible for a product metric to be influenced by the process used, and vice versa. A metric should be classified according to the factor that is believed to provide the major influence.

18.5   META-METRICS

Just as a meta-language is used to describe a language, a meta-metric is a measure of a software metric. It has already been stated that a useful metric should be measured objectively and algorithmically. The following are some meta-metrics that can be used to evaluate a proposed metric:

- Simplicity – does the metric lead to a simple result that is easily interpreted?
- Validity – does the metric measure what it purports to measure?
- Robustness – is the metric sensitive to the artificial manipulation of some factors that do not affect the performance of the software?
- Prescriptiveness – can the metric be used to guide the management of software development or maintenance?
- Analyzability – can the value of the metric be analyzed using standard statistical tools?

The goal is metrics that are simple, valid, robust, useful for development, and that can be analyzed properly.

18.6   SIZE METRICS

The size of a computer program used to be easily determined by the number of punched cards it took to contain the program. This metric, which was almost a weight measure for people who had to carry their programs to and from the computing center, is roughly equivalent to the lines of code metric that survives to this day. There are many possibilities for representing the size of a program, including the amount of memory required to contain the compiled version of it.

The size of a program is an important measure for several reasons:

- It is easy to compute after the program is completed
- It is the most important factor for many models of software development
- Productivity is normally based on a size measure

18.6.1   LINES OF CODE

The most familiar software measure is the count of the lines of code. It is represented by the symbol S_s, and the whole unit is LOC. For large programs it is appropriate to measure the size in thousands of lines of code (KLOC), which is represented by S. Although this may seem to be a simple metric that can be counted algorithmically, there is no general agreement about what constitutes a line of code. For example, are comments and bland lines included in the count? To do so may encourage programmers to introduce artificially many such lines in project development in order to create the illusion of high productivity. Furthermore, if the main interest is the size of the program that supports a certain function, it may be reasonable to include only executable statements. In addition, the advantages of programming languages that permit free-format coding create yet another problem. These languages often allow compounding with two or more statements on one line. To solve this dilemma, a definition of a line of code is required.

A line of code is any line of program text that is not a comment or blank line, regardless of the number of statements or fragments of statements on the line. This specifically includes all lines containing program headers, declarations, and executable and non-executable statements. This is the predominant definition for line of code used today by researchers.

18.6.2   TOKEN COUNT

As discussed above, a major problem with the S_s measure is that it is not consistent because some lines are more difficult to code than others. One solution to this problem is to give more weight to lines that have more detail in them. A natural weighting scheme to handle this problem is to use the number of "tokens," which are basic syntactic units distinguishable by a compiler. Halstead used this notion in calculating his metrics.

A computer program is considered to be a collection of tokens that can be classified as either operators or operands. The basic metrics are defined as:

- $\eta_1 =$ the number of unique operators
- $\eta_2 =$ the number of unique operands
- $N_1 =$ the total occurrences of operators
- $N_2 =$ total occurrences of operands

Generally, any symbol or keyword in a program that specifies an action is considered an operator, while a symbol used to represent data is considered an operand. Most punctuation marks are also considered as operators. Variables, constants, and even labels are operands. Operators consist of arithmetic symbols, command names, special symbols and even function names.

The size of a program in terms of the total number of tokens used is:

$$N = N_1 + N_2$$

Other metrics using these basic terms are vocabulary:

$$\eta = \eta_1 + \eta_2$$

Vocabulary accentuates the fact that, if you have a programming vocabulary consisting of only these η operators and operands, you could successfully construct this program. From a programmer's large vocabulary of operators and operands, these η have been chosen as the set to be used in writing this program.

Another measure is called the volume:

$$V = N(\log_2 \eta)$$

The unit of measurement of volume is the bit, the common unit for measuring the actual size of a program in a computer if a uniform binary encoding for the vocabulary is used.

18.6.3 FUNCTION COUNT

For large programs, it may be easier to predict the number of modules than the number of lines of code. However, unless there are strict guidelines about the way a program is divided into modules, this metric may give us little information.

A function in a program is defined as a collection of executable statements that performs a certain task, together with declarations of the formal parameters and local variables manipulated by those statements. A function is an abstraction of part of the tasks that the program is to perform. This idea is based on the observation that a programmer may think in terms of building a program from functions, rather than from statements or even modules.

The number of lines of code for any function will usually not be very large. One reason for this observation may be the limit on the human mental capacity. A programmer cannot manipulate information efficiently when the amount is much greater than that value.

18.7   McCABE'S COMPLEXITY

McCabe's metric is based on the complexity of the flow-of-control in the system. Suppose we could depict a software system as a directed graph, or graphs, where each block of sequential code represents a node, and each synchronous change in flow-of-control is depicted as a directed arc or edge.

In a multi-tasking or multi-processing system, each separate task would be represented by a separate flow graph. These graphs could be determined directly from the flow charts, dataflow diagrams, Petri nets, or finite state automata used to model the system.

The cyclomatic complexity would then be represented by:

$$C = e - n + 2p \tag{18.1}$$

where
C = the complexity number
e = the number of edges in the program
n = the number of nodes
p = the number of separate tasks

As an example, consider the software flow graph in Figure 18.1. Thus:

$$e = 4$$
$$n = 4$$
$$p = 1$$

Thus equation 18.1 becomes:

$$\begin{aligned} C &= e - n + 2p \\ &= 3 - 4 - 2(1) \\ &= 1 \end{aligned}$$

The higher the complexity of the software module, as indicated by C, the more difficult it will be to build, test, and maintain and the lower the reliability. In this case, $C = 1$. A high reliability can thus be expected.

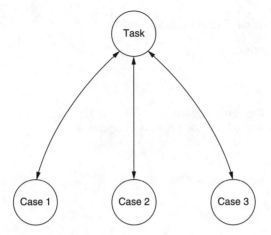

FIGURE 18.1 Software flow graph

Although the McCabe's metric provides some non-abstract measure of system reliability, it cannot depict asynchronous changes in flow-of-control, and thus has limited utility in real-time systems.

18.8 HALSTEAD MEASURES

These metrics provide a measure of the quality of the software development process by accounting for two factors, the number of distinct operators (instruction types) and the number of distinct operands (variables and constraints). Halstead defines a number of characteristics that can be quantified about the software and then relates these in different ways to describe the various aspects of the software. Such measures are:

- Vocabulary of the software
- Length of the program
- Volume of the software
- The potential volume
- The program level
- The effort

18.8.1 VOCABULARY OF THE SOFTWARE

This metric is defined as:

$$n = n1 + n2 \tag{18.2}$$

where
$n1$ = the number of distinct operators
$n2$ = the number of distinct operands

18.8.2 LENGTH OF THE PROGRAM

This metric is defined as:

$$N = N1 + N2 \tag{18.3}$$

where
$N1 =$ the total number of occurrences of operators
$N2 =$ the total number of occurrences of operands

18.8.3 VOLUME OF THE SOFTWARE

This metric is defined as:

$$V = N \log_2 n \tag{18.4}$$

where
$N =$ length of the program
$n =$ vocabulary of the software

V represents the volume of information required to specify a program and will vary with the programming language.

18.8.4 THE POTENTIAL VOLUME

This metric is defined as:

$$V^* = (2 + n2)(\log 2(2 + n2)) \tag{18.5}$$

18.8.5 THE PROGRAM LEVEL

This metric is defined as:

$$L = V^*/V$$

L is an attempt to measure the level of abstraction of the program. It is believed that increasing this number will increase system reliability.

18.8.6 EFFORT

This metric is defined as:

$$E = V/L$$

E is an attempt to measure the amount of mental effort required in the development of the code. Decreasing the effort level is believed to increase reliability as well as ease of implementation.

18.9   OTHER METRICS

Other metric techniques have been developed that measure the total process of the software development through a complete set of attribute descriptors, including:

- Complexity
- Correctness
- Efficiency
- Flexibility
- Integrity
- Interoperability
- Maintainability
- Portability
- Testability
- Usability

18.10   COMPUTER-AIDED METRICS

There are programs available that will analyze a software program by module and produce metric measurements. These measurements include call graphs, Kiviat diagrams of metric measurements, and module maps indicating the number of entrances, exits, and statement types within a module. These graphic measurements are particularly useful in reviewing revision level changes to the software and their effect on each module.

18.11   SOFTWARE METRICS METHODOLOGY

The software metrics methodology is a systematic approach to establishing quality requirements and identifying, implementing, and analyzing product software quality metrics. The methodology consists of the following steps, which are applied iteratively because insight gained from applying one step may show the need for further evaluation of the results of prior steps. The methodology includes the following.

18.11.1   ESTABLISH SOFTWARE QUALITY REQUIREMENTS

A list of quality factors is selected, prioritized, and quantified at the outset of system development or system change. These requirements shall be used to guide and control the development of the system and, on delivery of the system, to assess whether the system met the quality requirements specified in the contract.

Documentation produced:

- Quality requirements

18.11.2 IDENTIFY SOFTWARE QUALITY METRICS

The software quality metrics framework is applied in the selection of relevant metrics.
Documentation produced:

- Approved quality metrics framework
- Metrics set
- Cost–benefit analysis

18.11.3 IMPLEMENT THE SOFTWARE QUALITY METRICS

Tools are procured or developed, data are collected, and metrics are applied at each phase of the software life cycle.
Documentation produced:

- Description of data items
- Metrics/data item
- Traceability matrix
- Training plan and schedule

18.11.4 ANALYZE THE SOFTWARE QUALITY METRICS RESULTS

The metrics results are analyzed and reported to help control the development and assess the final product.
Documentation produced:

- Organization and development process changes

18.11.5 VALIDATE THE SOFTWARE QUALITY METRICS

Predictive metrics results are compared to the direct metrics results to determine whether the predictive metrics accurately "measure" their associated factors.
Documentation produced:

- Validation results

18.12 ESTABLISH SOFTWARE QUALITY REQUIREMENTS

Quality requirements are usually represented in either of the following ways:

- Direct metric value – a numerical target for a factor to be met in the final product

- Predictive metric value – a numerical target related to a factor to be met during system development

18.13 IDENTIFY A LIST OF POSSIBLE QUALITY REQUIREMENTS

Identifies quality requirements that may be applicable to the software system. In addition, list other general requirements that may affect.

REFERENCES

Buckley, F.J., *Implementing Configuration Management: Hardware, Software, and Firmware*, The Institute of Electrical and Electronics Engineers, Inc., New York, 1993.

Conte, S.D., Dunsmore, H.E., and Shen, V.Y., *Software Engineering Metrics and Models*, The Benjamin/Cummings Publishing Company, Inc., Menlo Park, CA, 1986.

Fries, R.C., *Reliability Assurance for Medical Devices, Equipment and Software*, Interpharm Press Inc., Buffalo Grove, IL, 1991.

Fries, R.C., *Reliable Design of Medical Devices*, Marcel-Dekker, Inc., New York, 1997.

Fries, R.C., *Handbook of Medical Device Design*, Marcel-Dekker, Inc., New York, 2001.

Halstead, M.H., *Elements of Software Science*, Elsevier, New York, 1977.

Institute of Electrical and Electronic Engineers, *IEEE Standard 1045: IEEE Standard for Software Productivity Metrics*, The Institute of Electrical and Electronic Engineers, Inc., New York, 1992.

Institute of Electrical and Electronic Engineers, *IEEE Standard 1061: Standard for a Software Quality Metrics Methodology*, The Institute of Electrical and Electronic Engineers, Inc., New York, 1992.

King, P.H. and Fries, R.C., *Design of Biomedical Devices and Systems*, Marcel-Dekker, Inc., New York, 2002.

Laplante, P., *Real-Time Systems Design and Analysis: An Engineer's Handbook*, The Institute of Electrical and Electronic Engineers, Inc., New York, 1993.

McCabe, T., A complexity measure, *IEEE Transactions of Software Engineering*, SE-2(4), December, 1976.

Möller, K.H. and Paulish, D.J., *Software Metrics: A Practitioner's Guide to Improved Product Development*, Chapman & Hall Computing, London, 1993.

Pressman, R.S., *Software Engineering: A Practitioner's Approach*, McGraw-Hill Book Company, New York, 1982.

19 Human factors

CONTENTS

19.1   What are human factors?...................................... 300
19.2   The human element in human factors engineering............... 301
19.3   The hardware element in human factors 302
19.4   The software element in human factors 304
19.5   The human factors process 307
19.6   Planning 307
19.7   Analysis 307
19.8   Conduct user studies 308
    19.8.1   Observations 308
    19.8.2   Interviews 308
    19.8.3   Focus groups.. 309
    19.8.4   Task analysis.. 309
    19.8.5   Benchmark usability test.............................. 310
    19.8.6   Write user profile..................................... 310
    19.8.7   Set up an advisory panel 310
19.9   Set usability goals 310
19.10   Design user interface concepts............................... 311
    19.10.1   Develop conceptual model............................. 311
    19.10.2   Develop user interface structure 311
    19.10.3   Define interaction style.............................. 312
    19.10.4   Develop screen templates............................. 312
    19.10.5   Develop hardware layout.............................. 312
    19.10.6   Develop a screenplay................................. 312
    19.10.7   Develop a refined design 312
    19.10.8   Develop a final design............................... 312
19.11   Model the user interface..................................... 313
19.12   Test the user interface 313
19.13   Specify the user interface 314
    19.13.1   Style guide 314
    19.13.2   Screen hierarchy map 314
    19.13.3   Screenplay 314
    19.13.4   Specification prototype............................... 314
    19.13.5   Hardware layouts 315
19.14   Additional human factors design considerations 315
    19.14.1   Consistency and simplicity........................... 315

19.14.2   Safety.. 315
19.14.3   Environmental/organizational considerations.......... 316
19.14.4   Documentation...................................... 316
19.14.5   Anthropometry...................................... 317
19.14.6   Functional dimensions 317
19.14.7   Psychological elements 319
19.14.8   Workstation design considerations.................... 320
19.14.9   Alarms and signals 320
19.14.10   Labeling 323
19.14.11   Software 324
19.14.12   Data entry 325
19.14.13   Displays 325
19.14.14   Interactive control................................ 327
19.14.15   Feedback 328
19.14.16   Prompts.. 328
19.14.17   Defaults... 329
19.14.18   Error management/data protection 329
References.. 329

Human factors engineering, also called ergonomics, can trace its roots to early industrial engineering studies of work efficiency and task performance using, for example, time-motion techniques. Human factors engineering emerged as a recognized discipline during the Second World War, while focusing primarily on military system performance, including problems in signal detection, workspace constraints, and optimal task training. The widespread recognition of the importance of applying human factors engineering in the design of tools, devices, tasks, and other human activities is reflected in the increasing number of disparate professionals interested in human factors. Their work products can be found in lay and professional publications, standards, and other documents. Human factors activities have improved the quality of personal and professional life across many domains. Public and professional interest in patient safety issues has promoted increased application of human factors engineering to the medical domain.

Numerous medical device companies have established human factors engineering programs to ensure the usability and safety of their devices. These companies also believe that their human factors engineering efforts enhance the marketability of their products. National and international regulations with respect to the safety of medical devices now require that human factors engineering principles be applied to the design of medical devices, and that this process be documented.

19.1 WHAT ARE HUMAN FACTORS?

Human factors is defined as the application of the scientific knowledge of human capabilities and limitations to the design of systems and equipment to produce products with the most efficient, safe, effective, and reliable operation. This definition includes several interesting concepts.

Although humans are capable of many highly technical, complex or intricate activities, they also have limitations to these activities. Of particular interest to the medical designer are limitations due to physical size, range of motion, visual perception, auditory perception, and mental capabilities under stress. Although the user may be characterized by these limitations, the designer cannot allow them to adversely affect the safety, effectiveness, or reliability of the device. The designer should therefore identify and address all possible points of interface between the user and the equipment, characterize the operating environment, and analyze the skill level of the intended users.

Interface points are defined as those areas that the user must control or maintain in order to derive the desired output from the system. Interface points include control panels, displays, operating procedures, operating instructions, and user training requirements.

The environment in which the device will be used must be characterized to determine those areas that may cause problems for the user, such as lighting, noise level, temperature, criticality of the operation, and the amount of stress the user is experiencing while operating the system. The design must then be adjusted to eliminate any potential problems.

The skill level of the user is an important parameter to be analyzed during the design process and includes such characteristics as educational background, technical expertise, and computer knowledge. To assure the user's skill levels have been successfully addressed, the product should be designed to meet the capabilities of the least-skilled potential user. Designing to meet this worst-case situation will assure the needs of the majority of the potential users will be satisfied.

The final and most important activity in human factors engineering is determining how these areas interact within the particular device. The points of interface are designed based on the anticipated operating environment and on the skill level of the user. The skill level may depend not only on the education and experience of the user, but on the operating environment as well. To design for such interaction, the designer must consider the three elements that comprise human factors: the human element, the hardware element, and the software element.

19.2   THE HUMAN ELEMENT IN HUMAN
FACTORS ENGINEERING

The human element addresses several user characteristics, including memory and knowledge presentation, thinking and reasoning, visual perception, dialogue construction, individual skill level, and individual sophistication. Each is an important factor in the design consideration.

A human being has two types of memory. Short-term memory deals with sensory input, such as visual stimuli, sounds, and sensations of touch. Long-term memory is composed of our knowledge database. If the human–machine interface makes undue demands on either short- or long-term memory, the performance of the individual in the system will be degraded. The speed of this degradation depends on the amount of data presented, the number of commands the user must remember, and/or the stress involved in the activity.

When a human performs a problem-solving activity, they usually apply a set of guidelines or strategies based on their understanding of the situation and their experiences with similar types of problems, rather than applying formal inductive or deductive reasoning techniques. The human–machine interface must be specific in a manner enabling the user to relate to their previous experiences and develop guidelines for a particular situation.

The physical and cognitive constraints associated with visual perception must be understood when designing the human–machine interface. For example, studies have shown that since the normal line of sight is within 15° of the horizontal line of sight, the optimum position for the instrument face is within a minimum of 45° of the normal line of sight (Figure 19-1). Other physical and cognitive constraints have been categorized and are available in references located at the end of this chapter.

When people communicate with one another, they communicate best when the dialogue is simple, easy to understand, direct, and to the point. The designer must assure device commands are easy to remember, error messages are simple, direct, and not cluttered with computer jargon and help messages are easy to understand and pointed. The design of dialogue should be addressed to the least-skilled potential user of the equipment.

The typical user of a medical device is not familiar with hardware design or computer programming. They are more concerned with the results obtained from using the device than about how the results were obtained. They want a system that is convenient, natural, flexible, and easy to use. They don't want a system that looks imposing, is riddled with computer jargon, requires them to memorize many commands, or has unnecessary information cluttering the display areas.

In summary, the human element requires a device which has inputs, outputs, controls, displays, and documentation that reflect an understanding of the user's education, skill, needs, experience, and the stress level when operating the equipment.

19.3   THE HARDWARE ELEMENT IN HUMAN FACTORS

The hardware element considers size limitations, the location of controls, compatibility with other equipment, the potential need for portability, and possible user training. It also addresses the height of the preferred control area and the preferred display area when the operator is standing (Figure 19-2), when the operator is sitting (Figure 19-3) and the size of the human hand in relation to the size of control knobs or switches (Figure 19-4).

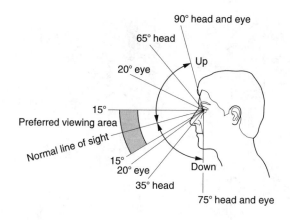

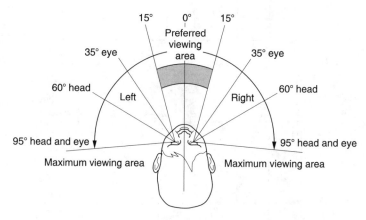

		Maximum*		
	Preferred	Eye rotation	Head rotation	Head and eye rotation
Up	15°	40°	65°	90°
Down	15°	20°	35°	75°
Right	15°	35°	60°	95°
Left	15°	35°	60°	95°

* Display area on the console defined by the angles measured from the normal line of sight

FIGURE 19-1 Normal line of sight

Hardware issues are best addressed by first surveying potential customers of the device to help determine the intended use of the device, the environment in which the device will be used, and the optimum location of controls and displays. Once the survey is completed and the results analyzed, a cardboard, foam, or wooden model of the device is built and reviewed with the potential customers. The customer can then get personal, hands-on experience

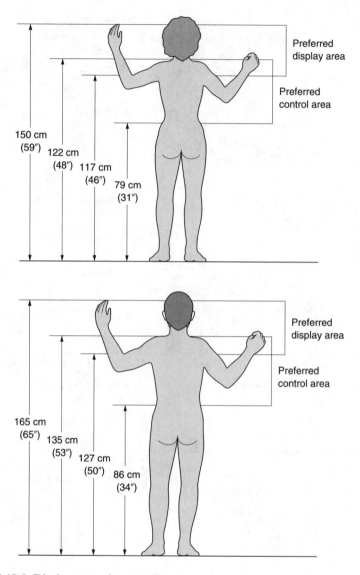

FIGURE 19-2 Display area when standing

with the controls, displays, the device framework, and offer constructive criticism on the design. Once all changes have been made, the model can be transposed into a prototype, using actual hardware.

19.4   THE SOFTWARE ELEMENT IN HUMAN FACTORS

The software element of the device must be easy to use and understand. It must have simple, reliable data entry, it should be menu driven if there are many

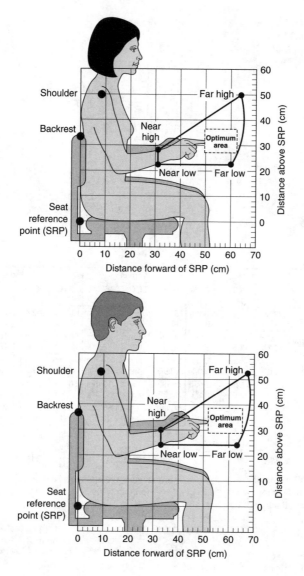

FIGURE 19-3 Display area when sitting

commands to be learned, displays must not be overcrowded, and dialogue must not be burdened with computer jargon. The software must provide feedback to the user through error messages and help messages. An indication that the process is involved in some activity is also important, as a blank screen leads to the assumption that nothing is active, and the user starts pushing keys or buttons.

Software must consider the environment in which it is to be used, especially with regard to colors of displays, type of data to be displayed, format

Hand data: Men, women and children

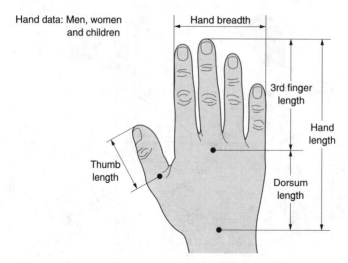

	Men			Women			Children			
Hand data	2.5% tile	50.0% tile	97.5% tile	2.5% tile	50.0% tile	97.5% tile	6 yr.	8 yr.	11 yr.	14 yr.
Hand length	173 mm (6.8")	191 mm (7.5")	208 mm (8.2")	157 mm (6.2")	175 mm (6.9")	191 mm (7.5")	130 mm (5.1")	142 mm (5.6")	160 mm (6.3")	178 mm (7.0")
Hand breadth	81 mm (3.2")	89 mm (3.5")	97 mm (3.8")	66 mm (2.6")	74 mm (2.9")	79 mm (3.1")	58 mm (2.3")	64 mm (2.5")	71 mm (2.8")	–
3rd finger lg.	102 mm (4.0")	114 mm (4.5")	127 mm (5.0")	91 mm (3.6")	100 mm (4.0")	112 mm (4.4")	74 mm (2.9")	81 mm (3.2")	89 mm (3.5")	102 mm (4.0")
Dorsum lg.	71 mm (2.8")	75 mm (3.0")	81 mm (3.2")	66 mm (2.6")	74 mm (2.9")	79 mm (3.1")	56 mm (2.2")	61 mm (2.4")	71 mm (2.8")	75 mm (3.0")
Thumb length	61 mm (2.4")	69 mm (2.7")	75 mm (3.0")	56 mm (2.2")	61 mm (2.4")	66 mm (2.6")	46 mm (1.8")	51 mm (2.0")	56 mm (2.2")	61 mm (2.4")

Additional data: Average man

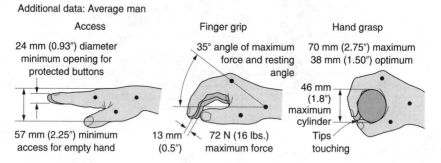

FIGURE 19-4 Hand sizes

of the data, alarm levels to be used, etc. Stress and fatigue can be reduced by consideration of color and the intensity of the displayed data. Operator effectiveness can be improved by optimizing the location of function keys, displaying more important data in the primary viewing area, and placing secondary data in the secondary display area. The inclusion of device checkout procedures and menus also improves operator effectiveness and confidence.

19.5 THE HUMAN FACTORS PROCESS

Human factors is the sum of several processes including the analytic process that focuses on the objectives of the proposed device and the functions that should be performed to meet those objectives; the design and development process that converts the results of the analyses into detailed equipment design features; the test and evaluation process which verifies that the design and development process has resolved issues identified in the analytic process.

Human factors engineering integrations begin with early planning and may continue throughout the life cycle of the device. As a minimum, human factors should continue until the device is introduced commercially. Human factors efforts following commercial introduction are important to the enhancement of the device and the development of future devices.

19.6 PLANNING

A human factors plan should be developed as an integral part of the overall plan for device development. The plan should guide human factors efforts in the interrelated processes of analysis, design and development, and test and evaluation. The plan should describe human factors tasks necessary to complete each process, the expected results of those tasks, the means of coordinating those tasks with the overall process for device development, and the schedule for that coordination. The plan should address the resources necessary for its accomplishment including levels of effort necessary for its management and coordination as well as for accomplishment of its individual tasks.

The plan should assure that results of human factors tasks are available in time to influence the design of the proposed device as well as the conduct of the overall project. Analysis tasks should begin very early. Iterations of analysis tasks that refine earlier products may continue throughout the project. Design and development build on the products of early analysis, and iterations may also continue throughout the project. Test and evaluation should begin with the earliest products of design and development. The results of test and evaluation should influence subsequent iterations of analysis, design and development, and test and evaluation tasks.

19.7 ANALYSIS

Successful human factors is predicated on careful analyses. Early analyses should focus on the objectives of the proposed device and the functions that should be performed to meet those objectives. Later analysis should focus on the critical human performance required of specific personnel as a means of establishing the human factors parameters for design of the device and associated job aids, procedures, and training and for establishing human factors test and evaluation criteria for the device. Analyses should be updated as required to remain current with the design effort.

19.8   CONDUCT USER STUDIES

The goal of user studies is to learn as much as possible within a reasonable time frame about the customer's needs and preferences as they relate to the product under development. Several methods are available for getting to know the customer.

19.8.1   OBSERVATIONS

Observations are a productive first step toward getting to know the user. By observing people at work, a rapid sense for the nature of their jobs is developed, including the pace and nature of their interactions with the environment, co-workers, patients, equipment, and documents. Such observations may be conducted in an informal manner, possibly taking notes and photographs. Alternatively, a more formal approach may be taken that includes rigorous data collection. For example, it may be important to document a clinician's physical movements and the time they spend performing certain tasks to determine performance benchmarks. This latter approach is referred to as a time-motion analysis and may be warranted if one of the design goals is to make the customer more productive.

Enough time should be spent observing users to get a complete sense for how they perform tasks related to the product under development. A rule of thumb in usability testing is that five to eight participants provide 80 to 90% of the information you seek. The same rule of thumb may be applied to observations, presuming that you are addressing a relatively homogeneous user population. Significant differences in the user population (i.e., a heterogeneous user population) may warrant more extensive observations. For example, it may become necessary to observe people who have different occupational backgrounds and work in different countries.

Designers and engineers should conduct their own observations. For starters, such observations increase empathy for the customer. Also, first-hand experience is always more powerful than reading a marketing report.

19.8.2   INTERVIEWS

Similar to observations, interviews provide a wealth of information with a limited investment of time. Structured interviews based on scripted questions are generally better than unstructured interviews (i.e., a free-flowing conversation). This is because a structured interview assures that the interviewer will ask everyone the same question, enabling a comparison of answers. Structured interviews may include a few open-ended questions to produce evoked comments and suggestions that could not be anticipated. The interview script should be developed from a list of information needs. Generally, questions should progress from general to more specific design issues. Care should be taken to avoid mixing marketing- and engineering-related concerns with usability concerns.

Interviews can be conducted just after observations are completed. Conducting the interviews prior to the observations can be problematic as it tends to alter the way people react.

19.8.3 FOCUS GROUPS

Conducting interviews with people in their working environment (sometimes referred to as contextual interviewing) is generally best. Interviewees are likely to be more relaxed and opinionated. Interviews conducted at trade shows and medical conferences, for example, are more susceptible to bias and may be less reliable.

Conducting interviews with a group of five to ten people at a time enables easy determination of a consensus on various design issues. In preparation for such a focus group, a script should be developed from a set of information requirements. Use the script as a guide for the group interview, but feel free to let the discussion take a few tangents if they are productive ones. Also, feel at liberty to include group exercises, such as watching a video or ranking and rating existing products, as appropriate.

Conduct enough focus groups to gain confidence that an accurate consensus has been developed. Two focus groups held locally may be enough if regional differences of opinion are unlikely and the user group is relatively homogenous. Otherwise, it may be appropriate to conduct up to four groups at each domestic and international site that provides a reasonable cross-section of the marketplace.

Document the results in a focus groups report. The report can be an expanded version of the script. Begin the report with a summary section to pull together the results. Findings (i.e., answers to questions) may be presented after each question. The findings from various sites may be integrated or presented separately, depending on the design issue and opportunity to tailor the product under development to individual markets. Results of group exercises may be presented as attachments and discussed in the summary.

19.8.4 TASK ANALYSIS

The purpose of task analysis is to develop a detailed view of customer interactions with a product by dividing the interactions into discrete actions and decisions. Typically, a flow chart is drawn that shows the sequence and logic of customer actions and decisions. The task analysis is extended to include tables that define information and control requirements associated with each action and decision. In the course of the task analysis, characterize the frequency, urgency, and criticality of integrated tasks, such as "checking the breathing circuit."

19.8.5 BENCHMARK USABILITY TEST

The start of a new product development effort is a good time to take stock of the company's existing products. An effective way to do this is to conduct a benchmark usability test that yields, in a quantitative fashion, both objective and subjective measures of usability. Such testing will identify the strengths and weaknesses of the existing products, as well as help establish usability goals for the new product.

19.8.6 WRITE USER PROFILE

To culminate the user study effort, write a so-called user profile. A user specification (two to five pages) summarizes the important things learned about the customers. The profile should define the user populations' demographics (age, gender, education level, occupational background, language), product-related experience, work environment, and motivation level. The user profile is a major input to the user specification that describes the product under development from the customer's point of view.

19.8.7 SET UP AN ADVISORY PANEL

To assure early and continued customer involvement, set up an advisory panel that equitably represents the user population. The panel may include three to five clinicians for limited product development efforts, or be twice as large for larger efforts. The panel participants are usually compensated for their time. Correspond with members of the panel on an as-needed basis and meet with them periodically to review the design in progress. Note that advisory panel reviews are not an effective replacement for usability testing.

19.9 SET USABILITY GOALS

Usability goals are comparable to other types of engineering goals in the sense that they are quantitative and provide a basis for acceptance testing. Goals may be objective or subjective. A sample objective goal might be: on average, users shall require 3 seconds to silence an alarm. This goal is an objective goal because the user's performance level can be determined simply by observation. For example, you can use a stop watch to determine task times. Other kinds of objective goals concentrate on the number of user errors and the rate of successful task completion.

A sample subjective goal is: on average, 75% of users shall rate the intuitiveness of the alarm system as 5 or better, where 1 = poor and 7 = excellent. This goal is subjective because it requires asking the user's opinion about their interaction with the given product. A rating sheet can be used to record their answers. Other kinds of subjective goals concentrate on mental processing and emotional response attributes, such as learning, frustration level, fear of making mistakes, etc.

Every usability goal is based on a usability attribute, e.g., task, speed or intuitiveness, includes a metric such as time or scale and sets a target performance level, such as 3 seconds or a rating of 5 or better.

Typically, up to 50 usability goals may be written, two-thirds of which are objective and one-third which are subjective. The target performance level on each goal is based on findings from preceding user studies, particularly the benchmark usability testing. If there is no basis for comparison, i.e., there are no comparable products, then engineering judgement must be used to set the initial goals and adjust them as necessary to assure they are realistic.

19.10   DESIGN USER INTERFACE CONCEPTS

Concurrent design is a productive method of developing a final user interface design. It enables the thorough exploration of several design concepts before converging on a final solution. In the course of exploring alternative designs, limited prototypes should be built of the most promising concepts and user feedback obtained on them. This gets users involved in the design process at its early stages and assures that the final design will be closely matched to user's expectations.

Note that the design process steps described below assume that the product includes both hardware and software elements. Some steps would be moot if the product has no software user interface.

19.10.1   DEVELOP CONCEPTUAL MODEL

When users interact with a product, they develop a mental model of how it works. This mental model may be complete and accurate or just the opposite. Enabling the user to develop a complete and accurate mental model of how a product works is a challenge. The first step is developing so-called conceptual models of how to represent the product's functions. This exercise provides a terrific opportunity for design innovation. The conceptual model may be expressed as a bubble diagram, for example, that illustrates the major functions of the product and functional interrelationships as you would like the users to think of them. You can augment the bubble diagram with a narrative description of the conceptual model.

19.10.2   DEVELOP USER INTERFACE STRUCTURE

Develop alternative user interface structures that compliment the most promising two or three conceptual models. These structures can be expressed in the form of screen hierarchy maps that illustrate where product functions reside and how many steps it will take users to get to them. Such maps may take the form of a single element, a linear sequence, a tree structure (cyclic or acyclic) or a network. In addition to software screens, such maps should show which functions are allocated to dedicated hardware controls.

19.10.3   DEFINE INTERACTION STYLE

In conjunction with the development of the user interface structures, alternative interaction styles should be defined. Possible styles include question and answer dialogs, command lines, menus, and direct manipulation.

19.10.4   DEVELOP SCREEN TEMPLATES

Determine an appropriate size display based on the user interface structure and interaction style, as well as other engineering considerations. Using computer-based drawing tools, draw the outline of a blank screen. Next, develop a limited number (perhaps three to five) of basic layouts for the information that will appear on the various screens. Normally, it is best to align all elements, such as titles, windows, prompts, numerics according to a grid system.

19.10.5   DEVELOP HARDWARE LAYOUT

Apply established design principles in the development of hardware layouts that are compatible with the evolving software user interface solutions. Assure that the layouts reinforce the overall conceptual model.

19.10.6   DEVELOP A SCREENPLAY

Apply established design principles in the development of a detailed screenplay. Do not bother to develop every possible screen at this time. Rather, develop only those screens that would enable users to perform frequently used, critical and particularly complex functions. Base the screen designs on the templates. Create new templates or eliminate existing templates as required while continuing to limit the total number of templates. Assure that the individual screens reinforce the overall conceptual model. You may choose to get user feedback on the screenplay (what some people call a paper prototype).

19.10.7   DEVELOP A REFINED DESIGN

Steps 5 and 6 describe prototyping and testing the user interface. These efforts will help determine the most promising design concept or suggest a hybrid of two or more concepts. The next step is to refine the preferred design. Several reiterations of the preceding steps may be necessary, including developing a refined conceptual model, developing a refined user interface structure and developing an updated set of screen templates. Then, a refined screenplay and hardware layout may be developed.

19.10.8   DEVELOP A FINAL DESIGN

Once again, steps 5 and 6 describe prototyping and testing the user interface. These efforts will help you determine any remaining usability problems with the refined design and opportunities for further improvement. It is likely that design changes at this point will be limited in nature. Most can be made directly to the prototype.

19.11 MODEL THE USER INTERFACE

Build a prototype to evaluate the dynamics of the user interface. Early proto-types of competing concepts may be somewhat limited in terms of their visual realism and how many functions they perform. Normally, it is best to develop a prototype that (1) presents a fully functional top-level that allows users to browse their basic options, and (2) enables users to perform a few sample tasks, i.e., walkthrough a few scenarios. As much as possible, include tasks that relate to the established usability goals.

User interface prototypes may be developed using conventional program-ming languages or rapid prototyping languages, such as SuperCard, Altia Design, Visual Basic, Toolbook, and the like. The rapid prototyping languages are generally preferable because they allow for faster prototyping and they are easier to modify based on core project team and user feedback.

Early in the screenplay development process, it may make sense to proto-type a small part of the user interface to assess design alternatives or to conduct limited studies, such as how frequently to flash a warning. Once detailed screenplays of competing concepts are available, build higher-fidelity proto-types that facilitate usability testing. Once a refined design is developed, build a fully functional prototype that permits a verification usability test. Such prototypes can be refined based on final test results and serve as a specification.

19.12 TEST THE USER INTERFACE

There are several appropriate times to conduct a usability test, including:

- At the start of a development effort to develop benchmarks
- When you have paper-based or computer-based prototypes of competing design concepts
- When you have a prototype of your refined design
- When you want to develop marketing claims regarding the performance of the actual product

While the rigor of the usability test may change, based on the timing of the test, the basic approach remains the same. You recruit prospective users to spend a concentrated period of time interacting with the prototype product. The users may undertake a self-exploration or perform directed tasks. During the course of such interactions you note the test participants' comments and document their performance. At intermittent stages, you may choose to have the test participant complete a questionnaire or rating/ranking exercise. Videotaping test proceedings is one way to give those unable to attend the test a first-hand sense of user-product interactions. Sometimes it is useful to create a 10 to 15 minute highlight tape that shows the most interesting moments of all test sessions.

During testing, collect the data necessary to determine if you are meeting the established usability goals. This effort will add continuity and objectivity to the usability engineering process.

19.13   SPECIFY THE USER INTERFACE

19.13.1   STYLE GUIDE

The purpose of a style guide is to document the rules of the user interface design. By establishing such rules, you can check the evolving design to determine any inconsistencies. Also, it assures the consistency of future design changes. Style guides, usually 10 to 15 pages in length, normally include a description of the conceptual model, the design elements, and elements of style.

19.13.2   SCREEN HIERARCHY MAP

The purpose of a screen hierarchy map is to provide an overview of the user interface structure. It places all screens that appear in the screenplay in context. It enables the flow of activity to be studied in order to determine if it reinforces the conceptual model. It also helps to determine how many steps users will need to take to accomplish a given task. Graphical elements of the screen hierarchy map should be cross-indexed to the screenplay.

19.13.3   SCREENPLAY

The purpose of a screenplay is to document the appearance of all major screens on paper. Typically, screen images are taken directly from the computer-based prototype. Ideally, the screenplay should present screen images in their actual scale and resolution. Each screen should be cross-indexed to the screen hierarchy map.

19.13.4   SPECIFICATION PROTOTYPE

The purpose of the specification prototype is to model accurately the majority of user interface interactions. This provides the core project team with a common basis for understanding how the final product should work. It provides a basis for writing the user documentation. It may also be used to orient those involved in marketing, sales, and training.

19.13.5 HARDWARE LAYOUTS

The hardware layout may be illustrated by the specification prototype. However, the hardware may not be located proximal to the software user interface. If this is the case, develop layout drawings to document the final hardware layout.

19.14 ADDITIONAL HUMAN FACTORS DESIGN CONSIDERATIONS

The design of medical devices should reflect human factors engineering design features that increase the potential for successful performance of tasks and for satisfaction of design objectives.

19.14.1 CONSISTENCY AND SIMPLICITY

Where common functions are involved, consistency is encouraged in controls, displays, markings, codings, and arrangement schemes for consoles and instrument panels.

Simplicity in all designs is encouraged. Equipment should be designed to be operated, maintained, and repaired in its operational environment by personnel with appropriate but minimal training. Unnecessary or cumbersome operations should be avoided when simpler, more efficient alternatives are available.

19.14.2 SAFETY

Medical device design should reflect system and personnel safety factors, including the elimination or minimization of the potential for human error during operation and maintenance under both routine and non-routine or emergency conditions. Machines should be designed to minimize the consequences of human error. For example, where appropriate, a design should incorporate redundant, diverse elements, arranged in a manner that increases overall reliability when failure can result in the inability to perform a critical function.

Any medical device failure should immediately be indicated to the operator and should not adversely affect safe operation of the device. Where failures can affect safe operation, simple means and procedures for averting adverse effects should be provided.

When the device failure is life-threatening or could mask a life-threatening condition, an audible alarm and a visual display should be provided to indicate the device failure. Wherever possible, explicit notification of the source of failure should be provided to the user. Concise instructions on how to return to operation or how to invoke alternate backup methods should be provided.

19.14.3 ENVIRONMENTAL/ORGANIZATIONAL CONSIDERATIONS

The design of medical devices should consider the following:

- The levels of noise, vibration, humidity, and heat that will be generated by the device and the levels of noise, vibration, humidity, and heat to which the device and its operators and maintainers will be exposed in the anticipated operational environment
- The need for protecting operators and patients from electric shock, thermal, infectious, toxicologic, radiologic, electromagnetic, visual, and explosion risks, as well as from potential design hazards, such as sharp edges and corners, and the danger of the device falling on the patient or operator
- The adequacy of the physical, visual, auditory, and other communication links among personnel and between personnel and equipment
- The importance of minimizing psychophysiological stress and fatigue in the clinical environment in which the medical device will be used
- The impact on operator effectiveness of the arrangement of controls, displays and markings on consoles and panels
- The potential effects of natural or artificial illumination used in the operation, control, and maintenance of the device
- The need for rapid, safe, simple, and economical maintenance and repair
- The possible positions of the device in relation to the users as a function of the user's location and mobility
- The electromagnetic environment(s) in which the device is intended to be used.

19.14.4 DOCUMENTATION

Documentation is a general term that includes operator manuals, instruction sheets, online help systems, and maintenance manuals. These materials may be accessed by many types of users. Therefore, the documentation should be written to meet the needs of all target populations.

Preparation of instructional documentation should begin as soon as possible during the specification phase. This assists device designers in identifying critical human factors engineering needs and in producing a consistent human interface. The device and its documentation should be developed together.

During the planning phase, a study should be made of the capabilities and information needs of the documentation users, including:

- The user's mental abilities
- The user's physical abilities

- The user's previous experience with similar devices
- The user's general understanding of the general principles of operation and potential hazards associated with the technology
- The special needs or restrictions of the environment

As a minimum, the operator's manual should include detailed procedures for setup, normal operation, emergency operation, cleaning, and operator troubleshooting.

The operator manual should be tested on models of the device. It is important that these test populations be truly representative of end-users and that they do not have advance knowledge of the device.

Maintenance documentation should be tested on devices that resemble production units.

Documentation content should be presented in language free of vague and ambiguous terms. The simplest words and phrases that will convey the intended meaning should be used. Terminology within the publication should be consistent. Use of abbreviations should be kept to a minimum but defined when they are used.

Information included in warnings and cautions should be chosen carefully and with consideration of the skills and training of intended users. It is especially important to inform users about unusual hazards and hazards specific to the device.

Human factors engineering design features should assure that the device functions consistently, simply, and safely, that the environment, system organization and documentation are analyzed and considered in the design, thus increasing the potential for successful performance of tasks and for satisfaction of design objectives.

19.14.5 ANTHROPOMETRY

Anthropometry is the science of measuring the human body and its parts and functional capacities. Generally, design limits are based on a range of values from the 5th percentile female to the 95th percentile male for critical body dimensions. The 5th percentile value indicates that 5% of the population will be equal to or smaller than that value and 95% will be larger. The 95th percentile value indicates that 95% of the population will be equal to or smaller than that value and 5% will be larger. The use of a design range from the 5th to the 95th percentile values will theoretically provide coverage for 90% of the user population for that dimension.

19.14.6 FUNCTIONAL DIMENSIONS

The reach capabilities of the user population play an important role in the design of the controls and displays of the medical device. The designer should

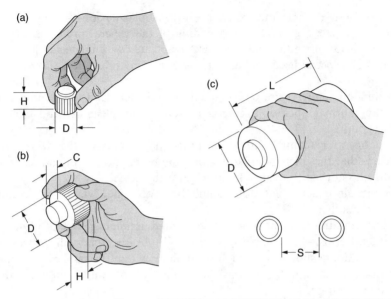

	Dimensions						
	(a) Finger grasp		(b) Thumb and fingers encircled			(c) Palm/hand grasp	
	'H' Height	'D' Diameter	'H' Height	'D' Diameter	'C' Clearance	'D' Diameter	'L' Length
Minimum	13 mm (0.50″)	10 mm (0.375″)	13 mm (0.50″)	25 mm (1.0″)	16 mm (0.625″)	38 mm (1.5″)	75 mm (3.0″)
Maximum	25 mm (1.0″)	100 mm (4.0″)	25 mm (1.0″)	75 mm (3.0″)	–	75 mm (3.0″)	–

	Torque		'S' Separation
	*	**	One hand individually
Minimum	–	–	25 mm (1.0″)
Preferred	–	–	50 mm (2.0″)
Maximum	32 mN-m (4.5 in.-oz.)	42 mN-m (6.0 in.-oz.)	–

* To and including 25 mm (1.0″) diameter knobs.
** Greater than 25 mm (1.0″) diameter knobs.

FIGURE 19-5 Example of functional dimensions

take into consideration both one- and two-handed reaches in the seated and standing positions (Figures 19-5 and 19-6).

Body mobility ranges should be factored into the design process. Limits of body movement should be considered relative to the age diversity and gender of the target user population.

The strength capacities of the device operators may have an impact on the design of the system controls. The lifting and carrying abilities of the

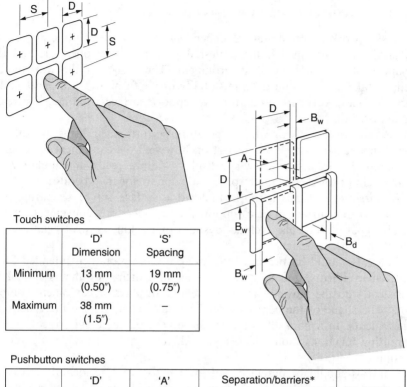

Touch switches

	'D' Dimension	'S' Spacing
Minimum	13 mm (0.50″)	19 mm (0.75″)
Maximum	38 mm (1.5″)	–

Pushbutton switches

	'D' Dimension	'A' Displacement	Separation/barriers*		Resistance
			'B$_w$'	'B$_d$'	
Minimum	19 mm (0.75″)	3 mm** (0.125″)	3 mm (0.125″)	5 mm (0.187″)	280 mN (10 oz.)
Maximum	38 mm (1.5″)	6 mm (0.250″)	6 mm (0.250″)	6 mm (0.250″)	16.6 N (60 oz.)

* Barriers shall have rounded edges.
** 5 mm (0.188″) for positive position switches.

FIGURE 19-6 Example of functional dimensions

personnel responsible for moving and/or adjusting the device need to be considered to assure the device can be transported and adjusted efficiently and safely.

19.14.7 PSYCHOLOGICAL ELEMENTS

It is crucial to consider human proficiency in perception, cognition, learning, memory, and judgement when designing medical devices to assure that operation of the system is as intuitive, effective, and safe as possible. This is discussed in Chapter 1.

19.14.8 WORKSTATION DESIGN CONSIDERATIONS

Successful workstation design is dependent on considering the nature of the tasks to be completed, the preferred posture of the operator, and the dynamics of the surrounding environment. The design of the workstation needs to take into account the adjustability of the furniture, clearances under work surfaces, keyboard and display support surfaces, seating, footrests, and accessories.

The effectiveness with which operators perform their tasks at consoles or instrument panels depends in part on how well the equipment is designed to minimize parallax in viewing displays, allow ready manipulation of controls, and provide adequate space and support for the operator.

A horizontal or nearly horizontal work surface serves primarily as a work or writing surface or as a support for the operator's convenience items. Certain types of controls, such as joysticks or tracking controls, can also be part of the surface design.

Controls should have characteristics appropriate for their intended functions, environments, and user orientations, and their movements should be consistent with the movements of any related displays or equipment components. The shape of the control should be dictated by its specific functional requirements. In a bank of controls, those controls affecting critical or life-supporting functions should have a special shape and, if possible, a standard location.

Controls should be designed and located to avoid accidental activation. Particular attention should be given to critical controls whose accidental activation might injure patients or personnel or might compromise device performance. Feedback on control response adequacy should be provided as rapidly as possible.

19.14.9 ALARMS AND SIGNALS

The purpose of an alarm is to draw attention to the device when the operator's attention may be focused elsewhere. Alarms should not be startling but should elicit the desired action from the user. When appropriate, the alarm message should provide instructions for the corrective action that is required. In general, alarm design will be different for a device that is continuously attended by a trained operator, such as an anesthesia machine, than for a device that is unattended and operated by an untrained operator, such as a patient-controlled analgesia device. False alarms, loud and startling alarms, or alarms that recur unnecessarily can be a source of distraction for both an attendant and the patient and thus be a hindrance to good patient care.

Alarm characteristics are grouped in the following three categories:

- High priority: a combination of audible and visual signals indicating that immediate operator response is required

- Medium priority: a combination of audible and visual signals indicating that prompt operator response is required
- Low priority: a visual signal, or a combination of audible and visual signals indicating that operator awareness is required

A red flashing light should be used for a high-priority alarm condition unless an alternative visible signal that indicates the alarm condition and its priority is employed. A red flashing light should not be used for any other purpose.

A yellow flashing light should be used for a medium-priority alarm condition unless an alternative visible signal that indicates the alarm condition and its priority is employed. A yellow flashing light should not be used for any other purpose.

A steady yellow light should be used for a low-priority alarm condition unless an alternative visible signal that indicates the alarm condition and its priority is employed.

Audible signals should be used to alert the operator to the status of the patient or the device when the device is out of the operator's line of sight. Audible signals used in conjunction with visual displays should be supplementary to the visual signals and should be used to alert and direct the user's attention to the appropriate visual display.

Design of equipment should take into account the background noise and other audible signals and alarms that will likely be present during the intended use of the device. The lowest volume control settings of the critical life support audible alarms should provide sufficient signal strength to preclude masking by anticipated ambient noise levels. Volume control settings for other signals should similarly preclude such masking. Ambient noise levels in hospital areas can range from 50 dB in a private room to 60 dB in intensive care units and emergency rooms, with peaks as high as 65 to 70 dB in operating rooms due to conversations, alarms, or the activation of other devices. The volume of monitoring signals normally should be lower than that of high-priority or medium-priority audible alarms provided on the same device. Audible signals should be located so as to assist the operator in identifying the device that is causing the alarm.

The use of voice alarms in medical applications should normally not be considered for the following reasons:

- Voice alarms are easily masked by ambient noise and other voice messages
- Voice messages may interfere with communications among personnel who are attempting to address the alarm condition
- The information conveyed by the voice alarm may reach individuals who should not be given specific information concerning the nature of the alarm
- The types of messages transmitted by voice tend to be very specific, possibly causing complication and confusion to the user

- In the situation where there are multiple alarms, multiple voice alarms would cause confusion
- Different languages may be required to accommodate various markets

The device's default alarm limits should be provided for critical alarms. These limits should be sufficiently wide to prevent nuisance alarms, and sufficiently narrow to alert the operator to a situation that would be dangerous in the average patient.

The device may retain and store one or more sets of alarm limits chosen by the user. When more than one set of user default alarm limits exists, the activation of user default alarm limits should require deliberate action by the user. When there is only one set of user default alarm limits, the device may be configured to activate this set of user default alarm limits automatically in place of the factory default alarm limits.

The setting of adjustable alarms should be indicated continuously or on user demand. It should be possible to review alarm limits quickly. During user setting of alarm limits, monitoring should continue and alarm conditions should elicit the appropriate alarms. Alarm limits may be set automatically or upon user action to reasonable ranges and/or percentages above and/or below existing values for monitored variables. Care should be used in the design of such automatic setting systems to help prevent nuisance alarms or variables that are changing within an acceptable range.

An audible high- or medium-priority signal may have a manually operated, temporary override mechanism that will silence it for a period of time, e.g., 120 seconds. After the silencing period, the alarm should begin sounding again if the alarm condition persists or if the condition was temporarily corrected but has now returned. New alarm conditions that develop during the silencing period should initiate audible and visual signals. If momentary silencing is provided, the silencing should be visually indicated.

An audible high-, or medium-priority signal may be equipped with a means of permanent silencing that may be appropriate when a continuous alarm is likely to degrade user performance of associated tasks to an unacceptable extent and in cases when users would otherwise be likely to disable the device altogether. If provided, such silencing should require that the user either confirm the intent to silence a critical life support alarm or take more than one step to turn the alarm off. Permanent silencing should be visually indicated and may be signalled by a periodic audible reminder. Permanent silencing of an alarm should not affect the visual representation of the alarm and should not disable the alarm.

Life support devices and devices that monitor a life-critical variable should have an audible alarm to indicate a loss of power or failure of the device. The characteristics of this alarm should be the same as those of the highest-priority alarm that becomes inoperative. It may be necessary to use battery power for such an alarm.

19.14.10 LABELING

Controls, displays, and other equipment items that need to be located, identified, or manipulated should be appropriately and clearly marked to permit rapid and accurate human performance. The characteristics of markings should be determined by such factors as the criticality of the function labeled, the distance from which the labels have to be read, the illumination level, the colors, the time available for reading, the reading accuracy required, and consistency with other markings.

Receptacles and connectors should be marked with their intended function or their intended connection to a particular cable. Convenience receptacles should be labeled with maximum allowable load in amperes or watts. The current rating of fuses should be permanently marked adjacent to the fuse holder. Fuse ratings should be indicated either in whole number, common fractions, or whole number plus common fractions. Labeling of fuses and circuit breakers should be legible in the ambient illumination range anticipated for the maintainer's location.

Operators and maintenance personnel should be warned of possible fire, radiation, explosion, shock, infection or other hazards that may be encountered during the use, handling, storage, or repair of the device. Electromedical instruments should be labeled to show whether they may be used in the presence of flammable gases or oxygen-rich atmospheres. Hazard warnings should be prominent and understandable.

Normally, labels should be placed above panel elements that users grasp, press, or otherwise handle so the label is not obscured by the hand. However, certain panel element positions, user postures and handling methods may dictate other label placements. Labels should be positioned to ensure visibility and readability from the position in which they should be read.

Labels should be oriented horizontally so that they may be read quickly and easily from left to right. Although not normally recommended, vertical orientation may be used, but only where its use is justified in providing a better understanding of intended function. Vertical labels should be read from top to bottom. Curved labels should be avoided except when they provide setting delimiters for rotary controls.

Labels should not cover any other information source. They should not detract from or obscure figures or scales that should be read by the operator. Labels should not be covered or obscured by other units in the equipment assembly. Labels should be visible to the operator during control activation. All markings should be permanent and should remain legible throughout the life of the equipment under anticipated use and maintenance conditions.

The words employed in the label should express exactly what action is intended. Instructions should be clear and direct. Words that have a commonly accepted meaning for all intended users should be utilized. Unusual technical terms should be avoided. Labels should be consistent within and across pieces of equipment in their use of words, acronyms, abbreviations, and part/system numbers. No mismatch should exist between the nomenclature used in documentation and that printed on the labels.

Symbols should be used only if they have a commonly accepted meaning for all intended users. Symbols should be unique and distinguishable from one another. A commonly accepted standard configuration should be used.

Human factors engineering hardware design considerations should include functional dimensions, workstation architecture considerations, alarms and signals, and labeling, and should always take the operator's psychological characteristics into account. Chapter 3 discusses human factors engineering software design considerations.

19.14.11 SOFTWARE

Computerized systems should provide a functional interface between the system and users of that system. This interface should be optimally compatible with the intended user and should minimize conditions that can degrade human performance or contribute to human error. Thus, procedures for similar or logically related transactions should be consistent. Every input by a user should consistently produce some perceptible response or output from the computer. Sufficient online help should be provided to allow the intended but uninitiated user to operate the device effectively in its basic functional mode without reference to a user's manual or experienced operator. Users should be provided appropriate information at all times on system status either automatically or upon request. Provision of information about system dysfunction is essential.

In applications where users need to log-on to the system, log-on should be a separate procedure that should be completed before a user is required to select among any operational options. Appropriate prompts for log-on should be displayed automatically on the user's terminal with no special action required other than turning on the terminal. Users should be provided feedback relevant to the log-on procedure that indicates the status of the inputs. Log-on processes should require minimum input from the user, consistent with system access security.

In the event of a partial hardware/software failure, the program should allow for orderly shutdown and establishment of a checkpoint so restoration can be accomplished without loss of data.

Where two or more users need to have simultaneous access to a computer system, under normal circumstances, operation by one person should not interfere with the operations of another person. For circumstances in which certain operators require immediate access to the system, an organized system for insuring or avoiding preemption should be provided. Provisions should be made so that preempted users are notified and can resume operations at the point of interference without data loss.

19.14.12 DATA ENTRY

Manual data entry functions should be designed to establish consistency of data entry transactions, minimize user's input actions and memory load, ensure compatibility of data entry with data display, and provide flexibility of user control of data entry. The system should provide feedback to the user about acceptance or rejection of an entry.

When a processing delay occurs, the system should acknowledge the data entry and provide the user with an indication of the delay. If possible, the system should advise the user of the time remaining for process completion. Data entry should require an explicit completion action, such as the depression of an ENTER key to post an entry into memory. Data entries should be checked by the system for correct format, acceptable value, or range of values. Where repetitive entry of data sets is required, data validation for each set should be completed before another transaction can begin.

Data should be entered in units that are familiar to the user. If several different systems of units are commonly used, the user should have the option of selecting the units either before or after data entry. Transposition of data from one system of units to another should be accomplished automatically by the device. When mnemonics or codes are used to shorten data entry, they should be distinctive and have a relationship or association to normal language or specific job-related terminology.

Data deletion or cancellation should require an explicit action, such as the depression of a DELETE key. When a data delete function has been selected by a user, a means of confirming the delete action should be provided, such as a dialogue box with a delete acknowledgement button or a response to a question such as Are you sure? (Y/N). In general, requiring a second press of the DELETE key is not preferred because of the possibility of an accidental double press. Similarly, after data have been entered, if the user fails to enter the data formally, for instance by pressing an ENTER key, the data should not be deleted or discarded without confirmation from the user.

Deleted data should be maintained in a memory buffer from which they can be salvaged, such as the UNDELETE option. The size and accessibility of this buffer should depend on the value of the data that the user can delete from the system.

The user should always be given the opportunity to change a data entry after the data have been posted. When a user requests change or deletion of a data item that is not currently being displayed, the option of displaying the old value before confirming the change should be presented. Where a data archive is being created, the system should record both the original entry and all subsequent amendments.

19.14.13 DISPLAYS

Visual displays should provide the operator with a clear indication of equipment or system status under all conditions consistent with the intended use and maintenance of the system. The information displayed to a user should be sufficient to allow the user to perform the intended task but should be limited to what is necessary to perform the task or to make decisions. Information necessary for performing different activities, such as equipment operation versus troubleshooting, should not appear in a single display unless the activities are related and require the same information to be used simultaneously. Information should be displayed only within the limits of precision required for the intended user activity or decision making and within the limits of accuracy of the measure.

Graphic displays should be used for the display of information when perception of the pattern of variation is important to proper interpretation. The choice of a particular graphic display type can have significant impact on user performance. The designer should consider carefully the tasks to be supported by the display and the conditions under which the user will view the device before selecting a display type.

Numeric digital displays should be used where quantitative accuracy of individual data items is important. They should not be used as the only display of information when perception of the variation pattern is important to proper interpretation or when rapid or slow digital display rates inhibit proper perception.

Displays may be coded by various features, such as color, size, location, shape, or flashing lights. Coding techniques should be used to help discriminate among individual displays and to identify functionally related displays, the relationship among displays, and critical information within a display.

Display formats should be consistent within a system. When appropriate for users, the same format should be used for input and output. Data entry formats should match the source document formats. Essential data, text, and formats should be under computer, not user, control. When data fields have a naturally occurring order, such as chronological or sequential, such order should be reflected in the format organization of the fields. Where some displayed data items are of great significance, or require immediate user response, those items should be grouped and displayed prominently. Separation of groups of information should be accomplished through the use of blanks, spacing, lines, color coding, or other similar means consistent with the application.

The content of displays within a system should be presented in a consistent, standardized manner. Information density should be held to a minimum in displays used for critical tasks. When a display contains too much data for presentation in a single frame, the data should be partitioned into separately displayable pages. The user should not have to rely on memory to interpret new data. Each data display should provide the needed context, including the recapitulation of prior data from prior displays, as necessary.

An appropriate pointing device, such as a mouse, trackball, or touch screen, should be used in conjunction with applications that are suited to direct manipulation, such as identifying landmarks on a scanned image or selecting graphical elements from a palette of options. The suitability of a given pointing device to user tasks should be assessed.

19.14.14 INTERACTIVE CONTROL

General design objectives include consistency of control action, minimized need for control actions, and minimized memory load on the user, with flexibility of interactive control to adapt to different user needs. As a general principle, the user should decide what needs doing and when to do it. The selection of dialogue formats should be based on anticipated task requirements and user skills.

System response times should be consistent with operational requirements. Required user response times should be compatible with required system response time. Required user response times should be within the limits imposed by the total user task load expected in the operational environment.

Control–display relationships should be straightforward and explicit, as well as compatible with the lowest anticipated skill levels of users. Control actions should be simple and direct, whereas potentially destructive control actions should require focused user attention and command validation/confirmation before they are performed. Steps should be taken to prevent accidental use of destructive controls, including possible erasures or memory dump.

Feedback responses to correct user input should consist of changes in the state or value of those elements of the displays that are being controlled. These responses should be provided in an expected and logical manner. An acknowledgement message should be employed in those cases where the more conventional mechanism is not appropriate. Where control input errors are detected by the system, error messages and error recovery procedures should be available.

Menu selection can be used for interactive controls. Menu selection of commands is useful for tasks that involve the selection of a limited number of options or that can be listed in a menu, or in cases when users may have relatively little training. A menu command system that involves several layers can be useful when a command set is so large that users are unable to commit all the commands to memory and a reasonable hierarchy of commands exists for the user.

Form-filling interactive control may be used when some flexibility in data to be entered is needed and when the users will have moderate training. A form-filling dialogue should not be used when the computer has to handle multiple types of forms and computer response is slow.

Fixed-function key interactive control may be used for tasks requiring a limited number of control inputs or in conjunction with other dialogue types.

Command language interactive control may be used for tasks involving a wide range of user inputs and when user familiarity with the system can take advantage of the flexibility and speed of the control technique.

Question and answer dialogues should be considered for routine data entry tasks when data items are known and their ordering can be constrained, when users have little or no training, and when the computer is expected to have moderate response speed.

Query language dialogue should be used for tasks emphasizing unpredictable information retrieval with trained user. Query languages should reflect a data structure or organization perceived by the users to be natural.

Graphic interaction as a dialogue may be used to provide graphic aids as a supplement to other types of interactive control. Graphic menus may be used that display icons to represent the control options. This may be particularly valuable when system users have different linguistic backgrounds.

19.14.15 FEEDBACK

Feedback should be provided that presents status, information, confirmation, and verification throughout the interaction. When system functioning requires the user to standby, WAIT or similar type messages should be displayed until interaction is again possible. When the standby or delay may last a significant period of time, the user should be informed. When a control process or sequence is completed or aborted by the system, a positive indication should be presented to the user about the outcome of the process and the requirements for subsequent user action. If the system rejects a user input, feedback should be provided to indicate why the input was rejected and the required corrective action.

Feedback should be self-explanatory. Users should not be made to translate feedback messages by using a reference system or code sheets. Abbreviations should not be used unless necessary.

19.14.16 PROMPTS

Prompts and help instructions should be used to explain commands, error messages, system capabilities, display formats, procedures, and sequences, as well as to provide data. When operating in special modes, the system should display the mode designation and the file(s) being processed. Before processing any user requests that would result in extensive or final changes to existing data, the system should require user confirmation. When missing data are detected, the system should prompt the user. When data entries or changes will be nullified by an abort action, the user should be requested to confirm the abort.

Neither humor nor admonishment should be used in structuring prompt messages. The dialogue should be strictly factual and informative. Error messages should appear as close as possible in time and space to the user entry that caused the message. If a user repeats an entry error, the second error message should be revised to include a noticeable change so that the user may be certain that the computer has processed the attempted correction.

Prompting messages should be displayed in a standardized area of the display. Prompts and help instructions for system-controlled dialogue should be clear and explicit. The user should not be required to memorize lengthy sequences or refer to secondary written procedural references.

19.14.17 DEFAULTS

Manufacturer's default settings and configurations should be provided in order to reduce user workload. Currently defined default values should be displayed automatically in their appropriate data fields with the initiation of a data entry transaction. The user should indicate acceptance of the default values. Upon user request, manufacturers should provide a convenient means by which the user may restore factory default settings.

Users should have the option of setting their own default values for alarms and configurations on the basis of personal experience. A device may retain and store one or more sets of user default settings. Activation of these settings should require deliberate action by the user.

19.14.18 ERROR MANAGEMENT/DATA PROTECTION

When users are required to make entries into a system, an easy means of correcting erroneous entries should be provided. The system should permit correction of individual errors without requiring re-entry of correctly entered commands or data elements.

REFERENCES

ANSI/AAMI HE74, *Human Factors Design Process for Medical Devices*, Association for the Advancement of Medical Instrumentation, Arlington, VA, 2001.

Association for the Advancement of Medical Instrumentation (AAMI), *Human Factors Engineering Guidelines and Preferred Practices for the Design of Medical Devices*, Association for the Advancement of Medical Instrumentation, Arlington, VA, 1993.

Backinger, C. and Kingsley, P., *Write It Right: Recommendations for Developing User Instruction Manuals for Medical Devices Used in Home Health Care*, U.S. Department of Health and Human Services, Rockville, MD, 1993.

Bogner, M.S., *Human Error in Medicine*, Lawrence Erlbaum Associates, Hillsdale, NJ, 1994.

Brown, C.M., *Human–computer Interface Design Guidelines*, Ablex Publishing Company, Norwood, NJ, 1989.

Fries, R.C., Human factors and system reliability, in *Medical Device Technology*, 3(2), March, 1992.

Fries, R.C., *Reliable Design of Medical Devices*, Marcel-Dekker, Inc., New York, 1997.

Fries, R.C., *Handbook of Medical Device Design*, Marcel-Dekker, Inc., New York, 2001.

Hartson, H.R., *Advances in Human–Computer Interaction*, Ablex Publishing Corporation, Norwood, NJ, 1985.

King, P.H. and Fries, R.C., *Design of Biomedical Devices and Systems*, Marcel-Dekker, Inc., New York, 2002.

Le Cocq, A.D., Application of human factors engineering in medical product design, *Journal of Clinical Engineering*, 12(4), July–August, 1987, pp. 271–277.

Mathiowetz, V., et al., Grip and pinch strength: normative data for adults, in *Archives of Physical Medicine and Rehabilitation*, 66, 1985.

MIL-HDBK-759, *Human factors Engineering Design for Army Material*, Department of Defense, Washington, DC, 1981.

MIL-STD-1472, *Human Engineering Design Criteria for Military Systems, Equipment and Facilities*, Department of Defense, Washington, DC, 1981.

Morgan, C.T., *Human Engineering Guide to Equipment Design*, Academic Press, New York, 1984.

Philip, J.H., Human factors design of medical devices: the current challenge, *First Symposium on Human Factors in Medical Devices*, December 13–15, 1989, ECRI, Plymouth Meeting, PA, 1990.

Pressman, R.S., *Software Engineering*, McGraw Hill, New York, 1987.

Weinger, M.B. and Englund, C.E., Ergonomic and human factors affecting anesthetic vigilance and monitoring performance in the operating room environment, *Anesthesiology*, 73(5), November, 1990, pp. 995–1021.

Wiklund, M.E., How to implement usability engineering, *Medical Device and Diagnostic Industry*, 15(9), 1993.

Wiklund, M.E., *Medical Device and Equipment Design – Usability Engineering and Ergonomics*, Interpharm Press, Inc., Buffalo Grove, IL, 1995.

Woodson, W.E., *Human Factors Design Handbook*, McGraw Hill, New York, 1981.

Yourdon, E., *Modern Structured Analysis*, Yourdon Press, Englewood Cliffs, NJ, 1989.

Section 5

Testing and data analysis

20 The basis and types of testing

CONTENTS

20.1   Testing defined.. 334
20.2   Parsing test requirements....................................... 335
20.3   Test protocol.. 337
20.4   Test methodology 337
     20.4.1   Time testing... 337
     20.4.2   Event testing 337
     20.4.3   Stress testing 337
     20.4.4   Environmental testing 338
     20.4.5   Time related... 338
     20.4.6   Failure related...................................... 339
20.5   Purpose of the test 339
20.6   Failure definition... 339
20.7   Determining sample size and test length 339
     20.7.1   Example 20-1... 340
     20.7.2   Example 20-2... 341
20.8   Types of testing 342
     20.8.1   Verification 342
     20.8.2   Validation... 342
     20.8.3   Black box 342
     20.8.4   White box.. 343
     20.8.5   Hardware testing 343
     20.8.6   Software testing 343
     20.8.7   Functional testing 344
     20.8.8   Robustness testing................................... 345
     20.8.9   Stress testing 345
     20.8.10   Safety testing...................................... 346
     20.8.11   Regression testing 347
References... 348

Testing may be defined as subjecting a device to conditions that indicate its weaknesses, behavior characteristics, and modes of failure. It is a continuous operation throughout the development cycle that provides pertinent information to the development team. Testing may be performed for three basic reasons: basic information, verification, and validation.

Basic information testing may include vendor evaluation, vendor comparison, and component limitability. Verification is the process of evaluating the products of a given phase to ensure correctness and consistency with respect to the products and standards provided as input to that phase. Validation includes proving the subsystems and system meet the requirements of the product specification.

Testing is an essential part of any engineering development program. If the development risks are high, the test program becomes a major component of the overall development effort. To provide the basis for a properly integrated development test program, the design specification should cover all criteria to be tested including function, environment, reliability, and safety. The test program should be drawn up to cover assurance of all these design criteria.

The ultimate goal of testing is assuring that the customer is satisfied. It is the customer who pays the bills, and if we are to be successful in business we have to solve their problems. We aim for quality, but quality isn't just an abstract ideal. We are developing systems to be used, and used successfully, not to be admired on the shelf. If quality is to be a meaningful and useful goal in the real world, it must include the customer.

20.1 TESTING DEFINED

Definitions matter, although consensus as to what testing really is is less important than being able to use these definitions to focus our attention on the things that should happen when we are testing. Historically, testing has been defined in several ways:

- Establishing confidence that a device does what it is supposed to do
- The process of operating a device with the intent of finding errors
- Detecting specification errors and deviations from the specification
- Verifying that a system satisfies its specified requirements or identifying differences between expected and actual results
- The process of operating a device or component under specified conditions, observing or recording the results, and making an evaluation of some aspect of the system or component

All these definitions are useful but in different ways. Some focus on what is done while testing, others focus on more general objectives like assessing quality and customer satisfaction, while others focus on goals like expected results. If customer satisfaction is a goal, this satisfaction, or what would constitute it, should be expressed in the requirements. Identifying differences between expected and actual results is valuable because it focuses on the fact that, when we are testing, we need to be able to anticipate what is supposed to happen. It is then possible to determine what actually does happen and compare the two.

If a test is to find every conceivable fault or weakness in the system or component, then a good test is one that has a good probability of detecting an as yet undiscovered error, and a successful test is one that detects an as yet undiscovered error. The focus on showing the presence of errors is the basic attitude of a good test.

Testing is a positive and creative effort of destruction. It takes imagination, persistence and a strong sense of mission to systematically locate the weaknesses in a complex structure and to demonstrate its failures. This is one reason why it is so hard to test our own work. There is a natural real sense in which we don't want to find errors in our own material.

Errors are in the work product, not in the person who made the mistake. With the "test to destroy" attitude, we are not attacking an individual in an organization or team of developers but rather are looking for errors in those developers' work products.

Everyone on the development team needs to understand that tests add value to the product by discovering errors and getting them on the table as early as possible – to save the developers from building products based on error-ridden sources, to ensure the marketing people can deliver what the customer wants, and to ensure management gets the bottom line on the quality and finance they are looking for.

20.2   PARSING TEST REQUIREMENTS

No matter what type of test is conducted, there are certain requirements that must be proven as a result of the test. Before testing begins, it is helpful to place all requirements into a database where they may be sorted on a variety of attributes, such as a responsible subsystem. The purpose of the database is to assure all requirements are addressed in the test protocol as well as providing a convenient tracking system for the requirements. Where the number of requirements is small, manual collation of the requirements is effective. Where the number of requirements is large, the use of a software program to parse requirements is most helpful.

Once the requirements are listed, they can be used to develop the various test protocols necessary for testing. In addition, the list of requirements can be made more useful by turning them into a checklist, as seen in Figure 20-1, by adding space for additional information, such as reference to the location of a particular requirement, location of the test protocol, location of the test results, the initials of the person performing and completing the test, and the date of test completion. This checklist is also invaluable in tracking all requirements

Requirement	Requirement number	Document location	Protocol location	Results location	Initials of tester	Test date
The unit must operate according to specification after exposure to an ambient temperature of 65° Centigrade	12	Product Specification Paragraph 10.2.1	Lab notebook # R232, Page 44	Lab notebook # R232, Page 45-46	JR	6/12/96
The unit must operate according to specification after exposure to an ambient temperature of −40° Centigrade	13	Product Specification Paragraph 10.2.2	Lab notebook # R232, Page 47	Lab notebook # R232, Page 48-49	JR	6/15/96
The unit must operate according to specification after exposure to an ambient temperature of +40° Centigrade and a relative humidity of 95%	14	Product Specification Paragraph 10.2.3	Lab notebook # R232, Page 54	Lab notebook # R232, Page 55-57	JL	7/13/96

FIGURE 20-1 Sample requirements table and checklist

to satisfy Quality Assurance and Regulatory departments as well as FDA and ISO auditors.

20.3 TEST PROTOCOL

It has been said that testing without a plan is not testing at all, but an experiment. Therefore, it is essential that each test performed be detailed in a test protocol that includes:

- The name of the device under test
- The type of test being performed
- The purpose of the test
- A definition of potential failures during the test
- Any special requirements
- The number of units on test
- The length of the test in hours or cycles
- A detailed procedure for running the test or reference to a procedure in another document, such as a standard
- The parameters to be recorded

20.4 TEST METHODOLOGY

Types of testing may include time testing, event testing, stress testing, environmental testing, time-related testing, and failure-related testing.

20.4.1 TIME TESTING

Time testing is conducted primarily to determine long-term reliability parameters, such as failure rate and mean time between failure. Time testing can also be conducted to determine what part or component fails, when it fails, the mode of failure at that particular time, the mechanism of failure and how much more or less life the equipment has that is required for operational use. This allows priorities of criticality for reliability improvement to be established.

20.4.2 EVENT TESTING

Event testing consists of repeated testing of equipment through its cycle of operation until failure. This type of testing is analogous to time-to-failure testing. One important parameter developed from this type of test is the number of cycles to failure.

20.4.3 STRESS TESTING

Stress testing has an important place in reliability assessment, but care must be taken in its application. Too much overstress may cause the test results to be inconclusive, as overstress may precipitate a failure that the product would not normally experience during normal usage. Care should also be taken to overstress in steps, rather than getting to the maximum value immediately. If the device fails, the step method allows the determination of where in the progression the failure occurred.

20.4.4 ENVIRONMENTAL TESTING

Environmental testing represents a survey of the reaction of a device to the environmental and shipping environments it should experience in its daily usage. By investigating a broad spectrum of the environmental space, greater confidence is developed in the equipment than if it was merely subjected to ambient conditions. As with overstress testing, avoid unusually extreme or unrealistic environmental levels because of the difficulty in their interpretation. Table 20-1 lists some typical environmental tests and the standard associated with its execution.

20.4.5 TIME RELATED

Time-related testing is conducted until a certain number of hours of operation or a certain number of cycles has been completed, e.g., a switch test conducted

TABLE 20-1
List of typical environmental tests

Environment	Applicable standard
Operating temperature	IEC 68-2-14
Storage temperature	IEC 68-2-1
	IEC 68-2-2
Operating humidity	IEC 68-2-30
Storage humidity	IEC 68-2-3
	IEC 68-2-30
Operating ambient pressure	IEC 68-2-13
Storage ambient pressure	IEC 68-2-13
Transportation	NSTA
Radiated electrical emissions	CISPR 11
Radiated magnetic emissions	VDE 871
Radiated electrical field	IEC 601-1-2
Electrical fast transient	IEC 601-1-2
Radiated magnetic immunity	IEC 1000-4-8
Line conducted immunity	IEC 1000-4-6
Operating vibration	IEC 68-2-6
	IEC 68-2-34
Unpackaged shock	IEC 68-2-27
Stability	UL 2601
Ingress of liquids	IEC 529
	IEC 601-1
Pneumatic supply	CEN-TC215

for 100 000 ON/OFF cycles or a monitor operated for 100 000 hours. This type of test will be important in choosing the correct formula to calculate MTBF from the test data.

20.4.6 FAILURE RELATED

A test may be conducted until all test units or a certain percentage of units have failed, e.g., ventilators operated until the first unit fails or power supplies power cycled until all have failed. This type of test will be important in choosing the correct formula to calculate MTBF from the test data.

20.5 PURPOSE OF THE TEST

The purposes for testing may include the feasibility of a design, comparing two or more vendors, comparing two or more configurations, testing the response to environmental stresses, developing reliability parameters, failure analysis, or validation of the device.

All testing, except the reliability demonstration, which is performed at the end of the product development cycle, is performed at a confidence level of 90%. This means one is 90% confident that the reliability parameters established in the test will be characteristic of units in the field. A 90% confidence level also yields a risk factor of (1 − confidence level) or 10%. The reliability demonstration should be conducted at a confidence level of 95%, giving a risk factor of 5%. These levels will be important in determining the number of test units and the length of test time.

20.6 FAILURE DEFINITION

For each test and for each device, a failure must be defined. This definition depends on the intended application and the anticipated environment. What is considered a failure for one component or device may not be a failure for another. The test protocol should be as detailed as possible in defining the failure.

20.7 DETERMINING SAMPLE SIZE AND TEST LENGTH

Once you determine the type of test to be performed, you need to decide on the test sample size and the length of time necessary to accomplish your testing goal. Sample size and test time are dependent upon the MTBF goal, originally defined in the product specification and on the confidence level at which the test will be conducted.

The formula for determining the sample size and test time is derived from the following equation:

$$\text{MTBF goal} = (\text{sample size})(\text{test time})(2)/\chi^2_{\alpha;2r+2} \qquad (20.1)$$

The equation thus becomes:

$$(\text{sample size})(\text{test time}) = \text{MTBF goal } (\chi^2_{\alpha;2r+2})/2 \qquad (20.2)$$

To complete the equation, we must first understand the Chi square chart included in Appendix 1. To use this chart first find the risk factor that the chart is based upon. As mentioned earlier, the risk factor is derived from the confidence level:

$$\text{Confidence level} = 1 - \alpha$$
$$\text{where } \alpha \text{ is the risk factor}$$

Thus, a confidence level of 90% yields a risk factor of 10%, while a confidence level of 95% yields a risk factor of 5%. Using the 90% confidence level, $\alpha = 0.10$ in equation 20.2.

The "r" in equation 20.2 is the number of failures. When calculating sample size and test time, it is assumed there will be no failures. This results in the minimal test time. Thus $r = 2(0)+2$ or 2 and equation 20.2 becomes

$$(\text{sample size})(\text{test time}) = (\text{MTBF goal})(\chi^2_{\alpha;2})/2$$

Looking at the Chi square chart in Appendix 1, go across the top row of the chart and find 0.10, or *. Go down that column to the line for $v = 2$. There you will find the number 4.605, or 4.61. Put this into the equation:

$$(\text{sample size})(\text{test time}) = \text{MTBF goal } (4.61)/2 \qquad (20.3)$$

Inserting the MTBF goal into the equation and solving it yields the unit test time or (sample size)(test time).

20.7.1 EXAMPLE 20-1

We want to test some power supplies to prove a MTBF goal of 50 000 hours of operation. How many units do we test and for how long, assuming no failures?

$$(\text{sample size})(\text{test time}) = \text{MTBF goal}(4.61)/2$$
$$(\text{sample size})(\text{test time}) = 50\,000(4.61)/2$$
$$= 115\,250 \text{ unit-hours}$$

From these data, we can calculate the possibilities listed in Table 20-2. These data are based on the statistical law that states that 1 unit tested for 10 000 hours is statistically equal to 10 units tested for 1000 hours each and 50 units tested for 200 hours each.

TABLE 20-2
Example 20-1: Sample size versus test time possibilities

Sample size	Test time (hours)
3	38 417
5	23 050
10	11 525
15	7 683
20	5 763
25	4 610
50	2 305
100	1 153

20.7.2 EXAMPLE 20-2

We want to test some power supplies to prove a MTBF goal of 50 000 hours of operation. How many units do we test and for how long, assuming one failure?

$$(\text{sample size})(\text{test time}) = (\text{MTBF goal})(\chi^2_{\alpha;2})/2$$

In this case, using the 90% confidence level, $\alpha = 0.10$ and $r = 2(1)+2$ or 4. Looking at the Chi square chart in Appendix 1, go across the top row of the chart and find 0.10. Go down that column to the line for $v = 4$. There you will find the number 7.779. Put this into the equation:

$$(\text{sample size})(\text{test time}) = \text{MTBF goal } (7.779)/2$$
$$(\text{sample size})(\text{test time}) = 50\,000\,(7.779)/2$$
$$= 194\,475 \text{ unit-hours}$$

From these data, we can calculate the possibilities listed in Table 20-3. Again, these data are based on the statistical law that states that 1 unit tested for 10 000 hours is statistically equal to 10 units tested for 1000 hours each and 50 units tested for 200 hours each.

An interesting observation is that one failure increased the test time by 69%. A second failure would yield the equation:

$$(\text{sample size})(\text{test time}) = 50\,000(10.645)/2$$
$$= 266\,125$$

This is an increase in time of 37% over the one failure example and 131% over zero failures. This proves that unreliability is costly in time and effort.

TABLE 20-3
Example 20-2: Sample size versus test time

Sample size	Test time (hours)
3	64 825
5	38 895
10	19 448
15	12 965
20	9 724
25	7 779
50	3 890
100	1 945

20.8 TYPES OF TESTING

20.8.1 VERIFICATION

Procedures that attempt to determine that the product of each phase of the development process is an implementation of a previous phase, i.e., it satisfies it. Each verification activity is a phase of the testing life cycle. The testing objective in each verification activity is to detect as many errors as possible. The testing team should leverage its efforts by participating in any inspections and walkthroughs conducted by development and by initiating verification, especially at the early stages of development.

20.8.2 VALIDATION

Validation is the process of evaluating a system or component during or at the end of the development process to determine whether it satisfies specified requirements.

20.8.3 BLACK BOX

The easiest way to understand black box testing is to visualize a black box with a set of inputs coming into it and a set of outputs coming out of it. The black box test is performed without any knowledge of the internal structure. The black box test verifies that the end-user requirements are met from the end-user's point of view.

Black box testing is a data-driven testing scheme. The tester views the device or program as a black box, i.e., the tester is not concerned about the internal behavior and structure. The tester is only interested in finding circumstances in which the device or program does not behave according to its specification. Black box testing that is used to detect errors leads to exhaustive input testing, as every possible input condition is a test case.

20.8.4 WHITE BOX

White box testing is the opposite of black box testing. It is performed by personnel who are knowledgeable of the internal structure and are testing from the developer's point of view.

White box testing is a logic-driven testing scheme. The tester examines the internal structure of the device or program and derives test data from an examination of the internal structure. White box testing is concerned with the degree to which test cases exercise or cover the structure of the device or program. The ultimate white box test is an exhaustive path test.

20.8.5 HARDWARE TESTING

Hardware testing includes various types of tests depending on the intended use of the device. Testing that occurs during almost every product development cycle includes:

- Vendor evaluation
- Component variation
- Environmental testing
- Safety evaluation
- Shipping tests
- Standards evaluation
- Product use/misuse
- Reliability demonstration

Often, hardware testing, especially that associated with the calculation of reliability parameters is performed twice during the development process. The first occurs immediately after the design phase and evaluates the robustness and reliability of the design. The second occurs after production of customer units begins. This testing evaluates the robustness and reliability of the manufacturing process.

Hardware testing is discussed in detail in Chapter 21.

20.8.6 SOFTWARE TESTING

Software testing consists of several levels of evaluation. Initially, module testing occurs, where the individual modules of the software program are evaluated and stress tested. This testing consists of verifying the design and implementation of the specification at the smallest component of the program. Testing involves running each module independently to assure it works, and then inserting errors, possibly through the use of an emulator. The test is basically an interface between the programmer and the software environment.

Integration testing occurs after each of the modules has been successfully tested. The various modules are then integrated with each other and tested to assure they work together.

System testing consists of merging the software with the hardware to assure both will work as a system. Testing involves verifying the external software interfaces, assuring the system requirements are met, and assuring the system, as a whole, is operational.

Acceptance testing is the final review of all the requirements specified for the system and assuring both hardware and software address them.

20.8.7 FUNCTIONAL TESTING

Functional testing (Table 20-4) is designed to verify that all the functional requirements have been satisfied. This type of testing verifies that given all the expected inputs then all of the expected outputs are produced. This type of testing is termed success-oriented testing because the tests are expected to produce successful results.

Testing of the functional capabilities involves the exercising of the operational modes and the events that allow a transition between the various software operational states. These tests are performed to verify that proper mode transitions are executed and proper outputs are generated given the correct inputs. These tests also verify that the software generates the expected output given the expected user input. A communication test tool should be utilized to test the proper operation of the remote communications protocol and functionality of the communications software located in the product under test. Timing tests should be performed for system critical functions relating to the system critical time and the operational window. Battery tests should be performed whenever a software change to the software that monitors the battery levels has been made. In addition, if new functionality is pushing the product to the absolute performance edge, then battery tests should also be performed because of its potential effect on any power down software routines.

TABLE 20-4
Examples of functional testing

Test type	Example
Functional modes	Transitions between operational modes
	Correct inputs generate correct outputs
	Inputs and outputs include switches, tones, messages and alarms
Remote communications	Connect and disconnect tests
	Valid commands and inquiries tests
	Handling of invalid commands and inquiries
	Tests for all baud rates supported
	Corrupted frames tests
	Error handling in general and the interface to the error handler
	Control mode testing with emphasis on safety
	Monitor mode testing with emphasis on fidelity of values reported
Timing	Active failure tests are completed within the system critical time
	Passive failure tests are completed within the operational window
Battery	Ramp up and ramp down of voltages
	Test the various levels of warnings, alarms, and errors

TABLE 20-5
Examples of robustness testing

Test type	Example
Boundary	Over and under specified limits
	Numerical values which determine logic flow based on a maximum or minimum value
	Negative numerical values
Overflow and underflow	Values too large for all algorithms
	Values too small for all algorithms
User interface	Enter unexpected values
	Enter unexpected sequences
Execution time line processing	Routines which have execution time limits are altered to introduce delays
	Tasks which have execution time limits are altered to introduce delays
	Routines with execution constraints due to parametric calculations are altered
Data transmission	Unexpected commands are transmitted to the remote communications handler
	Unexpected data are transmitted to the remote communications handler

20.8.8 ROBUSTNESS TESTING

Robustness testing (Table 20-5) is designed to determine how the software performs given unexpected inputs. Robustness testing determines whether the software recovers from an unexpected input, locks the system in an indeterminate state or continues to operate in a manner which is unpredictable. This type of testing is termed failure oriented because the test inputs are designed to cause the product to fail given foreseeable and reasonably unforeseeable misuse of the product.

Robustness testing is performed in order to determine software responses at the boundary limits of the product or test and manufacturing equipment and the test cases should include negative values.

As a part of robustness testing, algorithms are tested for overflow and underflow. The user interface is tested by entering unexpected values and sequences. Routines, tasks, or processes that are time constrained are altered to introduce reasonable delays in order to determine the reaction of the product or equipment. Communication software is given unexpected commands and data that are then transmitted to the remote communications handler.

20.8.9 STRESS TESTING

Stress testing (Table 20-6) is designed to ascertain how the product reacts to a condition in which the amount or rate of data exceeds the amount or rate

TABLE 20-6
Example of stress testing

Test type	Example
Duration	Overnight runs
	Weekend runs
	Other types of software burn-in tests
Buffer overload	Global buffers tested under loaded and overflow conditions
	Global data structures tested under loaded and overflow conditions
Remote communications	Verify the transfer at the maximum transfer rate
	Verify the transfer at the maximum transfer rate under maximum load conditions
Worst case scenario	Verify the product and test and manufacturing equipments operating capability under projected worst case
	Highest execution rate
	Event overload for event driven system

expected. Stress tests can help determine the margin of safety that exists in the product or equipment.

Stress tests are performed which exercise the equipment continuously over varying periods of time and operating parameters if latent errors exist in the software. Generally, these tests consist of overnight runs and weekend runs that gain the optimum benefit of the allotted test time. Global buffers and data structures are tested under loaded and overflow conditions in order to determine the response of the software. Remote communications load tests should be performed which verify the remote communications interface transfer rate at the maximum transfer rate under worst-case and maximum-load conditions. Worst-case scenario tests verify the product or equipment operating capability under the projected worst-case scenario. The worst-case scenario for products generally includes highest execution rate and event overload for event-driven systems. These tests should be limited to reasonable environmental tests which do not include temperature and vibration testing.

20.8.10 SAFETY TESTING

Safety testing (Table 20-7) is designed to verify that the product performs in a safe manner and that a complete assessment of the safety design has been accomplished.

Fail-safe tests should be performed specifically to verify the fail-safe provisions of the software design. These tests cover the error conditions only and do not address warnings or alarms which are more appropriately tested under the functional tests. Limited, non-destructive fault insertion tests should be performed by the software verification and validation engineers. Products require an analysis of the error handling routines as well as data corruption

TABLE 20-7
Examples of safety testing

Test type	Example
Fail-safe	Verify fail safe provisions of the software design
	Test error conditions and handling
	Test data corruption
Active failure	Tests completion within system critical time
	ROM testing via CRC computation and comparison to a stored value
	RAM testing for stuck bits in data and address paths
	RAM testing for address decoding problems
	LED indicators voltage tests
	Processor and controller tests
Passive failure	Watchdog timer test
	Watchdog disable tests
	Hardware RAM tests
	CRC generator
	Battery test
	Audio generators and speaker tests
	EEPROM tests
Safety	Critical parameters and their duplicates
	Events that lead to a loss of audio indicators
	Events that lead to a loss of visual indicators
	Events that lead to tactile errors, such as a key press
	Error handling for corrupted vectors and structures
	Error handling for corrupted sanity checks
	Sufficiency of periodic versus aperiodic tests
From hazard analysis	Single point failures
	Normal power up, run-time and power down safety tests

tests to ensure an acceptable level of safety. The analysis must include a review of the products active failure tests so that they are completed within the system critical time and within the product-defined operational window. A number of safety aspects that must also be addressed are the protection of critical parameters and events that lead to a loss of safety critical indicators. Safety testing of the product must utilize the hazards analysis in relation to failures. In addition, validation safety tests and internal product safety self tests that were performed on past products should be compiled, executed, and compared against the new product under test in order to arrive at a consistent and growing list of mandatory safety tests.

20.8.11 REGRESSION TESTING

Regression testing (Table 20-8) is performed whenever a software change or a hardware change that affects the software has occurred. Regression testing verifies that the change produces the desired effect on the altered component

TABLE 20-8
Regression testing sequence

Sequence step	Activity
1	Compare the new software to the existing baseline
2	Generate a cross reference listing to assess changes and to ensure no unintended side effects
3	Assess the amount of changes and the criticality
4	Determine the level of effort required and assess the risk
5	Test the new functions and the debug fixes
6	Execute a predetermined set of core tests to confirm no new unintended changes
7	Devote special attention to the safety implications

and that no other component that relies on the altered component is adversely affected.

Regression testing is performed on products and test and manufacturing equipment that have made a change to an established, validated baseline. Regression testing begins by comparing the new software to the existing baseline with a version difference tool and the generation of a cross-reference listing to assess the changes and to ensure that no unintended side effects are introduced. From this, an assessment of the amount of changes and their criticality is made, the level of effort that is required to perform the regression is estimated and the risk is assessed. The alterations are tested and a compiled list of core tests are executed in order to establish that no new unintended changes have been introduced. Special attention must be made to the safety implications.

REFERENCES

Fries, R.C., *Reliability Assurance for Medical Devices, Equipment and Software*, Interpharm Press, Buffalo Grove, IL, 1991.

Fries, R.C., *Reliable Design of Medical Devices*, Marcel-Dekker, Inc., New York, 1997.

Fries, R.C., *Handbook of Medical Device Design*, Marcel-Dekker, Inc., New York, 2001.

King, P.H. and Fries, R.C., *Design of Biomedical Devices and Systems*, Marcel-Dekker, Inc., New York, 2002.

Kit, E., *Software Testing in the Real World – Improving the Process*, Addison-Wesley Publishing Company, Reading, MA, 1995.

Laplante, P., *Real-Time Systems Design and Analysis – An Engineer's Handbook*, The Institute of Electrical and Electronic Engineers, Inc., New York, 1993.

Myers, G.J., *The Art of Software Testing*, John Wiley & Sons, New York, 1979.

Neufelder, A.M., *Ensuring Software Reliability*, Marcel-Dekker, Inc., New York, 1993.

21 Hardware verification and validation

CONTENTS

21.1 Standard tests.. 350
    21.1.1 Cycle testing.. 350
    21.1.2 Typical use testing..................................... 350
    21.1.3 10 × 10 testing....................................... 350
21.2 Environmental testing....................................... 351
    21.2.1 Operating temperature testing........................ 352
    21.2.2 Storage temperature testing.......................... 352
    21.2.3 Thermal shock testing............................... 352
    21.2.4 Humidity testing..................................... 353
    21.2.5 Mechanical shock testing............................ 353
    21.2.6 Mechanical vibration testing......................... 354
    21.2.7 Impact testing....................................... 354
    21.2.8 Electrostatic discharge............................... 355
    21.2.9 Electromagnetic compatibility........................ 355
21.3 Accelerated testing.. 356
    21.3.1 Increasing sample size............................... 356
    21.3.2 Increasing test severity.............................. 356
    21.3.3 Example 21-1... 357
    21.3.4 Example 21-2... 358
21.4 Sudden death testing.. 359
    21.4.1 Weibull testing and plotting.......................... 359
        21.4.1.1 Example 21-3.............................. 359
        21.4.1.2 Confidence limits......................... 360
        21.4.1.3 The shape of Weibull plots................ 361
21.5 The sudden death test....................................... 362
    21.5.1 Sudden death example............................... 365
References.. 369

The heart of the product development process is the verification and validation phase. During this time, testing indicates how well the product has been designed. The parts count reliability prediction had indicated whether the

349

design would meet the reliability goal. It indicated what parts of the circuit had the potential for a high failure rate. Design and tolerance analysis had indicated whether the correct component was being used and if it had been specified properly. None of these exercises had indicated how well the components would work together, once the device became operational. To obtain this information, the device must be tested both in its intended application environment as well as in the worst-case condition.

21.1   STANDARD TESTS

Standard tests are conducted at room temperature, with no acceleration of any parameters. Standard tests are varied, dependent upon their purpose, and include:

- Cycle testing
- Typical use testing
- 10×10 testing

21.1.1   CYCLE TESTING

Cycle testing is usually conducted on individual components, such as switches, phone jacks, or cable. Testing consists of placing the component in alternating states, such as ON and OFF for a switch or IN and OUT for a phone plug, while monitoring the operation in each state. One cycle consists of one pass through each state.

Cycle testing could also consist of passing through the state of operation and non-operation of a component or device. Thus a power supply could be power-cycled, with a cycle consisting of going from zero power to maximum power and back to zero. For devices, a cycle could consist of 8 hours ON and 16 hours OFF.

21.1.2   TYPICAL USE TESTING

Typical use testing consists of operation of a device as it will be operated in its typical environment. This testing is usually incorporated when conducting a reliability demonstration or for calculating a long-term MTBF value.

The test unit is tested electrically and mechanically prior to testing and certain parameters are checked at periodic times, such as 2, 4, 8, 24, 48, 72, 96 and 128 hours after beginning the test and weekly thereafter. These recordings aid in determining drift or degradation in certain parameters.

21.1.3 10×10 TESTING

Ten samples of a component or device are subjected to a test where recordings of a particular parameter are taken at ten different time periods. A chart is

Unit	1	2	3	4	5	6	7	8	9	10	Mean	S.D.
1	350	380	400	360	340	370	330	340	360	340	357	20
2	200	130	190	200	130	150	250	230	240	160	188	41
3	270	250	270	240	300	230	330	330	300	350	287	39
4	270	140	160	170	160	140	430	130	130	130	186	90
5	230	180	170	150	260	240	210	230	240	210	212	33
6	280	180	70	390	300	210	400	440	370	230	287	110
7	180	210	270	190	210	170	170	270	190	200	206	34
8	190	220	180	190	170	190	200	120	170	130	176	29
9	200	180	160	180	200	120	90	170	140	170	161	33
10	230	190	260	180	290	170	280	220	260	170	225	43
Mean	240	206	213	225	236	199	269	248	240	209		
S.D.	50	66	85	78	67	67	100	95	80	74		

FIGURE 21-1 10 × 10 test matrix

created with the ten units listed in the left column and the ten recordings listed across the top (Figure 21-1). Mean and standard deviation values are calculated for each of the ten recordings and ten units.

By reading the horizontal rows of data, the repeatability of the results can be determined. By analyzing the vertical columns, the variability among the units can be measured.

21.2 ENVIRONMENTAL TESTING

Environmental testing is conducted on a device to assure its ability to withstand the environmental stresses associated with its shipping and operational life. Testing is usually conducted on the first devices built in the manufacturing area under manufacturing processes. Environmental testing includes:

- Operating temperature
- Storage temperature
- Thermal shock
- Humidity
- Mechanical shock
- Mechanical vibration
- Impact
- Electrostatic discharge
- Electromagnetic compatibility

Prior to each test, the device is tested electrically and mechanically to assure it is functioning according to specification. At the conclusion of each environmental test, the device is again tested electrically and mechanically to determine if the environmental test has affected the specified operation. Any observed failures will be fixed and a decision to rerun the test made, based on the type of change made and the inherent risk.

21.2.1   OPERATING TEMPERATURE TESTING

The operating temperature test assures the device will operate according to specification at the extremes of the typical operating temperature range. The test also analyzes the internal temperatures of the device to ensure none exceed the temperature limits of any components.

After the functional checkout, the device has thermocouples placed inside at locations that are predicted to be the hottest. The device is turned ON and placed in a temperature chamber for 4 hours at each of the operating temperature limits as specified in the Product Specification or at $0°$ Centigrade and $+55°$ Centigrade if no limits are specified. Between temperatures, the device should be removed from the chamber until it has reached the appropriate temperature. Thermocouple readings are recorded continuously on a chart recorder throughout the test. Where a chart recorder is not available, the readings should be taken every 30 minutes.

The unit is functionally tested after the temperature exposure. The thermocouple readings are evaluated with regard to the upper extreme of component temperatures.

21.2.2   STORAGE TEMPERATURE TESTING

The storage temperature test assures the device will withstand the stresses of the shipping and storage environment. After the functional checkout, the device is turned OFF and placed in a temperature chamber for 8 hours at each of the storage temperature limits as specified in the Product Specification or at $-40°$ Centigrade and $+65°$ Centigrade if no limits are specified. Between temperatures, the device should be removed from the chamber, allowed to come to room temperature and then functionally tested. The unit is functionally tested after the temperature exposure.

21.2.3   THERMAL SHOCK TESTING

The thermal shock test assures the device will withstand the stresses of alternate exposure to hot and cold temperatures. After the functional checkout, the device is turned OFF and placed in a thermal shock chamber with one chamber set at $-20°$ Centigrade, the second chamber set at $+55°$ Centigrade and the transition time between chambers set at less than 5 minutes. The minimum time spent at each temperature is one hour. The device should be cycled through a minimum of five cycles of temperature extremes. The unit is functionally tested after the temperature exposure.

21.2.4 HUMIDITY TESTING

The humidity test assures the device will withstand the stresses of exposure to a humid environment. After the functional checkout, the device is turned off and placed in a humidity chamber with the environment set to 40° Centigrade and 95% relative humidity. The chamber and accessories are so constructed that condensate will not drip on the device. The chamber shall also be trans-vented to the atmosphere to prevent the buildup of total pressure. The device will be exposed for a maximum of 21 days.

The unit is allowed to dry following exposure. It is then opened and examined for moisture damage. All observations are documented with photographs if possible. The unit is then functionally tested.

21.2.5 MECHANICAL SHOCK TESTING

The mechanical shock test assures the device is able to withstand the stresses of handling, shipping, and everyday use. Devices may be tested in the packaged or unpackaged state. Devices may also be tested on a shock table where parameters are set, such as in Table 21-1, to meet the anticipated environment. When using the shock table, several types of waveforms are ordinarily available, depending on the type of impact expected. The haversine waveform simulates impact with a rebound while a sawtooth waveform simulates impact with no rebound. The device may also be dropped the designated distance, from Table 21-1, on to a hard surface by measuring the height above the floor and dropping the device. One disadvantage of the drop test is the inability to adjust the shock pulse to match the surface and the rebound. With either type of test, the device is usually shocked a maximum of three times in each axis. Following testing, the device is examined for any internal damage. The device is also functionally tested.

TABLE 21-1
Mechanical shock parameters

Device Weight (lbs)	Device Greatest dimension (inches)	Effective free fall height (in.)	Typical Values Acceleration (Gs)	Pulse duration (msec)
<100	<36	48	500	2
	>36	30	400	2
100–200	<36	30	400	2
	>36	24	350	2
200–1000	<36	24	350	2
	36–60	36	430	2
	>60	24	350	2
>1000		18	300	2

21.2.6 MECHANICAL VIBRATION TESTING

The mechanical vibration test assures the device is able to withstand the vibration stresses of handling, shipping, and everyday use, especially where the device is mobile.

Devices may be tested in the packaged or unpackaged state. In the unpackaged state, holes are cut in the device for observation of the internal hardware with a strobe light or for insertion of accelerometers for measuring vibration. Accelerometers are attached to the desired components and their frequencies and amplitudes recorded on an X–Y plotter.

Vibrate the device via a frequency sweep or via random vibration. The random vibration more closely simulates the actual field environment, although resonant frequencies and the frequencies of component damage are more easily obtained with the frequency sweep.

When using the frequency sweep, the sweep should be in accordance with the suggested parameters listed in Table 21-2. Subject the device to three sweeps in one axis at a sweep rate of 0.5 octave/min. An octave is defined as the interval of two frequencies having a basic ratio of 2. During the sweeps, the acceleration, as listed in Table 21-2, is the maximum acceleration observed at any point on the device.

Resonant frequencies are determined either through accelerometer readings or through observation of the internal hardware. Resonances are defined as board or component movement of a minimum of twice the difference between the device and table acceleration. Severe resonance is usually accompanied by a steady drone from the resonating component. Once resonant frequencies are determined, a dwell at each resonant frequency for 15 minutes follows the frequency sweeps.

The above tests are repeated until all three orthogonal axes have been tested. The unit is examined for physical damage and functionally tested after each axis is completed.

21.2.7 IMPACT TESTING

Impact testing assures the ability of the device to withstand the collision stresses of shipping and everyday use for mobile devices. The test simulates large, mobile devices bumping into walls or door frames while being moved.

TABLE 21-2
Mechanical vibration parameters

Locale	Format	Frequency sweep	Acceleration
Domestic	Unpackaged	5–200–5 Hz	1.5 G
International	Unpackaged	5–300–5 Hz	2.0 G
Domestic	Packaged	5–300–5 Hz	1.5 G
International	Packaged	5–500–5 Hz	2.0 G

The test is conducted by rolling a device down an inclined ramp and allowing it to slam into a solid wall or by attaching the device to an adjustable piston drive, which is set to slam the device into a solid wall with a predetermined force. The unit is functionally tested following impact.

21.2.8 ELECTROSTATIC DISCHARGE

Electrostatic discharge testing assures the ability of the device to withstand short-duration voltage transients caused by static electricity, capacitive or inductive effects, and load switching. For software-controlled devices, a differentiation between hard failures (failures that cause the device to become inoperable and not rebootable) and soft failures (failures that cause the device to become inoperable but rebootable) must be made and the acceptability of each defined, according to risk.

The device is placed on a grounded metal plane. Static discharges are delivered to the four quadrants of the plane and to appropriate places on the device, such as front panel, back panel, keyboard, etc., from a static generator or a current injector. One-shot static charges should be delivered directly to the device and to the air surrounding the device. Where the device is connected to accessory equipment via cables, such as analog or RS-232 cables, static discharges should be delivered in the area of the cable connections, on both pieces of equipment. All discharges should be one-shot and should begin at 2000 volts and increase in 2000 volt increments until the maximum of 20 000 volts is reached. The unit is functionally tested following application of ESD.

21.2.9 ELECTROMAGNETIC COMPATIBILITY

Electromagnetic compatibility (EMC) testing is conducted to determine the maximum levels of electromagnetic emissions the device is allowed to produce and to determine the minimum levels of electromagnetic interference to which the device must not be susceptible. Medical devices, especially those used in the operating room environment, must not interfere with the operation of other devices or have its operation interfered with by other devices through electromagnetic radiations.

It is particularly important to conduct EMC testing on products containing:

- Digital circuitry, especially microprocessor-based devices
- Circuits containing clock or crystal oscillators
- Devices where data information is transmitted via a telemetric or radio frequency link
- Monitors used in close proximity to other devices, or where they cause feedback to other devices

Tests should be conducted in a testing laboratory containing an anechoic chamber or shielded chamber of sufficient size to adequately contain the test.

The device is configured and operated in a manner that approximates its use in a medical facility. When necessary, a dummy load and/or signal simulator may be employed to duplicate actual equipment operation.

It is a known that most Bovie units, especially older ones, produce radiation that is worse than that called out in any standard. Thus, as a practical approach to EMC, many companies use a Bovie unit in the vicinity of the test device to check its susceptibility. In the laboratory environment, the test device can be used in the presence of other devices to test its radiation. Subject all devices to conducted and radiated emissions and to conducted and radiated susceptibility testing. Monitor the functionality of the unit throughout the test.

A new concern in the EMC area is the use of cellular phones in the hospital. It is felt these phones put out emissions to which other devices are susceptible. The FDA is currently researching this area. It is expected that this area will be included in required EMC testing.

21.3 ACCELERATED TESTING

The length of time available to conduct a test determines whether the test is performed in a standard or an accelerated mode. In the standard mode, tests are run at ambient temperature and typical usage parameters. The test time is the actual time of operation. In the accelerated mode, test time is reduced by varying parameters, such as temperature, voltage, or frequency of cycling, above their normal levels, or performing a test, such as sudden death testing.

Accelerated testing is a shortening of the length of the test time by varying the parameters of the test. Testing can be accelerated in several ways:

- Increase the sample size
- Increase the test severity
- Use sudden death testing

21.3.1 INCREASING SAMPLE SIZE

Reliability tests are accelerated by increasing the sample size, provided the life distribution does not show a wearout characteristic during the anticipated life. Test time is inversely proportional to the sample size, so that increasing the sample size reduces the test time.

Large sample size reliability test conducted to provide a high total operating time should be supported by some long-duration tests if there is a reason to suspect that failure modes exist which have high times to failure.

21.3.2 INCREASING TEST SEVERITY

Increasing test severity is a logical approach to reducing test time when large sample sizes cannot be used.

The severity of tests may be increased by increasing the stresses acting on the test unit. These stresses can be grouped into two categories:

- Operational, such as temperature and humidity
- Application, such as voltage, current, self-generated heat or self-generated mechanical stresses

Increasing the temperature severity is the usual method of accelerating testing.

It is important, in accelerated testing, to assure that unrealistic failure modes are not introduced by the higher stresses. It is also possible that interactions may occur between separate stresses, so that the combined weakening effect is greater that would be expected from a single additive process.

When conducting accelerated testing, an essential calculation is acceleration factor, that is the parameter that indicates how much acceleration was conducted. To calculate the acceleration factor, the following equation is used:

$$\text{acceleration factor} = \exp(-(EA/K)(1/TA - 1/TU)) \qquad (21.1)$$

where

EA = energy of activation (0.5 eV)

K = Boltzman's constant (0.0000863 eV/degree Kelvin)

TU = temperature in degrees Kelvin

TA = accelerate temperature in degrees Kelvin.

21.3.3 EXAMPLE 21-1

Ten power supplies are tested to failure at 150° Centigrade. The units are expected to be used at 85° Centigrade. What is the minimum life (time of the first failure) at 85° Centigrade? What is the MTBF at 85° Centigrade?

The failure rates in hours are listed as:

2750 3100 3400 3800 4100
4400 4700 5100 5700 6400

Calculation of acceleration factor:

$$EA = 0.5$$
$$K = 0.0000863$$
$$TU = 85 + 273 = 358° \text{ Kelvin}$$
$$TA = 150 = 273 = 423° \text{ Kelvin}$$
$$\text{Acceleration factor} = \exp(-(EA/K)(1/TA - 1/TU))$$
$$= e(-(0.5/0.0000863)(1/423 - 1/358))$$
$$= 12$$

Calculation of minimum life at 85° Centigrade:

$$\text{minimum life} = (\text{acceleration factor}) \times (\text{failure at } 85°)$$
$$= (12) \times (2750)$$
$$= 33\,000 \text{ hours}$$

Calculation of MTBF at 150° Centigrade:

$$\text{MTBF} = \text{sum of the times of operation/number of errors}$$
$$= 2750 + 3100 + 3400 + 3800 + 4100 + 4400 + 4700 + 5100$$
$$+ 5700 + 6400/10$$
$$= 43\,450/10$$
$$= 4345 \text{ hours}$$

Calculation of MTBF at 85° Centigrade:

$$\text{MTBF} = \text{acceleration factor (MTBF at } 150°)$$
$$= 12(4345)$$
$$= 52\,140 \text{ hours}$$

21.3.4   EXAMPLE 21-2

Integrated circuits are to be burned-in to eliminate infant mortality failures. We want the burn-in to be equivalent to 1000 hours of operation at ambient temperature (24° Centigrade). How long do we run the units at 50° Centigrade? How long do we run the units at 100° Centigrade?

Calculation at 50° Centigrade:

$$\text{acceleration factor} = \exp(-(EA/K)(1/TA - 1/TU))$$
$$= e(0.5/0.0000863)(1/323 - 1/297)$$
$$= 4.8$$
$$\text{length of run time} = \text{run time at } 24°/\text{acceleration factor}$$
$$= 1000/4.8$$
$$= 208 \text{ hours}$$

Calculation at 100° Centigrade:

$$\text{acceleration factor} = e((0.5/0.0000863)(1/297 - 1/373))$$
$$= 53$$
$$\text{length of time} = 1000/53$$
$$= 19 \text{ hours}$$

21.4   SUDDEN DEATH TESTING

Sudden death testing is a form of accelerated testing where the total test sample is arbitrarily divided into several, equally numbered groups. All units in each group are started simultaneously. When the first unit in a group fails, the whole group is considered to have failed. Testing is stopped on the remaining un-failed units in the group as soon as the first one fails. The entire test is terminated when the first unit in the last group fails.

To understand the analysis for this test, it is necessary to understand the concept of Weibull testing and plotting.

21.4.1   WEIBULL TESTING AND PLOTTING

Weibull paper is a logarithmic probability plotting paper constructed with the y axis representing the cumulative probability of failure and the x axis representing a time value, in hours or cycles. Data points are established from failure data, with the failure times arranged in increasing order or value of occurrence. Corresponding median ranks are assigned from a percent rank table, based on the sample size. An example will illustrate the point.

21.4.1.1   Example 21-3

Six power supplies were placed on life test. The six units failed at 100, 45, 170, 340, 530 and 240 hours respectively. To plot the data, first arrange the failure times in increasing value, as listed below. Then determine the median ranks by using the table in Appendix 2, with $N =$ sample size $= 6$. Going to the column headed by 50.0, read the six median ranks as below:

Failure order number	Life in hours	Median ranks (%)
1	45	10.910
2	100	26.445
3	170	42.141
4	240	57.859
5	340	73.555
6	530	89.090

Figure 21-2 shows the resultant plot. The resultant line can be used to determine the MTBF and the percent that will fail at any given time. For $\beta = 1$, the MTBF is found by drawing a line from the 63.2% point on the y axis to the resultant line. Then, dropping a line from this point to the x axis gives the MTBF value. The MTBF is 262 hours.

To find the percentage of units that will have failed at 400 hours, draw a vertical line from the x axis to the resultant line. Then draw a horizontal line

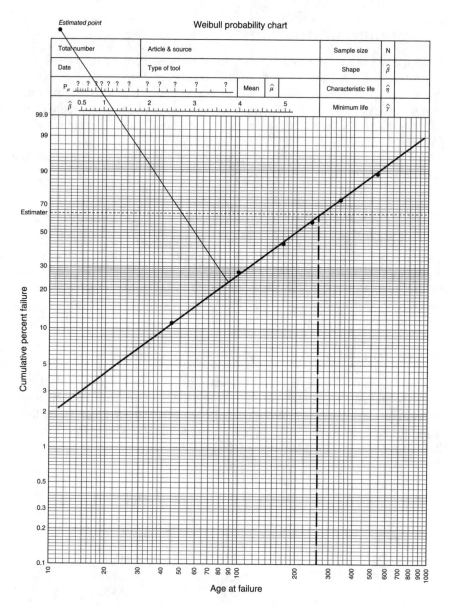

FIGURE 21-2 Weibull plot

from that point to the y axis. This is the failure percentage. In this case, 80% of all units produced will fail by 400 hours.

21.4.1.2 Confidence limits

The confidence limits for this example can be determined in a similar fashion. For example, if the 90% confidence level for the above test were desired, the

5% and 95% ranks would be obtained from the median rank table. Since a 90% confidence level means a 10% risk level, one-half the risk level is at each extreme.

Failure order	Life hours	Median ranks	5% Ranks	95% Ranks
1	45	10.910	0.851	39.304
2	100	26.445	6.285	58.180
3	170	42.141	15.316	72.866
4	240	57.859	27.134	84.684
5	340	73.555	41.820	93.715
6	500	89.090	60.696	99.149

The data are plotted in Figure 21-3. The confidence limits on the MTBF are obtained by reading the time values at the intersections of the 63.2% line with the 5% and 95% confidence bands. In this case, $m_{l2} = 110$ hours and $m_{u2} = 560$ hours.

21.4.1.3   The shape of Weibull plots

The type of plot obtained contains much valuable information on the test data. The shape parameter (β) value and the shape of the curve are very important.

On some Weibull papers, a perpendicular line is drawn from the plot to a point on the paper, called the estimation point. This perpendicular line passes through a scale that indicates a β value. On other papers, a line parallel to the plot is drawn through a scale to give the β value. When $\beta = 1$, the failure rate is constant and the test units are in their useful life period. Where $\beta < 1$, the failure rate is decreasing with time (early life period). When $\beta > 1$, the failure rate increases with time (wearout period). In reality, the unit may be in its useful life period and indicate a β value slightly above or below 1.

Weibull plots may be of two types:

- Linear
- Curved

Linear plots (Figure 21-4) indicate a single failure mode. The plot is used to determine the MTBF as well as the percentage of units that have failed at a particular time or number of cycles of operation. This is done by drawing a vertical line from the desired value on the x axis to the plot and then determining the corresponding intersectional point on the y axis.

Curved plots (Figure 21-5) are indicative of multiple failure modes. The curved plot can usually be separated into its component linear plots by fitting lines parallel to the curved portions. Once linear plots are obtained from the curved plot, information as noted in the previous paragraph can be obtained.

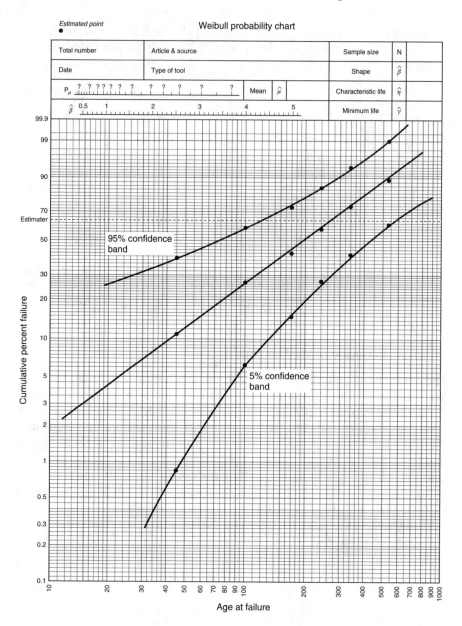

FIGURE 21-3 Weibull plot of confidence limits

21.5 THE SUDDEN DEATH TEST

Sudden death testing consists of dividing the test sample into equal groups of samples. Each group is tested until the first failure occurs in the group. At that time, all members of the group are taken off the test. Once all groups have

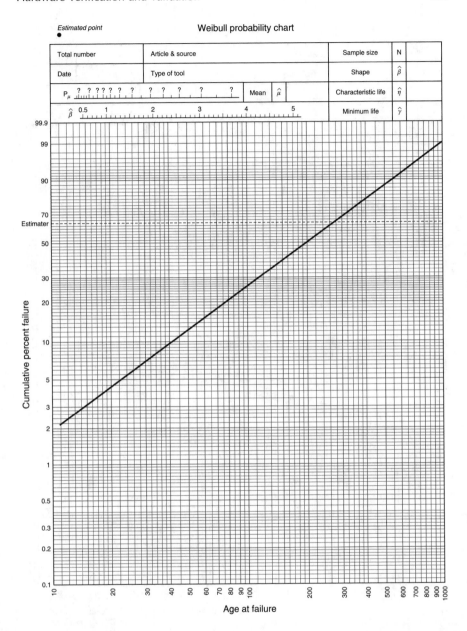

FIGURE 21-4 Weibull linear plot

failed, each group is considered as one failure. The data is plotted on Weibull paper as above. This produces the sudden death line that represents the distribution of lines at the median rank for the first failure.

The median rank for the first failure for N = the number of samples in a group is determined. A horizontal line is drawn from this point on the y axis

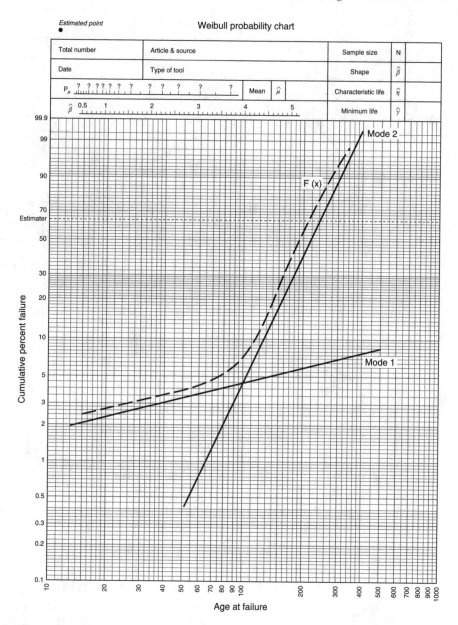

FIGURE 21-5 Weibull curved plot

and intersects a vertical line drawn from the sudden death line at the 50% level. A line parallel to the sudden death line is drawn at the intersection of these two lines. This is the population line that represents the distribution for all units in the test sample.

21.5.1 SUDDEN DEATH EXAMPLE

Forty power supplies are available for testing. Randomly divide the power supplies into five groups of eight pumps each. All pumps are put on test in each group simultaneously. The testing proceeds until any pump in each group fails, at which time the testing of all pumps in that group stops.

For our example,

Group	Unit number	Time of failure
1	4	235 hours
2	8	315
3	3	120
4	6	85
5	2	350

To analyze the data, first arrange the failures in ascending hours to failure. The median ranks are determined from the median rank tables in Appendix 2, based on a sample size of $N = 5$, since there were only five failures.

Failure order number	Life in hours	Median ranks (%)
1	85	12.95
2	120	31.38
3	235	50.00
4	315	68.62
5	350	87.06

The results are plotted on Weibull paper (Figure 21-6). The resulting line is called the sudden death line. It represents the cumulative distribution of the first failure in eight of the population of power supplies.

The median rank for the first failure in $N = 8$ is 8.30%, found by looking in the median rank table under $N = 8$ and Order number $= 1$. Thus the sudden death line represents the distribution of the lines at which 8.3% of the samples are most likely to fail.

To find the population line, draw a vertical line through the intersection of the sudden death line and the horizontal line at the 50% level. Then draw a horizontal line from the 8.3% point on the y axis until it meets this vertical line. This point is the 8.3% life point of the population. Next, draw a straight line through this point, parallel to the sudden death line, thus determining the population line (Figure 21-7). The MTBF of the population line can be determined by drawing a vertical line from the intersection of the population

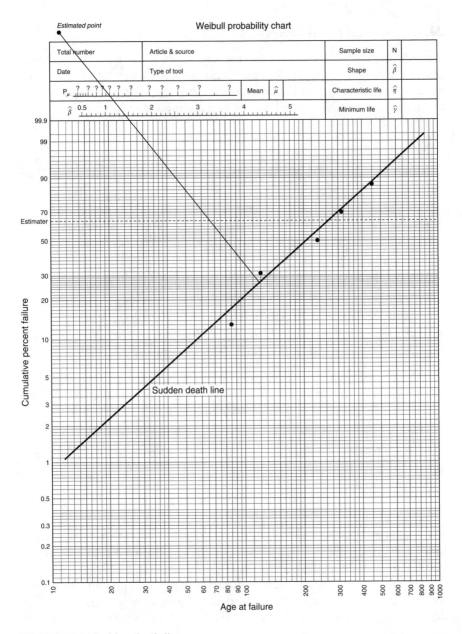

FIGURE 21-6 Sudden death line

line and the 63.2% level and reading the corresponding life in hours. In this case, MTBF = 950 hours. Obtain the confidence limits on this result by choosing the confidence level, e.g., 90%, obtaining the corresponding ranks from the median rank table, e.g., $N = 5$, 5% rank and 95% rank, and plotting

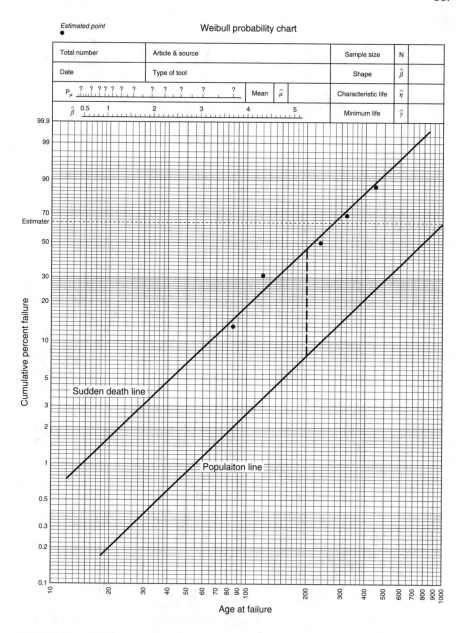

FIGURE 21-7 The population line

these to obtain the sudden death band lines. Then shift these bands vertically down by a distance equal to the vertical distance between the sudden death line and the population line. These new bands are the exact population confidence bands.

The bands are plotted in Figure 21-8.

Failure order	Life hours	Median ranks (%)	5% Rank	95% Rank
1	85	12.95	1.02	45.07
2	120	31.38	7.64	65.74
3	235	50.00	18.93	81.07
4	315	68.62	34.26	92.36
5	350	87.06	54.939	8.98

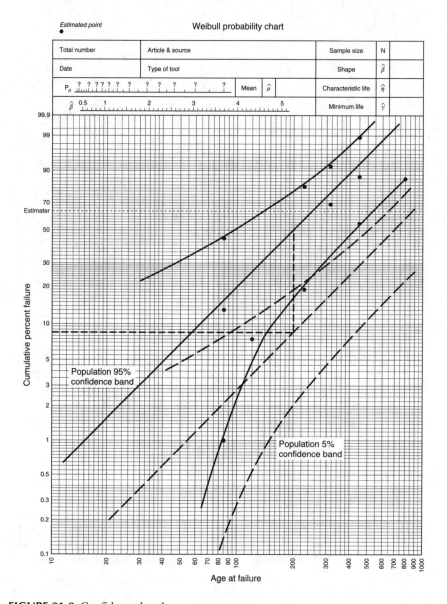

FIGURE 21-8 Confidence bands

REFERENCES

Frankel, E.G., *Systems Reliability and Risk Analysis*, Martinus Nijhoff Publishers, The Hague, 1984.

Fries, R.C., *Reliability Assurance for Medical Devices, Equipment and Software*, Interpharm Press, Inc., Buffalo Grove, IL, 1991.

Fries, R.C., *Reliable Design of Medical Devices*, Marcel-Dekker, Inc., New York, 1997.

Fries, R.C., *Handbook of Medical Device Design*, Marcel-Dekker, Inc., New York, 2001.

Ireson, W.G. and Coombs Jr., C.F., *Handbook of Reliability Engineering and Management*, McGraw-Hill Book Company, New York, 1988.

Jensen, F. and Peterson, N.E., *Burn-In*, John Wiley and Sons, New York, 1982.

King, P.H. and Fries, R.C., *Design of Biomedical Devices and Systems*, Marcel-Dekker, Inc., New York, 2002.

Lloyd, D.K. and Lipow, M., *Reliability Management, Methods and Management*, 2nd edition, American Society for Quality Control, Milwaukee, WI, 1984.

Logothetis, N. and Wynn, H.P., *Quality Through Design*, Oxford University Press, London, UK, 1990.

Mason, R.L., Hunter, W.G., and Hunter, J.S., *Statistical Design and Analysis of Experiments*, John Wiley & Sons, New York, 1989.

MIL-STD-202, *Test Methods for Electronic and Electrical Component Parts*, Department of Defense, Washington, DC, 1980.

MIL-STD-750, *Test Methods for Semiconductor Devices*, Department of Defense, Washington, DC, 1983.

MIL-STD-781, *Reliability Design Qualification and Production Acceptance Tests: Exponential Distribution*, Department of Defense, Washington, DC, 1977.

MIL-STD-883, *Test Methods and Procedures for Microelectronics*, Department of Defense, Washington, DC, 1983.

Montgomery, D.C., *Design and Analysis of Experiments*, 2nd edition, John Wiley & Sons, New York, 1984.

O'Connor, P.D.T., *Practical Reliability Engineering*, 3rd edition, John Wiley & Sons, Chichester, UK, 1991.

Reliability Analysis Center, *Nonelectronic Parts Reliability Data: 1995*, Reliability Analysis Center, Rome, NY, 1994.

Ross, P.J., *Taguchi Techniques for Quality Engineering*, McGraw-Hill, New York, 1988.

Taguchi, G., *Introduction to Quality Engineering*, Unipub/Asian Productivity Association, 1986.

Taguchi, G., *Systems of Experimental Design*, Unipub/Asian Productivity Association, 1978.

22 Software verification and validation

CONTENTS

22.1   Allocation of software testing.................................... 373
22.2   Verification and validation test method commonality 373
22.3   Validation and test overview.................................... 375
       22.3.1   Techniques, methodologies, and test approach 375
       22.3.2   Software testing requirements........................... 377
       22.3.3   Verification and validation reporting................... 378
22.4   The essentials of software testing 378
       22.4.1   The quality of the test process determines the success
                of the test effort...................................... 379
       22.4.2   Prevent defect migration by using early life-cycle
                testing techniques...................................... 379
       22.4.3   The time for software testing tools is now.............. 379
       22.4.4   A real person must take responsibility for improving
                the testing process 380
       22.4.5   Testing is a professional discipline requiring trained
                and skilled people 380
       22.4.6   Cultivate a positive team attitude of creative
                destruction 380
References 381

Software verification and validation requires that evidence be collected to demonstrate that specified requirements have been met by the process and the product. Verification is normally associated with and performed during product development to assure that the software development process, methodology, and design have been met by the current version of the software and product. Validation is a terminal activity to software development and demonstrates that the software design and implemented code satisfies the predetermined requirements and specifications for the product. There are other fundamental differences between software verification and validation, but the primary difference is that verification assures that the software was developed according to a documented process and validation assures that the product and software requirements were satisfied.

371

The application of the principles of quality control, quality assurance, safety and software verification, and validation in the medical product manufacturing industry has changed dramatically. Consumer expectations and international competition have increased the pressures to produce goods of the highest quality at a reasonable cost. This expectation for the highest-quality product at the most reasonable price is balanced against the consumer and government requirement that medical products must be safe, effective, and efficacious at any cost.

Testing the final product for compliance to predetermined specifications is no longer adequate to assure the quality of the product or its software. Manufacturers must assure the quality of the product through the design and development phases of the product life cycle. Software verification and validation should be designed to maximize the assurance of quality and minimize testing.

In the complex regulatory environment of medical products, the only way to satisfy the requirements of the myriad regulatory agencies, international communities, and corporate commitments is to establish a systematic approach to medical product software development. This systematic approach must adhere to the basic principles of quality assurance and provide efficient and effective management of commitments. A good software quality assurance program will minimize redundancy, assure access to information and integrate information from all disciplines and levels of the organization. It will also provide the advantage of flexibility, particularly when standards frequently change, where management can impose new directives and products and technologies evolve quickly. A rigorous yet flexible software quality assurance program provides the stability and assurance that can allow a corporation to respond proactively to its market and competition without risking product quality or patient safety.

Software verification and validation must be performed whenever the quality or effectiveness of the product cannot be adequately tested or evaluated in the final product. Verification and validation is also appropriate for (1) utility systems, support software, or test equipment and software whose failure could directly affect the safety of the product, patient, consumer, or user; (2) any software or equipment and its software that is unique or custom designed; (3) any software or equipment and its software whose reliability or reproducibility is unknown or suspect.

Software verification and validation requires that evidence be collected to demonstrate that specified requirements have been met by the process and the product. Verification is normally associated with and performed during product development to assure that the software development process, methodology, and design have been met by the current version of the software and product. Validation is a terminal activity to software development and demonstrates that the software design and implemented code satisfies the predetermined requirements and specifications for the product. There are other fundamental differences between software verification and validation but the primary difference is that verification assures that the software was developed according to a documented process and validation assures that the product and software requirements were satisfied.

22.1 ALLOCATION OF SOFTWARE TESTING

In order to achieve uniform, consistent and sufficient software test coverage it is of benefit to allocate the various aspects of software testing to corresponding software life cycle activities. During the design process and activities, the software designers perform their design activities and store the resultant design. While the design evolves, the designers should generate test information sheets that will specify the testing to be conducted in order to validate the implemented design. The test information sheets should be used and reviewed as a part of the design walk-throughs. Since these tests are at the discretion of the designer, they should be prioritized by safety, reliability, effectiveness, or performance, and then any other appropriate criteria. These tests should target the integrated software components, the interfaces between the integrated tasks or functions and path testing between the various tasks and functions.

When the design has been completed, it is given to the programmers who will create the source code. As the programmers generate the code, they should also generate test information sheets that specify the testing to be conducted in order to validate the implemented design and requirements. The test information sheets should be used and reviewed as a part of the code walk-throughs. Since these tests are at the discretion of the programmer, they should be prioritized by safety, reliability, effectiveness, or performance, and then any other appropriate criteria. These tests should target the individually completed components for functionality, robustness, and stress testing. The code that is constructed by the programmer will also undergo debug testing. This level of testing is at the function, routine, or component level and satisfies path testing, interface testing, and logic or branch testing.

After the code has been implemented and integrated the formal testing commences. This type of testing is performed by both the software development engineers as well as the software verification and validation engineers. The software developers will execute their testing based on the test information sheets that were generated as the design and code evolved. The software verification and validation engineers will have produced a second set of test information sheets based on the design and code that was documented in the software requirements and software design document. At the conclusion of this formal testing both types of test information sheets are reviewed for adequacy, completeness, and coverage, and signed off and archived.

22.2 VERIFICATION AND VALIDATION TEST METHOD COMMONALITY

The safety and performance characteristics of products and their software must be judged by methods that are reliable. Test method verification and validation is a fundamental building block of any software quality assurance program and it begins during the development of a new product or with the integration of new capabilities into an existing product. Not only do correct or passing test results get recorded, but unacceptable or failure results must not be ignored or discounted without adequate rationale or justification. Test results that do not meet their specification must be investigated and the investigation should be appropriate, competent, timely, and complete. Most important of all, the investigation results and rationale must be determined.

Software verification by definition requires a stable and defined life cycle. Any organization desiring to create a cohesive and efficient verification and validation effort must first define a software life cycle covering the "cradle to grave" development of the software produced. Once this is accomplished, its application to a project is made. Be prepared for setbacks but do not change the defined process unless absolutely necessary. One implementation of an industry-accepted life cycle is as good as another and allowing deviations while executing the new process causes inconsistency which, over time, places doubt in the minds of the users and ultimately erodes your confidence in the process. Validation requires and assumes that verification is working. In fact, it mandates that there is a defined process that is consistently being followed. It is possible to perform validation without verification, but if validation testing finds a design error late in the software development life cycle, then it is significantly costlier to correct than if it was found during the earlier verification phases.

An efficient verification and validation organization is capable of producing salient results during the validation effort and permeating a common test approach. The first step in establishing this effort requires performing a survey of each product line and the test equipment that the software verification and validation group will support. The outcome of this survey is the generation of two lists that identify the microprocessors and controllers and the software languages that were found. For example, the first list might show 80x86, 8051, and 8085 and the second list would be assembly language for each microprocessor and controller on the first list as well as any high-order-level languages, such as "C" and "QBASIC."

The second step is to implement a common test set (CTS) containing a suite of static and dynamic test tools that run on all products and equipment undergoing software verification and validation. This is the first step at promoting a commonality of verification and validation intent across the corporation's products and supporting test equipment. The CTS should be employed as soon as software becomes available and should be viewed as both a bench test and a run-time software test tool. The static branch of the CTS tools require only the source code and functions as the bench test effort. An example of a static tool would be the Lint for "C" software. The dynamic branch of the CTS tools provide the run-time test capability, which includes both the computer–host environment as well as the target hardware. In the computer–host environment, debuggers and simulators will dominate.

The tools for the target environment include in-circuit emulators, timing and event diagramming devices, and execution profilers.

The third branch of the CTS encompasses the data generator tools which could also be labeled as remote communications tools. Given the pervasive remote communications capability in most medical products, either through RS-232-C or GPIB, support must be provided for this area. A common tool for this is National Instruments LabVIEW which provides the capability to communicate via different protocols. This branch provides a wealth of opportunity to automate software testing of the product being developed because canned batch mode data files can be generated and executed in a fraction of the time that any other method of testing consumes. Taken one step further, a tool can be developed that acts as an editor in quickly creating a wide variety of test scenarios.

22.3   VALIDATION AND TEST OVERVIEW

Medical companies are faced with validating both products and test and manufacturing equipment. The test and manufacturing equipment spans the range from manufacturer-developed hardware and software support equipment at one end to software written or modified by the manufacturer which executes on a host PC or workstation at the other end. While there is a significant difference between products and test and manufacturing equipment, there are basic software standards that are applicable to both and a common approach to software validation should be applied. The only caveat is that the level of validation effort should be adjusted and based on the potential of harm to the customer or user and the view that some equipment will fall under process validation.

Within the phases of software development the generic activities concerned with testing are code and test, integrate and test, and software system testing. The code and test activities include development of the code and debugging the implemented code by the software developers. The integrate and test activities include the integration of software components and the testing of the integrated parts. The software system testing activity typically encompasses the verification and validation testing that is performed by the software verification and validation engineers on the fully integrated software and hardware.

22.3.1   TECHNIQUES, METHODOLOGIES, AND TEST
APPROACH

The software validation approach and the test categories to be applied to the product and test and manufacturing equipment should be selected based on the categorization of the life cycle that the product or test and manufacturing equipment belongs to. For example, if the product or test and manufacturing equipment is new and deemed to be a high level of concern, then a full software development life cycle process should be adhered to. If the product or test and manufacturing equipment to be produced is based on an existing baseline which has accumulated sufficient runtime to realize a high level of confidence that a majority of the faults have been detected, then an accelerated enhancement development life cycle should be followed.

The test approach to any product or test and manufacturing equipment should be a combination of requirements testing and safety testing. Requirements testing encompasses a rigorous development effort that includes the production of a requirements design specification. Once the requirements and design are solidified and approved, the software verification and validation engineers can systematically detail the requirements to be tested and trace them to the design in the design specification. The embodiment of this effort is the requirements traceability matrix. Completing the requirements traceability matrix requires that the software verification and validation engineers complete the final column of the requirements traceability matrix that details the testing performed to validate the requirement. This thorough and systematic approach to requirements testing provides high confidence that the test coverage was sufficient.

Safety testing takes a different approach to validation in that the focus is shifted to preventing harm to the user. This approach is aimed at producing a product or equipment that is safe for its intended use. When applied to medical products, a key element to this approach is the production of a hazard analysis. This analysis starts at the system level and decomposes the product into its mechanical, electrical, and software components. This analysis attempts to mitigate single-point failures or justify a single-error trap by calculating a low probability of occurrence. Safety testing of a medical product requires the utilization of the hazards analysis in the software validation effort. When applied to equipment validation, safety testing takes on a different meaning. Safety in this perspective requires surveying the environment and role that the equipment plays in supporting the production of a safe product. If the equipment is utilized to make a pass or fail determination of a product on a production line then the safety issue is elevated. Furthermore, if the test and manufacturing equipment is the sole check of a function of a product before it leaves the production line and is boxed for shipment, then the safety issue is elevated to the level of the product it supports. By contrast, if the equipment consists of a label generator, then safety testing ensures control of the software and validating that the process in place minimizes the chances of an error occurring due to human intervention.

The preferred software test approach to all products or test and manufacturing equipment is white box testing as opposed to black box testing, but this may not be warranted for all functions such as user interface testing. Furthermore, code inspection as the sole technique for validation is to be avoided unless the change is a hard-coded data change, such as strings or constants as opposed to a logic change, which alters the instruction order.

Software testing of a product or test and manufacturing equipment is normally performed at the software component level and software system level. Software component-level testing concentrates on individual components or grouping of components as opposed to software system-level testing where the focus is on the performance of the software as a complete entity. Software component-level testing is performed during the code and test activities and the integrate and test activities and is best performed by the software developers. Software system-level testing is performed during the software system testing activity and should be performed by the software verification and validation engineers.

22.3.2 SOFTWARE TESTING REQUIREMENTS

Software component-level testing is concerned with subsections of the software product and the integration of these subsections. This level of testing is the responsibility of the software engineers who develop the code. Products that fall into the full development life cycle should address this subject in a software development plan. Software system-level testing should be performed by the software verification and validation engineers.

The software systems-level testing begins with the software verification and validation engineers completing the requirements traceability matrix except for the test column. The software verification and validation engineers then validate the process that the developers used to create the software system. If necessary, all compiles and links must set the highest warning level flags to produce detailed listings. The verification and validation testing will be performed from a known and controlled test bed. The software verification and validation engineers now perform software fault insertion testing. For embedded software, the verification and validation engineers utilize the in-circuit emulator with the latest software and hardware to perform the functional, robustness, stress, and safety testing. The verification and validation engineers should then remove the in-circuit emulator and perform functional and robustness testing of the user interface and stress testing of the remote communications interface.

The software verification and validation engineers should then execute the appropriate CTS test suite in order to locate software design errors, suspicious coding practices, unused variables, improperly scoped variables and to reverse engineer software in generating test cases. For embedded software, the verification and validation engineers should validate the EPROM burn-in procedure. This should be conducted by using inconsistent memory fill techniques such as all ones, all zeros, halt OPCODE or a jump to an interrupt service routine that handles an illegal address error.

After all testing has been concluded, including the verification of any fixes due to errors produced by the software system tests, the software verification and validation engineers complete and review the requirements traceability matrix in order to verify that all requirements have been tested and satisfied.

The software verification and validation engineers then complete the requirements traceability matrix and any necessary reports in order to provide closure. The software verification and validation engineers then complete the software verification and validation report and submit it to a controlled environment. A software verification and validation report includes a version specific identifier, such as the cyclic redundancy check (CRC) identifier. In addition, the software verification and validation report lists all baselined items and specifications that were verified with this version of software.

22.3.3 VERIFICATION AND VALIDATION REPORTING

The test documentation that is generated for a particular product or equipment depends on the life cycle and its level of concern classification. The verification and validation report summarizes the results of the verification and validation activity. The summary should contain:

- Description of the tasks performed
- Time or number of cycles each activity was run
- Summary of task results
- Summary of errors found and their resolution
- Assessment of the software reliability

When summarizing the errors found, the report should include:

- Description and location
- Impact
- Criticality
- Rationale for resolution
- Results of retest

Any deviations from the test plan must be highlighted and justified in the test summary.

22.4   THE ESSENTIALS OF SOFTWARE TESTING

Kit lists six essentials of software testing:

- The quality of the test process determines the success of the test effort
- Prevent defect migration by using early life-cycle testing techniques
- The time for software testing tools is now
- A real person must take responsibility for improving the test process
- Testing is a professional discipline requiring trained, skilled people
- Cultivate a positive team attitude of creative destruction

22.4.1 THE QUALITY OF THE TEST PROCESS DETERMINES THE SUCCESS OF THE TEST EFFORT

The quality of a software system is primarily determined by the quality of the software process that produced it. Likewise, the quality and effectiveness of software testing are primarily determined by the quality of the test processes used.

Testing has its own cycle. The testing process begins with the product requirements phase and from there parallels the entire development process. In other words, for each phase of the development process, there is an important testing activity.

Test groups that operate within organizations having an immature development process will feel more pain than those that don't. But regardless of the state of maturity, the test group can and should focus on improving its own internal process. An immature test process within an immature development organization will result in an unproductive, chaotic, frustrating environment that produces low-quality results and unsatisfactory products. People effectively renovating a testing process within that same immature organization will serve as a catalyst for improving the development process as a whole.

22.4.2 PREVENT DEFECT MIGRATION BY USING EARLY LIFE-CYCLE TESTING TECHNIQUES

More than half the errors are usually introduced in the requirements phase. The cost of errors is minimized if they are detected in the same phase as they are introduced, and an effective test program prevents the migration of errors from any development phase to any subsequent phases.

While many of us are aware of this, in practice we often do not have mechanisms in place to detect these errors until much later – often not until function and system test, at which point we have entered "the Chaos Zone." Chances are that we are currently missing the best opportunity for improving the effectiveness of our testing if we are not taking advantage of the proven testing techniques that can be applied early in the development process.

22.4.3 THE TIME FOR SOFTWARE TESTING TOOLS IS NOW

After many years of observation, evaluation, and mostly waiting, we can now say the time for testing tools has arrived. There is a wide variety of tool vendors to choose from, many of which have mature, healthy products.

It is important to have a strategy for tool acquisition and a proper procedure for handling tool selection. While such procedures are based on common sense, they do need to be systematically implemented. Tool acquisition is an area where there may be a strong case for seeking independent expert advice.

22.4.4 A REAL PERSON MUST TAKE RESPONSIBILITY FOR IMPROVING THE TESTING PROCESS

If the testing group is feeling pain, start campaigning for improvements to a few of the key issues, such as better specifications, and better reviews and inspections. Management should appoint an architect or small core team to prioritize potential improvements and lead the testing improvement effort, and must make it clear that they will give their ongoing support. It is not rocket science – but it takes effort and time. Tools can help tremendously, but they must be used within an overall test process that includes effective test planning and design.

22.4.5 TESTING IS A PROFESSIONAL DISCIPLINE REQUIRING TRAINED AND SKILLED PEOPLE

The software testing process has evolved considerably and has reached the point where it is a discipline requiring trained professionals. To succeed today, an organization must be adequately staffed with skilled software testing professionals who get proper support from management. Testing should be independent, unbiased, and organized for the fair sharing of recognition and rewards for contributions made to product quality.

22.4.6 CULTIVATE A POSITIVE TEAM ATTITUDE OF CREATIVE DESTRUCTION

Testing requires disciplined creativity. Good testing, that is devising and executing successful tests, tests that discover the defects in a product, requires real ingenuity and may be viewed as destructive. Indeed, considerable creativity is needed to destroy something in a controlled and systematic way. Good testers are methodically taking the product apart, finding its weaknesses, pushing it up to and beyond its limits.

Establishing the proper "test to break" mental attitude has a profound effect on testing success. If the objective is to show that the product does what it shouldn't do, and doesn't do what it should, we're on the way to testing success. Although far from the norm today, the results that we get when practitioners and their managers together cultivate this attitude of disciplined, creative destruction are nothing less than astonishing.

Successful testing requires a methodological approach. It requires us to focus on the basic critical factors: planning, project and process control, risk, management, inspections, measurement, tools, organization, and professionalism. Remember that testers make a vital positive contribution throughout the development process to ensure the quality of the product.

REFERENCES

Evans, M.W. and Marciniak, J.J., *Software Quality Assurance & Management*, John Wiley & Sons, Inc., New York, 1987.

Fagan, M.E., Design and code inspections to reduce errors in program development, *IBM Systems Journal*, 15(3), p. 182–211.

Fairley, R.E., *Software Engineering Concepts*, McGraw-Hill Book Company, New York, 1985.

Fries, R.C., *Reliability Assurance for Medical Devices, Equipment and Software*, Interpharm Press, Inc., Buffalo Grove, IL, 1991.

Fries, R.C., Pienkowski, P. and Jorgens III, J., Safe, effective, and reliable software design and development for medical devices, *Medical Instrumentation*, 30(2), March/April, 1996.

Fries, R.C., *Reliable Design of Medical Devices*, Marcel-Dekker, Inc., New York, 1997.

Fries, R.C., *Handbook of Medical Device Design*, Marcel-Dekker, Inc., New York, 2001.

IEEE, *IEEE Standards Collection – Software Engineering*, The Institute of Electrical and Electronic Engineers, Inc., New York, 1993.

King, P.H. and Fries, R.C., *Design of Biomedical Devices and Systems*, Marcel-Dekker, Inc., New York, 2002.

Kit, E., *Software Testing in the Real World – Improving the Process*, Addison-Wesley Publishing Company, Reading, MA, 1995.

Laplante, P., *Real-Time Systems Design and Analysis – An Engineer's Handbook*, The Institute of Electrical and Electronic Engineers, Inc., New York, 1993.

Leveson, N.G., Software safety: why, what, and how, *Computing Surveys*, 18(2), June, 1986.

Myers, G.J., *The Art of Software Testing*, John Wiley and Sons, New York, 1979.

Neufelder, A.M., *Ensuring Software Reliability*, Marcel-Dekker, Inc., New York, 1993.

Pressman, R., *Software Engineering – A Practitioner's Approach*, McGraw-Hill Book Company, New York, 2005.

Yourdon, E., *Modern Structured Analysis*, Yourdon Press, Englewood Cliffs, NJ, 1989.

23 Analysis of test results

CONTENTS

23.1 Failure rate 384
    23.1.1 Example 23-1.. 384
    23.1.2 Example 23-2.. 384
23.2 Mean time between failures (MTBF)............................ 385
    23.2.1 Time-terminated, failed parts replaced 385
        23.2.1.1 Example 23-3............................... 385
    23.2.2 Time-terminated, no replacement 386
    23.2.3 Failure-terminated, failed parts replaced 387
        23.2.3.1 Example 23-4............................... 387
    23.2.4 Failure-terminated, no replacement 387
    23.2.5 No failures observed................................... 388
        23.2.5.1 Example 23-5............................... 388
23.3 Reliability... 388
    23.3.1 Example 23-6.. 389
    23.3.2 Example 23-7.. 389
23.4 Confidence level.. 390
    23.4.1 Example 23-8.. 390
23.5 Confidence limits... 390
    23.5.1 Time-terminated confidence limits 390
        23.5.1.1 Example 23-9............................... 391
    23.5.2 Failure-terminated confidence limits 391
23.6 Minimum life 392
23.7 Graphical analysis.. 392
    23.7.1 Pareto analysis 392
    23.7.2 Graphical plotting..................................... 393
        23.7.2.1 Example 23-10.............................. 393
    23.7.3 Weibull plotting 394
References... 394

The heart of reliability is the analysis of data, from which desired reliability parameters can be calculated. These parameters are calculated from testing throughout the product development process. Early calculations are updated as the program progresses and the presence or lack of reliability improvement becomes apparent.

Reliability parameter calculation assumes the product is in the useful life period of the bathtub curve. During this period, the failure rate is constant and the exponential distribution is used for calculations. In standards and handbooks where failure rates and MTBF values are listed, the same assumption is made and the exponential distribution is used.

Calculations of some parameters, such as MTBF, are dependent upon the termination mode of the test. Time-terminated tests, where tests are ended after a predetermined time period has elapsed, are calculated different than failure-terminated tests, where tests are ended after a predetermined number of units have failed.

The calculations necessary to determine the following parameters will be reviewed:

- Failure rate
- MTBF
- Reliability
- Confidence limits

In addition, graphical analysis will be discussed and its application to dealing with reliability data.

23.1 FAILURE RATE

Failure rate is the number of failures per million hours of operation. For devices in their useful life period, the failure rate is the reciprocal of the MTBF.

$$MTBF = 1/\lambda \qquad (23.1)$$

The failure rate is stated as failures per hour for this equation.

23.1.1 EXAMPLE 23-1

An EEG machine has a MTBF of 4380 hours. What is the failure rate?

$$\lambda = 1/MTBF$$
$$= 1/4380$$
$$= 0.000228 \text{ failures per hour}$$
$$= 228 \text{ failures per million hours}$$

23.1.2 EXAMPLE 23-2

Ten power supplies are put on test, to be terminated after each has completed 1000 hours of operation. Two power supplies fail, one at 420 hours and the other at 665 hours. What is the failure rate of the power supplies?

Eight units completed 1000 hours.

$$\text{Total test time} = 8(1000) + 420 + 665$$
$$= 9085 \text{ hours}$$
$$\lambda = \text{number of failures/total test time}$$
$$= 2/9085$$
$$= 0.000220 \text{ failures per hour}$$
$$= 220 \text{ failures per million hours}$$

23.2 MEAN TIME BETWEEN FAILURES (MTBF)

Mean time between failures is the time at which 63% of the operational devices in the field will have failed. MTBF is the reciprocal of the failure rate. It is also calculated from test data dependent upon the type of test run, e.g., time-terminated or failure-terminated, and upon whether the failed units were replaced or not. Five different methods of MTBF calculation are available:

- Time-terminated, failed parts replaced
- Time-terminated, no replacement
- Failure-terminated, failed parts replaced
- Failure-terminated, no replacement
- No failures observed during the test

23.2.1 TIME-TERMINATED, FAILED PARTS REPLACED

$$\text{MTBF} = N(td)/r \tag{23.2}$$

where

$N = $ number of units tested
$td = $ test duration
$r = $ number of failures

23.2.1.1 Example 23-3

The performance of ten pressure monitors is monitored while operating for a period of 1200 hours. The test results are listed below. Every failed unit is replaced immediately. What is the MTBF?

Unit number	Time of failure (hours)
1	650
2	420
3	130 and 725

4	585
5	630 and 950
6	390
7	No failure
8	880
9	No failure
10	220 and 675

$N = 10$
$r = 11$
$td = 1200$ hours

$$\text{MTBF} = N(td)/r$$
$$= 10(1200)/11$$
$$= 1091 \text{ hours}$$

23.2.2 TIME-TERMINATED, NO REPLACEMENT

$$\text{MTBF} = \left(\sum T_i\right) + (N - r)td/r \qquad (23.3)$$

where
    $N =$ number of units tested
    $td =$ test duration
    $r =$ number of failures
    $T_i =$ individual failure times

Using the data in Example 23.3

Unit number	Time of failure (hours)
1	650
2	420
3	130
4	585
5	630
6	390
7	No failure
8	880
9	No failure
10	220

$$\text{MTBF} = \left(\sum T_i\right) + (N - r)/td/r$$
$$= (650 + 420 + 130 + 585 + 630 + 390 + 880 + 220) + 2(1200)/8$$
$$= (3905 + 2400)/8$$
$$= 788 \text{ hours}$$

23.2.3 FAILURE-TERMINATED, FAILED PARTS REPLACED

$$\text{MTBF} = N(td)/r$$

where

N = Number of units tested
td = test duration
r = number of failures

23.2.3.1 Example 23-4

Six TENS units were placed on test until all units failed, the last occurring at 850 hours. The test results are listed below. Every failed unit, except the last one, is replaced immediately. What is the MTBF?

Unit number	Time of failure (hours)
1	130
2	850
3	120 and 655
4	440
5	725
6	580

$$\text{MTBF} = N(td)/r$$
$$= 6(850)/7$$
$$= 729 \text{ hours}$$

23.2.4 FAILURE-TERMINATED, NO REPLACEMENT

$$\text{MTBF} = \left(\sum T_i\right) + (N - r)td/r$$

Using the data from Example 23.4

Unit number	Time of failure (hours)
1	130
2	850
3	120
4	440
5	725
6	580

$$\text{MTBF} = \left(\sum T_i\right) + (N - r)td/r$$
$$= (130 + 850 + 120 + 440 + 725 + 580) + 0(850)/6$$
$$= 3965 + 0/6$$
$$= 658 \text{ hours}$$

23.2.5 NO FAILURES OBSERVED

For the case where no failures are observed, an MTBF value cannot be calculated. A lower one-sided confidence limit must be calculated and the MTBF stated to be greater than that value.

$$\text{ml} = 2(Ta)/\chi^2_{\alpha;2}$$

where

ml = lower one-sided confidence limit

Ta = total test time

$\chi^2_{\alpha;2}$ = the chi-square value from the table in Appendix 1,

where α is the risk level and 2 is the degrees

of freedom

23.2.5.1 Example 23-5

Ten ventilators are tested for 1000 hours without failure. What is the MTBF at a 90% confidence level?

$$N = 10$$
$$td = 1000$$
$$r = 0$$
$$1 - \% = 0.90$$
$$\% = 0.10$$
$$Ta = N(td) = 10(1000) = 10\,000$$
$$\text{ml} = 2(Ta)/\chi^2_{\alpha;2}$$
$$= 2(10\,000)/\chi^2_{10;2}$$
$$= 20\,000/4.605$$
$$= 4343 \text{ hours}$$

We can then state that the MTBF > 4343 hours, with 90% confidence.

23.3 RELIABILITY

Reliability has been defined as the probability that an item will perform a required function, under specified conditions, for a specified period of time, at a desired confidence level. Reliability may be calculated from either the failure rate or the MTBF. The resultant number is the percentage of units that will survive the specified time.

Reliability can vary between 0 (no reliability) and 1.0 (perfect reliability). The closer the value is to 1.0, the better the reliability will be. To calculate the parameter "reliability," two parameters are required:

- Either the failure rate or the MTBF
- The mission time or specified period of operation

$$\text{Reliability} = \exp(-\lambda t)$$
$$= \exp(-/\text{MTBF})$$

23.3.1 EXAMPLE 23-6

Using the data in Example 23.2, calculate the reliability of the power supplies for an operating period of 3200 hours.

$\lambda = $ failure rate $ = 220$ failures per million hours
for the equation, λ must be in failures per hour
thus, $220/1\,000\,000 = 0.000220$ failures per hour
$t = 3200$ hours

$$\text{Reliability} = \exp(-\lambda t)$$
$$= \exp - (0.000220)(3200)$$
$$= \exp - (0.704)$$
$$= 0.495$$

This states that, after 3200 hours of operation, one half of the power supplies in operation will not have failed.

23.3.2 EXAMPLE 23-7

Using the time-terminated, no replacement case, calculate the reliability of the pressure monitors for 500 hours of operation.

$$\text{Reliability} = \exp - (\lambda t)$$
$$= \exp - (t/\text{MTBF})$$
$$= \exp - (500/788)$$
$$= \exp - (0.635)$$
$$= 0.530$$

Thus, 53% of the pressure monitors will not fail during the 500 hours of operation.

23.4 CONFIDENCE LEVEL

Confidence level is the probability that a given statement is correct. Thus, when a 90% confidence level is used, the probability that the findings are valid for the device population is 90%.

Confidence level is designated as:

$$\text{Confidence level} = 1 - \alpha$$
$$\text{where}$$
$$\alpha = \text{the risk level}$$

23.4.1 EXAMPLE 23-8

Test sample size is determined using a confidence level of 98%. What is the risk level?

$$\text{Confidence level} = 1 - \alpha$$
$$\alpha = 1 - \text{confidence level}$$
$$= 1 - 0.98$$
$$= 0.02 \text{ or } 2\%$$

23.5 CONFIDENCE LIMITS

Confidence limits are defined as the extremes of a confidence interval within which the unknown has a designated probability of being included. If the identical test was repeated several times with different samples of a device, it is probable that the MTBF value calculated from each test would not be identical. However, the various values would fall within a range of values about the true MTBF value. The two values which mark the end points of the range are the lower and upper confidence limits. Confidence limits are calculated based on whether the test was time or failure terminated.

23.5.1 TIME-TERMINATED CONFIDENCE LIMITS

$$\text{mL} = 2(Ta)/\chi^2_{\alpha;2r+2}$$

where

$$\text{mL} = \text{lower confidence limit}$$
$$Ta = \text{total test time}$$
$$\chi^2_{\alpha;2r+2} = \text{Chi square value from Appendix 1 for } \alpha \text{ risk level}$$
$$\text{and } 2r + 2 \text{ degrees of freedom}$$
$$\text{mU} = 2(Ta)/\chi^2_{1-\alpha/2;2r}$$

23.5.1.1 Example 23-9

Using the data from the time terminated, no replacement data from Example 23.3, at a 90% confidence limit:

$$Ta = 6305 \, \text{hours}$$
$$@ = 1 - \text{confidence level} = 0.10$$
$$@/2 = 0.05$$
$$r = 8$$
$$2r + 2 = 18$$
$$mL = 2(6305)\chi^2_{0.05;18}$$
$$= 12\,610/28.869$$
$$= 437 \, \text{hours}$$
$$mU = 2(6305)/\chi^2_{0.95;16}$$
$$= 12\,610/7.962$$
$$= 1584 \, \text{hours}$$

We can thus say:

$$437 < \text{MTBF} < 1584 \, \text{hours}$$

or the true MTBF lies between 437 and 1584 hours.

23.5.2 FAILURE-TERMINATED CONFIDENCE LIMITS

$$mL = 2(Ta)/\chi^2\alpha/2; 2r$$
$$\text{and}$$
$$mU = 2(Ta)/\chi^2 1 - \alpha/2; 2r$$

Using the data from the failure-terminated, no replacement data from Example 23.4, at a 95% confidence limit:

$$Ta = 3945 \, \text{hours}$$
$$@ = 0.05$$
$$@/2 = 0.025$$
$$1 - @/2 = 0.975$$
$$r = 6$$
$$2r = 12$$
$$mL = 2(3945)/\chi^2_{0.025;12}$$
$$= 7890/23.337$$
$$= 338 \, \text{hours}$$

$$mU = 2(3945)/\chi^2_{0.975;12}$$
$$= 7890/4.404$$
$$= 1792 \, \text{hours}$$

Thus,

$$338 < \text{MTBF} < 1792$$

23.6   MINIMUM LIFE

The minimum life of a device is defined as the time of occurrence of the first failure.

23.7   GRAPHICAL ANALYSIS

Graphical analysis is a way of looking at test data or field information. It can show failure trends, determine when a manufacturing learning curve is nearly complete, indicate the severity of field problems or determine the effect of a burn-in program.

Several types of graphical analysis are advantageous in reliability analysis:

- Pareto analysis
- Graphical plotting
- Weibull analysis

23.7.1   PARETO ANALYSIS

Pareto analysis is a plot of individual failures versus the frequency of the failures. The individual failures are listed on the x- axis and the frequency of occurrence on the y- axis. The result is a histogram of problems and their severity. The problems are usually plotted with the most frequent on the left. Once the results are obtained, appropriate action can be taken. Figure 23-1 is an example of a pareto analysis based on the following data:

Problem	Frequency
Power supply problems	10
Leaks	8
Defective parts	75
Cable problems	3
Missing parts	42
Shipping damage	2

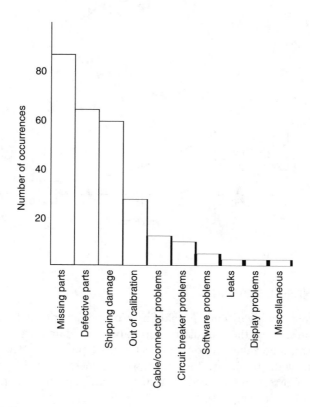

FIGURE 23-1 Pareto analysis

23.7.2   GRAPHICAL PLOTTING

When plotting data, time is usually listed on the x- axis and the parameter to be analyzed on the y- axis.

23.7.2.1   Example 23-10

Nerve stimulators were subjected to 72 hours of burn-in at ambient temperature prior to shipment to customers. Reports of early failures were grouped into 50-hour intervals and showed the following pattern:

Hourly increment	Number of failures
0–50	12
51–100	7
101–150	4
151–200	1
201–250	1

Figure 23-2 is a plot of the data. The data indicate the number of failures begins to level off at approximately 200 hours. The burn-in was changed to an accelerated burn-in, equal to 300 hours of operation.

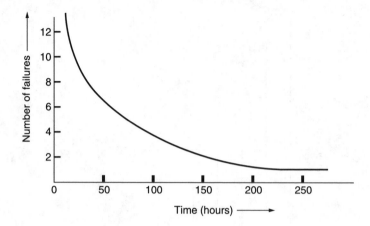

FIGURE 23-2 Plot of field data

23.7.3 WEIBULL PLOTTING

Weibull paper is a logarithmic probability plotting paper constructed with the y- axis representing the cumulative probability of failure and the x- axis representing a time value, in hours or cycles. Data points are established from failure data, with the failure times arranged in increasing order or value of occurrence. Corresponding median ranks are assigned from a percent rank table, based on the sample size.

REFERENCES

Frankel, E.G., *System Reliability and Risk Analysis*, Martinus Nijhoff Publishers, The Hague, 1984.

Fries, R.C., *Reliability Assurance for Medical Devices, Equipment and Software*, Interpharm Press, Inc., Buffalo Grove, IL, 1991.

Fries, R.C., *Reliable Design of Medical Devices*, Marcel-Dekker, Inc., New York, 1997.

Fries, R.C., *Handbook of Medical Device Design*, Marcel-Dekker, Inc., New York, 2001.

Ireson, W.G. and Coombs Jr., C.F., *Handbook of Reliability Engineering and Management*, McGraw-Hill Book Company, New York, 1988.

King, J.R., *Probability Charts for Decision Making*, Team, New Hampshire, 1971.

King, P.H. and Fries, R.C., *Design of Biomedical Devices and Systems*, Marcel-Dekker, Inc., New York, 2002.

Lloyd, D.K. and Lipow, M., *Reliability Management, Methods and Mathematics*, 2nd edition, The American Society for Quality Control, Milwaukee, WI, 1984.

Mann, N.R., et al., *Methods for Statistical Analysis of Reliability and Life Data*, John Wiley and Sons, New York, 1974.

Nelson, W., *Applied Life Data Analysis*, John Wiley and Sons, New York, 1982.

O'Connor, P.D.T., *Practical Reliability Engineering*, 3rd edition, John Wiley & Sons, Chichester, UK, 1991.

Section 6

The manufacturing and maintenance processes

24 GMPs and manufacturing

CONTENTS

24.1   A history of GMPs... 398
24.2   The GMP regulation 400
    24.2.1   Design controls... 400
    24.2.2   Purchasing controls..................................... 400
    24.2.3   Servicing controls....................................... 401
    24.2.4   Changes in critical device requirements.................. 401
    24.2.5   Harmonization 401
24.3   Design for manufacturability 402
    24.3.1   The DFM process 402
24.4   Design for assembly 403
    24.4.1   Overall design concept................................. 403
    24.4.2   Component mounting 403
    24.4.3   Test points 403
    24.4.4   Stress levels and tolerances 404
    24.4.5   PCBs.. 404
    24.4.6   Miscellaneous 404
    24.4.7   Design for assembly process 404
24.5   The manufacturing process 405
    24.5.1   Pre-production activity 405
    24.5.2   The pilot run build 406
    24.5.3   The production run...................................... 407
    24.5.4   Customer delivery 407
References... 407

The FDA promulgated the good manufacturing practices (GMP) for medical devices regulations in 1978, drawing authority from the Medical Devices Amendments to the Federal Food, Drug, and Cosmetic Act of 1976. The GMP regulations represented a total quality assurance program intended to control the manufacture and distribution of devices. It allows the FDA to periodically inspect medical device manufacturers for compliance to the regulations.

Manufacturers must operate in an environment in which the manufacturing process is controlled. Manufacturing excellence can only be achieved by designing products and processes to address potential problems before they occur. Manufacturers must also operate in an environment that meets GMP regulations. This requires proof of control over manufacturing processes.

24.1   A HISTORY OF GMPS

Two years after the Medical Device Amendments of 1976 were enacted, the FDA issued its final draft of the medical device good manufacturing practices (GMP) regulation, a series of requirements that prescribed the facilities, methods, and controls to be used in the manufacturing, packaging, and storage of medical devices. Except for an update of organizational references and revisions to the critical device list included in the 1978 final draft's preamble, these regulations have remained virtually unchanged since they were published in the *Federal Register* on July 21, 1978. That does not mean that their interpretation has not changed.

Several key events since that date have influenced the way the FDA has interpreted and applied these regulations. The first occurred in 1987 with the FDA's publication of the "Guidelines on General Principles of Process Validation," which not only provided guidance but advised industry that device manufacturers must validate other processes when necessary to assure that these processes would consistently produce acceptable results.

In 1989, the FDA published a notice of availability for design control recommendations titled "Preproduction Quality Assurance Planning: Recommendations for Medical Device Manufacturers." These recommendations fulfilled a promise made by the CDRH director to a congressional hearing committee to do something to prevent device failures that were occurring due to design defects, resulting in some injuries and deaths. It was also a warning to industry that the FDA was moving to add design controls to the GMP regulation.

The next year, the FDA moved closer to adding design controls, publishing the "Suggested Changes to the Medical Device Good Manufacturing Practices Regulation Information Document," which described the changes the agency was proposing to make to the GMP regulation. Comments asserted that the FDA did not have the authority to add design controls to the GMPs, a point that became moot later that year when the Safe Medical Devices Act of 1990 (SMDA) became law. SMDA amended section 520(f) of the Federal Food, Drug, and Cosmetic Act to add "preproduction design validation" controls to the device GMP regulation.

SMDA also added to the FD&C Act a new section 803, which encouraged the FDA to work with foreign countries toward mutual recognition agreements for the GMP and other regulations. Soon afterward, the FDA began to actively pursue the harmonization of GMP requirements on a global basis.

Over the following 2 years, the FDA took steps to assure that manufacturers with device applications under review at the agency were also in compliance with GMPs. The first step was taken in 1991, when CDRH established its "reference list" program for manufacturers with pending premarket approval (PMA) applications, ensuring that no PMA would be approved while the device maker had significant GMP violations on record. In 1992, the program was extended to all 510(k)s. Under this umbrella program, 510(k)s would not be processed if there was evidence on hand that the site where the 510(k) device would be manufactured was not in compliance with GMPs.

On November 23, 1993, the FDA acted on comments it had received 3 years earlier regarding its "Suggested Changes" document, publishing a proposed revision of the 1978 GMPs in the *Federal Register*. The proposal incorporated almost all of the 1987 version of ISO 9001, the quality systems standard compiled by the International Organization for Standardization. While supporting adoption of ISO 9001, most of the comments received from industry objected to the addition of proposals such as applying the GMP regulation to component manufacturers.

In July 1995, the FDA published a working draft of the proposed final revised GMP regulation. As stated in that draft, the two reasons for the revision were to bring about the addition of design and servicing controls, and to ensure that the requirements were made compatible with those of ISO 9001 and EN46001 (ISO 13485), the quality standard that manufacturers must meet if they select the European Union directives' total quality system approach to marketing.

Among the proposals in this version that drew the most fire from industry were the application of GMPs to component manufacturers and use of the term "end of life," which was intended to differentiate between servicing and reconditioning. The FDA agreed to delete most but not all of the objectionable requirements during an August, 1995 FDA–industry meeting and the GMP Advisory Committee meeting in September, 1995. The end-of life concept was deleted from the GMPs, but was retained in the medical device reporting regulation.

As the GMPs now stand, they are very similar to the proposed ISO 13485 standard. To further harmonize the two documents, the FDA's July 1995 working draft includes additions that incorporate the requirements of the 1994 version of ISO 9001 that were not in the 1987 version.

In addition, the FDA has indicated that GMP inspections might be made by third parties. If that happens, these inspections would probably begin on a small scale with third parties doing follow-up to non-violative inspections. But, eventually, third parties could play an important role in mitigating delays from the FDA's reference list, which, while not now referred to by that name, is still in effect and not likely to be dropped by the agency. Although review of a 510(k) is not affected by the manufacturer being on the list, a 510(k) will not be approved until the manufacturing site is found to be in GMP compliance. The availability of the third-party auditors to inspect those sites might speed up the review process under those circumstances.

Also in the future is a training course for GMP specialists being prepared by the Association for the Advancement of Medical Instrumentation (AAMI). If this course were incorporated into the FDA investigator certification training, it could help assure that the GMP regulation is interpreted and applied uniformly by FDA, consultants, and the device industry.

24.2 THE GMP REGULATION

The latest draft of the GMP regulation was published for comment in the Federal Register on November 23, 1993. They were established to replace quality assurance program requirements with quality system requirements that include design, purchasing, and servicing controls, clarify record-keeping requirements for device failure and complaint investigations, clarify requirements for qualifying, verifying, and validating processes and specification changes, and clarify requirements for evaluating quality data and correcting quality problems. In addition, the FDA has also revised the Current Good Manufacturing Practice (CGMP) requirements for medical devices to assure they are compatible with specifications for quality systems contained in international quality standard ISO 9001.

The following changes were made from previous regulations.

24.2.1 DESIGN CONTROLS

Over the past several years, the FDA has identified lack of design controls as one of the major causes of device recalls. The intrinsic quality of devices, including their safety and effectiveness, is established during the design phase. The FDA believes that unless appropriate design controls are observed during preproduction stages of development, a finished device may not be safe nor effective for its intended use. Based on experience with administering the CGMP regulations, which currently do not include preproduction design controls, the FDA is concerned that the current regulations provide less than an appropriate level of assurance that devices will be safe and effective. Therefore, the FDA is proposing to add general requirements for design controls to the device CGMP regulations for all Class III and II devices, and several Class I devices.

24.2.2 PURCHASING CONTROLS

The quality of purchased product and services is crucial to maintaining the intrinsic safety and effectiveness of a device. Many device failures due to problems with components that result in recall are due to unacceptable components provided by suppliers. The FDA has found during CGMP inspections that the use of unacceptable components is often due to the failure of the manufacturer of finished devices to adequately establish and define requirements for the device's purchased components, including quality requirements. Therefore, the FDA believes that the purchasing of components, finished devices, packaging, labeling, and manufacturing materials must be conducted with the same level of planning, control, and verification as internal activities. The FDA believes the appropriate level of control should be achieved through a proper mixture of supplier and in-house controls.

24.2.3 SERVICING CONTROLS

The FDA has found, as a result of reviewing service records, that the data resulting from the maintenance and repair of medical devices provide valuable insight into the adequacy of the performance of devices. Thus, the FDA believes that service data must be included among the data manufacturers used to evaluate and monitor the adequacy of the device design, the quality system, and the manufacturing process. Accordingly, the FDA is proposing to add general requirements for the maintenance of servicing records and for the review of these records by the manufacturer. Manufacturers must assure that the performance data obtained as a part of servicing product are fed back into the manufacturer's quality system for evaluation as part of the overall device experience data.

24.2.4 CHANGES IN CRITICAL DEVICE REQUIREMENTS

The FDA is proposing to eliminate the critical component and critical operation terminology contained in the present CGMP regulation. The increased emphasis on purchasing controls and on establishing the acceptability of component suppliers assures that the intent of the present critical component requirement is carried forward into the revised CGMP. The addition of a requirement to validate and document special processes further ensures that the requirements of the present critical operation requirements are retained. The FDA is proposing to retain the distinction between critical and non-critical devices for one regulatory purpose. Traceability will continue to be required only for critical devices.

24.2.5 HARMONIZATION

The FDA is proposing to reorganize the structure of the device CGMP regulations and modify some of their language in order to harmonize them with international quality standards. The FDA is also proposing to relocate and combine certain requirements to better harmonize the requirements with specifications for quality systems in the ISO 9001 quality standard and to use as much common language as possible to enhance conformance with ISO 9001 terminology. By requiring all manufacturers to design and manufacture devices under the controls of a total quality system, the FDA believes the proposed changes in the CGMP regulations will improve the quality of medical devices manufactured in the U.S. for domestic distribution or exportation as well as devices imported from other countries. The proposed changes should ensure that only safe and effective devices are distributed in conformance with the Act. Harmonization means a general enhancement of CGMP requirements among the world's leading producers of medical devices.

24.3   DESIGN FOR MANUFACTURABILITY

Design for manufacturability (DFM) assures that a design can be repeatably manufactured while satisfying the requirements for quality, reliability, performance, availability, and price. One of the fundamental principles of DFM is reducing the number of parts in a product. Existing parts should be simple and add value to the product. All parts should be specified, designed, and manufactured to allow 100% usable parts to be produced. It takes a concerted effort by design, manufacturing, and vendors to achieve this goal.

Design for manufacturability is desirable because it is less costly. The reduction in cost is due to:

- A simpler design with fewer parts
- Simple production processes
- Higher quality and reliability
- Easier to service

24.3.1   THE DFM PROCESS

The theme of DFM is to eliminate non-functional parts, such as screws or fasteners, while also reducing the number of functional parts. The remaining parts should each perform as many functions as possible. The following questions help in determining if a part is necessary:

- Must the part move relative to its mating part?
- Must the part be of a different material than its mating part or isolated from all other parts?
- Must the part be separate for disassembly or service purposes?

All fasteners are automatically considered candidates for elimination.

A process that can be expected to have a defect rate of no more that a few parts per million consists of:

- Identification of critical characteristics
- Determine product elements contributing to critical characteristics
- For each identified product element, determine the step or process choice that affects or controls required performance
- Determine a nominal value and maximum allowable tolerance for each product component and process step
- Determine the capability for parts and process elements that control required performance
- Assure that the capability index (Cp) is greater than or equal to 2, where

$$Cp = (\text{specification width})/\text{process capability}$$

24.4   DESIGN FOR ASSEMBLY

Design for assembly is a structured methodology for analyzing product concepts or existing products for simplification of the design and its assembly process. Reduction in parts and assembly operations, and individual part geometry changes to ease assembly are the primary goals. The analysis process exposes many other life cycle cost and customer satisfaction issues which can then be addressed. Design and assembly process quality are significantly improved by this process.

Most textbook approaches to design for assembly (DFA) discuss elimination of parts. While this is a very important aspect of DFA, there are also many other factors that affect product assembly. A few rules include the following.

24.4.1   OVERALL DESIGN CONCEPT

- The design should be simple with a minimum number of parts
- Assure the unit is light weight
- The system should have a unified design approach, rather than look like an accumulation of parts
- Components should be arranged and mounted for the most economical assembly and wiring
- Components that have a limited shelf life should be avoided
- The use of special tools should be minimized
- The use of wiring and harnesses to connect components should be avoided

24.4.2   COMPONENT MOUNTING

- The preferred assembly direction is top-down
- Repositioning of the unit to different orientations during assembly should be avoided
- All functional internal components should mount to one main chassis component
- Mating parts should be self-aligning
- Simple, foolproof operations should be used

24.4.3   TEST POINTS

- Pneumatic test points shall be accessible without removal of any other module
- Electrical test points shall include, but not be limited to:
  - Reference voltages
  - Adjustments
  - Key control signals
  - Power supply voltages
- All electronic test points shall be short-circuit protected and easily accessible

24.4.4 Stress levels and tolerances

- The lowest possible stress levels should be used
- The possible operating limits and mechanical tolerances should be maximized
- Operations of known capability should be used

24.4.5 PCBs

- Adequate clearance should be provided around circuit board mounting locations to allow for tools
- Components should be soldered, not socketed
- PCBs must be mechanically secured and supported
- There must be unobstructed access to test and calibration points
- Exposed voltages should be less than 40 volts

24.4.6 Miscellaneous

- All air intakes should be filtered and an indication that the filter needs to be changed should be given to the user
- The device shall be packed in a recyclable container so as to minimize the system installation time

24.4.7 Design for assembly process

Develop a multi-functional team before the new product architecture is defined. This team should foster a creative climate which will encourage ownership of the new product's design and delivery process. Establish product goals through a benchmarking process or by creating a model, drawing, or a conception of the product. Perform a design for assembly analysis of the product. This identifies possible candidates for elimination or redesign, as well as highlighting high-cost assembly operations. Segment the product architecture into manageable modules or levels of assembly. Apply design for assembly principles to these assembly modules to generate a list of possible cost opportunities. Apply creative tools, such as brainstorming, to enhance the emerging design and identify further design improvements. As a team, evaluate and select the best ideas, thus narrowing and focusing the team's goals. Make commodity and material selections. Start early supplier involvement to assure economical production. With the aid of cost models or competitive benchmarking, establish a target cost for every part in the new design. Start the detailed design of the emerging product. Model, test, and evaluate the new design for form, fit, and function.

Re-apply the process at the next logical point. Share the results.

24.5   THE MANUFACTURING PROCESS

The process of producing new product may be said to be a multi-phased process consisting of:

- Pre-production activity
- The pilot run build
- The production run
- Delivery to the customer

24.5.1   PRE-PRODUCTION ACTIVITY

Prior to the first manufacturing build, manufacturing is responsible for completing a myriad of activity.

Manufacturing and engineering should work together to identify proposed technologies and to assure that the chosen technology is manufacturable.

The selection of suppliers should begin by consulting the current approved suppliers listing to determine if any of the existing suppliers can provide the technology and/or parts. A new supplier evaluation would be necessary if a supplier is being considered as a potential source for a component, subassembly, or device.

A pilot run plan must be developed that specifies the quantity of units to be built during the pilot run, the yield expectations and contingency plans, the distribution of those units, the feedback mechanism for problems, the intended production location, staffing requirements, training plan, post production evaluation, and any other key issues specific to the project.

The manufacturing strategy needs to be developed. The strategy must be documented and communicated to appropriate personnel to ensure it is complete, meets the business objectives, and ultimately is reflected in the design for the product. Developing a strategy for producing the product involves work on five major fronts:

- The production plan
- The quality plan
- The test plan
- The materials plan
- The supplier plan

The production plan details how manufacturing will produce the product. The first step is defining the requirements of the production process. Some of these requirements will be found in the business proposal and product specification. A bill of materials structure is developed for the product which best meets the defined requirements. Based on this bill of materials, a process flow diagram can be developed along with specific details of inventory levels and locations, test points, skills, resources, tooling required, and processing times.

The quality plan details the control through all phases of manufacture, procurement, packaging, storage, and shipment which collectively assures that the product meets specifications. The plan should cover not only initial production, but also how the plan will be matured over time, using data collected internally and from the field.

The test plan specifies the "how" of the quality plan. This document must have enough technical detail to assure that the features are incorporated in the product design specification. Care must be taken to ensure that the manufacturer's test strategies are consistent with those of all suppliers.

The materials plan consists of defining the operating plan by which the final product, parts, accessories, and service support parts will be managed logistically to meet the launch plans. This involves product structure, lead times, inventory management techniques, inventory phasing/impact estimates, and identification of any special materials considerations that must be addressed. Any production variants which will be in production, as well as potentially obsolete products, would be detailed.

The supplier plan consists of a matrix of potential suppliers versus evaluation criteria. The potential suppliers have been identified using preliminary functional component specifications. The evaluation criteria should include business stability, quality systems, cost, engineering capabilities, and test philosophy.

The DFMA review should be held when a representative model is available. This review should be documented, with action items assigned.

24.5.2 THE PILOT RUN BUILD

The objective of this phase is to complete the pilot run and validate the manufacturing process against the objectives set forth in the manufacturing strategy and the product specification.

The pilot run build is the first build of devices using the manufacturing documentation. It is during this phase that training of the assembly force takes place. All training should be documented so no employee is given a task without the appropriate training prior to the task.

The pilot run build will validate the manufacturing process against the strategy and the manufacturing documentation. The validation will determine if manufacturing has met its objectives, including:

- Standard cost
- Product quality
- Documentation
- Tooling
- Training
- Process control

The validation will also determine if the production testing is sufficient to ensure that the product meets the specified requirements.

The pilot run build also validates the supplier plan and supplier contracts. The validation will determine if the manufacturing plan is sufficient to control the internal processes of the supplier. The method and ground rules for communication between the two companies must be well defined to ensure that both parties keep each other informed of developments which impact the other. It should also confirm that all points have been addressed in the supplier contract and that all the controls and procedures required by the agreement are in place and operating correctly.

Internal failure analysis and corrective action takes place, involving investigating to the root cause all failures during the pilot run. The information should be communicated to the project team in detail and in a timely manner. The project team determines the appropriate corrective action plans.

A pilot run review meeting is held to review all aspects of the build, including the manufacturing documentation. All remaining issues must be resolved and documentation corrected. Sufficient time should be allowed in the project schedule for corrective action to be completed before the production run.

24.5.3 THE PRODUCTION RUN

The objective of this phase is to produce high-quality product on time, while continuing to fine tune the process using controls which have been put in place.

During this phase, the first production order of units and service parts is manufactured. The training effort continues, as new employees are transferred in or minor refinements are made to the process. Line failures at any point in the process should be thoroughly analyzed and the root cause determined. Product cost should be verified at this time.

24.5.4 CUSTOMER DELIVERY

The objective of this phase is to deliver the first production units to the customer, refine the manufacturing process based on lessons learned during the first build, and finally to monitor field unit performance to correct any problems.

Following production and shipment of product, continued surveillance of the production process should take place to measure its performance against the manufacturing strategy. The production process should be evaluated for effectiveness as well as unit field performance. Feedback from the field on unit problems should be sent to the project team, where it may be disseminated to the proper area.

REFERENCES

Boothroyd Dewhurst, Inc., *Design for Manufacture and Assembly/Service/Environment and Concurrent Engineering (Workshop Manual)*, Boothroyd Dewhurst, Inc., Wakefield, RI, 1966.

Food and Drug Administration, *21 CFR Part 820 Medical Devices; Current Good Manufacturing Practice (CGMP Regulations; Proposed Revisions)* November 23, 1993.

Fries, R.C., *Handbook of Medical Device Design*, Marcel-Dekker, Inc., New York, 2001.

Fries, R.C., *Reliability Assurance for Medical Devices, Equipment and Software*, Interpharm Press, Inc., Buffalo Grove, IL, 1991.

Fries, R.C., *Reliable Design of Medical Devices*, Marcel-Dekker, Inc., New York, 1997.

Hooten, W.F., A brief history of FDA good manufacturing practices, *Medical Device & Diagnostic Industry*, 18(5), May, 1996.

King, P.H. and Fries, R.C., *Design of Biomedical Devices and Systems*, Marcel Dekker, Inc., New York, 2002.

25 Configuration management

CONTENTS

25.1 Configuration identification 410
    25.1.1 Functional baseline 410
    25.1.2 Allocated baseline 411
    25.1.3 Developmental configuration 412
    25.1.4 Product baseline 412
25.2 Configuration audits 412
    25.2.1 Functional configuration audits 413
    25.2.2 Physical configuration audits 413
    25.2.3 In-process audits 414
25.3 Configuration management metrics 414
25.4 The FDA's view of configuration management................... 414
25.5 Status accounting 415
References 416

Configuration management is a discipline applying technical and administrative direction and surveillance to:

- Identify and document the functional and physical characteristics of configuration items
- Audit the configuration items to verify conformance to specifications, interface control documents, and other contract requirements
- Control changes to configuration items and their related documentation
- Record and report information needed to manage configuration items effectively, including the status of proposed changes and the implementation status of approved changes

Based on the operations of configuration management, it may be said to consist of four major divisions:

- Configuration identification
- Configuration change control

409

- Configuration status accounting
- Configuration audits

The purpose of configuration management is to maintain the integrity of products as they evolve from specifications through design, development, and production. Configuration management is not an isolated endeavor. It exists to support product development and maintenance.

Applying configuration management techniques to a particular project requires judgements to be exercised. Too little configuration management causes products to be lost, requiring previous work to be redone. Too much configuration management and the organization will never produce any products, because everyone will be too busy shuffling paperwork.

Applying configuration management to a project depends on the value of the product, the perceived risks, and the impact on the product if one of the perceived risks actually materializes. The main question to be answered is, what is required to obtain a reasonable degree of assurance that the integrity of the product will be maintained?

25.1   CONFIGURATION IDENTIFICATION

The first step in managing a collection of items is to uniquely identify each one. As a process, configuration identification is the selection of the documents to comprise a baseline for the system and the configuration items involved, and the numbers to be affixed to the items and documents.

In the configuration management sense, a baseline is a document, or a set of documents, formally designated and fixed at a specific time during a configuration item's life cycle. By establishing baselines, we can extend the orderly development of the system from specifications into design documentation, and then into hardware and software items themselves. Typically, four baselines are established in each project:

- Functional
- Allocated
- Developmental configuration (software only)
- Product

The four baselines are summarized in Table 25-1.

25.1.1   FUNCTIONAL BASELINE

The functional baseline is the initially approved documentation that describes a system's or item's functional characteristics, and the verifications required to demonstrate the achievement of those specified functional characteristics. This is the initial baseline to be established on a project and usually consists of the system specification, a document that establishes the technical characteristics of what the total collection of all the hardware and software is to do.

TABLE 25-1
Summary of baselines

Baseline	Content	Implementation
Functional	System specification	Contract award or completion of the peer review
Allocated	Unit specifications	Not later than the critical design review
	Interface control document	Not later than the critical design review
	Software requirements specification	Software requirements review
	Interface requirements specifications	Software requirements review
Developmental	Software top-level design documents	Preliminary design review
configuration	Software detailed design documents	Critical design review
	Source, object, and executable code	Unit test
Product	Hardware technical data package	Physical configuration audit
	Software design requirements	Physical configuration audit
	Source, object, and executable code	
	User and maintenance manuals	
	Test plans, test procedures, and test reports	

The functional baseline is a part of the formal agreement between a customer and the developer. It is normally established at the time of contract award, although it can be established after contract award at a specified review.

25.1.2 ALLOCATED BASELINE

The allocated baseline is the initially approved documentation that describes:

- An item's functional and interface characteristics that are allocated from a higher-level configuration item
- Interface requirements with interfacing configuration items
- Design constraints
- The verification required to demonstrate the achievement of those specified functional and interface characteristics

The allocated baseline consists of two type of documents:

- Specifications for the items themselves
- Interface requirements documents

Specifications for the items themselves are called unit specifications for hardware and the software requirements specification for software. These specifications describe each of the essential requirements of each hardware and software configuration item, including functions, performances, design constraints, and attributes.

Interface requirements documents are of two types: interface control drawings and interface requirements specifications. The interface control drawings identify the hardware interfaces between the hardware configuration items. The interface requirements specifications identify the interfaces between the software configuration items.

25.1.3 DEVELOPMENTAL CONFIGURATION

The developmental configuration is the software and associated technical documentation, which defines the evolving configuration of a software configuration item under development. It is under the developer's control and describes the software configuration at any stage of the design, coding, and testing effort. Current practice is to implement the developmental configuration in a phased manner as the individual components achieve specific values.

The developmental configuration is established incrementally. Items of the developmental configuration are baselined when they are reviewed with peers. Substantial efforts have been made as part of these reviews and the results reflect agreements reached with others. Although the documents remain under the control of the originating organization, some means of identifying the reviewed documents and tracking their changes is required.

25.1.4 PRODUCT BASELINE

The product baseline is the initially approved documentation that describes all the necessary functional and physical characteristics of the configuration item, any required interoperability characteristics of a configuration item, and the selected functional and physical characteristics designated for production acceptance testing. Typically, for hardware, the product baseline consists of the technical data package, including engineering drawings and associated lists, and all the rest of the items necessary to ensure that the hardware products can be fabricated by a third party. For software, the product baseline includes the software code on electronic media and the other items required to assure the code can be reproduced and maintained.

The product baseline is established on completion of formal acceptance testing of the system and the completion of a physical configuration audit.

25.2 CONFIGURATION AUDITS

An audit is an independent evaluation of a product to ascertain compliance to specifications, standards, contractual agreements, or other criteria. In the area of configuration management, there are three types of audits:

- Functional configuration audits

- Physical configuration audits
- In-process audits

Each audit has a different purpose.

25.2.1 FUNCTIONAL CONFIGURATION AUDITS

The purpose of a functional configuration audit is to validate that the development of a configuration item has been completed satisfactorily, and that the configuration item has achieved the performance and functional characteristics specified in the functional or allocated configuration. The audits are held at the end of the development cycle, following completion of all the testing on items that have been developed. The goal of the audits is to obtain a reasonable degree of confidence that the items have met all their requirements.

There are a number of cautions that should be observed at this point. First, the functional configuration audit is not the time to review the test program itself for adequacy. The judgement that the test program was adequate for the intended purposes should have already been made.

Second, there is sometimes a viewpoint expressed that, if anything changed, the entire test program should be reinitiated. There are judgements to be made, and extreme calls on either end of the spectrum should be avoided. Regression or check tests should be used in doubtful cases.

Third, there are cases in which there has been only one test made, with one test report and a series of actions. In such circumstances, convening a functional configuration audit to review that one test may not be warranted. For this reason, in software, functional configuration audits are not usually held.

25.2.2 PHYSICAL CONFIGURATION AUDITS

The physical configuration audit is a technical examination of a designated configuration item to verify that the configuration item, as built, conforms to the technical documentation that defines it. On the hardware side, a physical configuration audit is an audit of the actual product itself against its technical data package. The reason for this audit for hardware is straightforward. It has been previously verified, at the functional configuration audit, that the item constructed as part of the development cycle met all the requirements in the specification. Now, if the technical data package provides accurate instructions on how to build identical items, then many of the items that meet those specifications can be produced without the exhaustive testing required for the initial item. Confirmatory and first-item testing will take place during production, but these can be done on a sampling basis, rather than on 100% of the production items.

25.2.3 IN-PROCESS AUDITS

In-process audits are performed to determine whether the configuration management process, established in an organization, is being followed and to ascertain what needs to be improved. The task of conducting an in-process audit is usually relegated to the quality assurance function.

25.3 CONFIGURATION MANAGEMENT METRICS

Configuration management metrics can be obtained from the configuration management library, which holds the source files, both documents and source code. By examining the documentation in the source file, the following can be obtained:

- Documentation sizes
- Documentation changes
- Size of documentation changes

Documentation sizes can be easily measured in words, using any standard word-counting program. Metrics can then be provided for individual documents, individual types of documents, and documents grouped by configuration item.

Documentation changes are the actual number of changes for each document identified above, where one change is defined as one formal issue of a set of page changes to an original document.

The size of document changes consists of the actual size, in words, for the changes for each document identified above.

In a similar manner to documentation metrics, the following source code metrics are also easily obtained:

- The number of source files of code
- The number of revisions to source file code
- Actual number of source line of code

25.4 THE FDA'S VIEW OF CONFIGURATION MANAGEMENT

In the March, 1996 draft of their design control guidance document, the FDA states that the procedures for controlling change include methods for:

- Controlling the identification of development status
- Requesting and approving changes
- Ensuring that changes are properly integrated through formal change control procedures
- Obtaining approval to implement a change
- Version identification, issue, and control

Change control procedures require the complete documentation of approved changes and the communication of configuration changes to all who are affected. Design changes are reviewed to determine whether they influence previously approved design verification or validation results. In general, for any approved document, subsequent changes to that document should be approved by the same authority that approved the original design. In addition, the request for a change should be accompanied by an assessment of the total impact of the change.

The FDA believes configuration management refers to the documentation to be controlled, the procedures for controlling it, and the responsibilities of those managing the documentation. It includes a system of traceability, including traceability of components, service manuals, and procedures that could be affected by a change. The controlled documents are configuration items and collectively form the device configuration.

Typically the device configuration includes specifications, design documents, test documents, and all other deliverables, including those documents required for regulatory records.

The draft document has been issued for review and comment by medical device manufacturers.

25.5   STATUS ACCOUNTING

Status accounting is the recording activity. It follows up on the results of configuration management activities. It keeps track of the current configuration identification documents, the current configuration of the delivered software, the status of changes being reviewed, and the status of implementation of approved changes.

Status accounting refers to the record-keeping functions inherent in the other configuration management activities and to the specialized management information system that must exist to provide all the technical information. Thus, for each document authored, reviewed, approved, and distributed, recordings are made of all the current data for a document, specification, or change in order to communicate this information to the project/users/support activities as fast as it becomes available. The data must be in a form to allow traceability from top to bottom and bottom to top.

The first step in establishing a configuration status accounting capability is to identify the overall reporting requirements. Then these reporting requirements are used to determine the detailed requirements for the supporting facility. Acquisition of the resources, including hardware, software, communications, space, and people, can then be initiated. The database can then be initialized and the initial reports produced. Establishing this capability requires substantial efforts and should be initiated as early as possible in the development process. Updating the database will be a continuing activity, and the reports themselves will change as the user's needs evolve.

REFERENCES

Berlack, H.R., *Software Configuration Management*, John Wiley & Sons, Inc., New York, 1992.

Buckley, F.J., *Implementing Configuration Management: Hardware, Software, and Firmware*, The Institute of Electrical and Electronic Engineers, Inc., New York, 1993.

Evans, M.W. and Marciniak, J.J., *Software Quality Assurance and Management*, John Wiley & Sons, Inc., New York, 1987.

Food and Drug Administration, *Draft of Design Control Guidance for Medical Device Manufacturers*, March, 1996.

Fries, R.C., *Reliable Design of Medical Devices*, Marcel-Dekker, Inc., New York, 1997.

Fries, R.C., *Handbook of Medical Device Design*, Marcel-Dekker, Inc., New York, 2001.

IEEE Std 1042, *IEEE Guide to Software Configuration Management*, The Institute of Electrical and Electronic Engineers, Inc., New York, 1986.

IEEE Std 828, *IEEE Standard for Software Configuration Management Plans*, The Institute of Electrical and Electronic Engineers, Inc., New York, 1990.

King, P.H. and Fries, R.C., *Design of Biomedical Devices and Systems*, Marcel Dekker, Inc., New York, 2002.

MIL-STD-483, *Configuration Management Practices for Systems, Equipment, Munitions, and Computer Programs*, Department of Defense, Washington, DC, 1979.

MIL-STD-973, *Configuration Management*, Department of Defense, Washington, DC, 1992.

O'Connor, P.D.T., *Practical Reliability Engineering*, 3rd edition, John Wiley & Sons, Chichester, UK, 1991.

26 Analysis of field data

CONTENTS

26.1   Analysis of field service reports 418
        26.1.1   The database 418
        26.1.2   Data analysis 419
26.2   Failure analysis of field units 421
26.3   Warranty analysis 422
References 422

The goal of the product development process is to put a safe, effective, and reliable medical device in the hands of a physician or other medical personnel where it may be used to improve health care. The device has been designed and manufactured to be safe, effective and reliable. The manufacturer warranties the device for a certain period of time, usually 1 year. Is this the end of the manufacturer's concern about the device? It should not be. There is too much valuable information to be obtained.

When a product is subjected to reliability activities during design and development, testing is performed to determine the degree of reliability present and the confidence in that determination. There is, however, no guarantee that the product, as manufactured and shipped, has that same degree of reliability. The most meaningful way to determine the degree of reliability within each device is to monitor its activity in the field.

Analysis of field data is the means of determining how a product is performing in actual use. It is a means of determining the reliability growth over time. It is a measure of how well the product was specified, designed, and manufactured. It is a source of information on the effectiveness of the shipping configuration. It is also a source for information for product enhancements or new designs.

Field information may be obtained in any of several ways, including:

- Analysis of field service reports
- Failure analysis of failed units
- Warranty analysis

26.1   ANALYSIS OF FIELD SERVICE REPORTS

The type of data necessary for a meaningful analysis of product reliability is gathered from field service reports. The reports contains such vital information as:

- Type of product
- Serial number
- Date of service activity
- Symptom of the problem
- Diagnosis
- List of parts replaced
- Labor hours required
- Service representative

The type of product allows classification by individual model. The serial number allows a history of each individual unit to be established and traceability to the manufacturing date. The date of service activity helps to indicate the length of time until the problem occurred.

The symptom is the problem, as recognized by the user. The diagnosis is the description of the cause of the problem from analysis by the service representative. The two may be mutually exclusive, as the cause of the problem may be remote from the user's original complaint. The list of parts replaced is an adjunct to the diagnosis and can serve to trend parts usage and possible vendor problems. The diagnosis is then coded, where it may later be sorted.

The required labor hours help in evaluating the complexity of a problem, as represented by the time involved in repair. It, along with the name of the service representative, acts as a check on the efficiency of the individual representative, as average labor hours for the same failure code may be compared on a representative-to-representative basis. The labor hours per problem may be calculated to assist in determining warranty cost as well as determining the efficiency of service methods.

The only additional data which are not included in the field service report are the date of manufacture of each unit and the length of time since manufacture that the problem occurred. The manufacturing date is kept on file in the device history record. The length of time since manufacture is calculated by subtracting the manufacturing date from the date of service.

26.1.1   THE DATABASE

Field service reports are sorted by product upon receipt. The report is scanned for completeness. Service representatives may be contacted where clarification of an entry or lack of information would lead to an incomplete database record. The diagnoses are coded, according to a list of failures, as developed by reliability assurance, design engineering and manufacturing engineering (Figure 26-1). Manufacturing date and the length of time since

Failure code	Failure
Base machine	
101	Missing parts
102	Shipping damage
103	Circuit breaker wiring damage
104	Regulator defect
105	Shelf latch broken
Monitor	
201	Display problems
202	Control cable defect
203	Power board problem
204	Control board problem
205	Unstable reference voltage

FIGURE 26-1 List of failure codes

manufacture are obtained. The data are then ready to be entered into the computer.

The data are entered into a computer database, where they may be manipulated to determine the necessary parameters. Each field service report is input to a single database record, unless the service report contains multiple failure codes. Figure 26-2 shows a sample database record.

The data are first sorted by service date, so trending can be accomplished by a predetermined time period, such as a fiscal quarter. Data within that time frame are then sorted by problem code, indicating the frequency of problems during the particular reporting period. A pareto analysis of the problems can then be developed. Data are finally sorted by serial number, which gives an indication of which devices experienced multiple service calls and/or experienced continuing problems.

Percentages of total problems are helpful in determining primary failures. Spreadsheets are developed listing the problems versus manufacturing dates and the problems versus time since manufacturing. The spreadsheet data can then be plotted and analyzed.

26.1.2 DATA ANALYSIS

The most important reason for collecting the field data is to extract the most significant problem information and put it in such a form that the cause of product problems may be highlighted, trended, and focused upon. The cause of the problem must be determined and the most appropriate solution implemented. A "band-aid" solution is unacceptable.

Field	Field content
1	Service date
2	Device serial number
3	Manufacturing date
4	Time in use (hours)
5	Failure code
6	Failed parts 1
7	Failed parts 2
8	Failed parts 3
9	Failed parts 4
10	Failed parts 5
11	Time to repair (hours)
12	Service representative ID

FIGURE 26-2 Sample database record

Pareto analysis is used to determine what the major problems are. The individual problems are plotted along the x- axis and the frequency on the y- axis. The result is a histogram of problems, where the severity of the problem is indicated, leading to the establishment of priorities in addressing solutions.

Several graphical plots are helpful in analyzing problems. One is the plot of particular problems versus length of time since manufacturing. This plot is used to determine the area of the life cycle in which the problem occurs. Peaks of problem activity indicate infant mortality, useful life or wearout, depending on the length of time since manufacture.

A second plot of interest is that of a particular problem versus the date of manufacture. This plot is a good indication of the efficiency of the manufacturing process. It shows times where problems occur, e.g., the rush to ship product at the end of a fiscal quarter, lot problems on components, or vendor problems. The extent of the problem is an indication of the correct or incorrect solution.

Another useful plot is that of the total number of problems versus the date of manufacture. The learning curve for the product is visible at the peaks of the curve. It can also be shown how the problems for subsequent builds decrease as manufacturing personnel become more familiar and efficient with the process.

Trending of problems, set against the time of reporting, is an indicator of the extent of a problem and how effective the correction is. Decreasing numbers indicate the solution is effective. Reappearing high counts indicate the initial solution did not address the cause of the problem.

The database is also useful for analyzing warranty costs. The data can be used to calculate warranty expenses, problems per manufactured unit, and warranty costs as a percentage of sales. A similar table can be established for installation of devices.

26.2 FAILURE ANALYSIS OF FIELD UNITS

Most failure analysis performed in the field is done at the board level. Service representatives usually solve problems by board swapping, since they are not equipped to troubleshoot at the component level. Boards should be returned to be analyzed to the component level. This not only yields data for trending purposes, but highlights the real cause of the problem. It also gives data on problem parts or problem vendors.

The most important process in performing field failure analysis is focusing on the cause of the problem, based on the symptom. It does no good to develop a fix for a symptom if the cause is not known. To do so only

Product code	Parameters	Cost 1/95	Cost 2/95	Cost year to date
4425	Normal warranty	$	$	$
	Recall warranty	$	$	$
	Total warranty	$	$	$
	Setup cost	$	$	$
	Total cost	$	$	$
	Sales	$	$	$
	Warranty/sales			
	Setup/sales			
	Total/sales			
	Number of units shipped			
	Number of units setup			
	Number warranty units			
	Number of recall units			
	Warranty/unit	$	$	$
	Recall/unit	$	$	$
	Setup/unit	$	$	$
	Total/unit	$	$	$

FIGURE 26-3 Warranty analysis

creates additional problems. Analysis techniques, such as fault tree analysis of FMEA, may help to focus on the cause.

Once the component level analysis is completed, pareto charts may be made, highlighting problem areas and prioritizing problem solutions. The major problems can be placed in a spreadsheet and monitored over time. Graphical plots can also be constructed to monitor various parameters over time.

26.3 WARRANTY ANALYSIS

Warranty analysis is an indication of the reliability of a device in its early life, usually the first year. Warranty analysis (Figure 26-3) is a valuable source of information on such parameters as warranty cost as a percentage of sales, warranty cost per unit, installation cost per unit, and percentage of shipped units experiencing problems. By plotting these data, a trend can be established over time.

REFERENCES

AAMI, *Guideline for Establishing and Administering Medical Instrumentation*, Association for the Advancement of Medical Instrumentation, Arlington, VA, 1984.

Fries, R.C., et al., A reliability assurance database for analysis of medical product performance, *Proceedings of the Symposium one Engineering of Computer-Based Medical Systems*, The Institute of Electrical and Electronic Engineers, New York, 1988.

Fries, R.C., *Reliable Design of Medical Devices*, Marcel-Dekker, Inc., New York, 1997.

Fries, R.C., *Handbook of Medical Device Design*, Marcel-Dekker, Inc., New York, 2001.

King, P.H. and Fries, R.C., *Design of Biomedical Devices and Systems*, Marcel-Dekker, Inc., New York, 2002.

MIL-HDBK-472, *Maintainability Prediction*, Department of Defense, Washington, DC, 1966.

Appendices

1 Chi square table

ν/γ	0.975	0.950	0.900	0.050	0.100	0.050	0.025
1	0.001	0.004	0.016	0.455	2.706	3.841	5.024
2	0.051	0.103	0.211	1.386	4.605	5.991	7.738
3	0.216	0.352	0.584	2.366	6.251	7.815	9.438
4	0.484	0.711	1.064	3.357	7.779	9.488	11.143
5	0.831	1.145	1.610	4.351	9.236	11.070	12.832
6	1.237	1.635	2.204	5.348	10.645	12.592	14.449
7	1.690	2.167	2.833	6.346	12.017	14.067	16.013
8	2.180	2.733	3.490	7.344	13.362	15.507	17.535
9	2.700	3.325	4.168	8.343	14.684	16.919	19.023
10	3.247	3.940	4.865	9.342	15.987	18.307	20.483
11	3.816	4.575	5.578	10.341	17.275	19.675	21.920
12	4.404	5.226	6.304	11.340	18.549	21.026	23.337
13'	5.009	5.892	7.042	12.340	19.812	22.362	24.736
14	5.629	6.571	7.790	13.339	21.064	23.685	26.119
15	6.262	7.261	8.547	14.339	22.307	24.996	27.488
16	6.908	7.962	9.312	15.338	23.542	26.296	28.845
17	7.564	8.672	10.085	16.338	24.769	27.587	30.191
18	8.231	9.390	10.865	17.338	25.989	28.869	31.526
19	8.907	10.117	11.651	18.338	27.204	30.144	32.852
20	9.591	10.851	12.443	19.337	28.412	31.410	34.170
21	10.283	11.591	13.240	20.337	29.615	32.671	35.479
22	10.982	12.338	14.041	21.337	30.813	33.924	36.781
23	11.688	13.091	14.848	22.337	32.007	35.172	38.076
24	12.401	13.848	15.659	23.337	33.196	36.415	39.364
25	13.120	14.611	16.473	24.337	34.382	37.652	40.646
26	13.844	15.379	17.292	25.336	35.563	38.885	41.923
27	14.573	16.151	18.114	26.336	36.741	40.113	43.194
28	15.308	16.928	18.939	27.336	37.916	41.337	44.461
29	16.047	17.708	19.768	28.336	39.087	42.557	45.722
30	16.791	18.493	20.599	29.336	40.256	43.773	46.979

2 Percent rank tables

Sample Size = 1

Order Number	2.5	5.0	10.0	50.0	90.0	95.0	97.5
1	2.50	5.00	10.00	50.00	90.00	95.00	97.50

Sample Size = 2

Order Number	2.5	5.0	10.0	50.0	90.0	95.0	97.5
1	1.258	2.532	5.132	29.289	68.377	77.639	84.189
2	15.811	22.361	31.623	71.711	94.868	97.468	98.742

Sample Size = 3

Order Number	2.5	5.0	10.0	50.0	90.0	95.0	97.5
1	0.840	1.695	3.451	20.630	53.584	63.160	70.760
2	9.430	13.535	19.580	50.000	80.420	86.465	90.570
3	29.240	36.840	46.416	79.370	96.549	98.305	99.160

Sample Size = 4

Order Number	2.5	5.0	10.0	50.0	90.0	95.0	97.5
1	0.631	1.274	2.600	15.910	43.766	52.713	60.236
2	6.759	9.761	14.256	38.573	67.954	75.140	80.588
3	19.412	24.860	32.046	61.427	85.744	90.239	93.241
4	39.764	47.287	56.234	84.090	97.400	98.726	99.369

Sample Size = 5

Order Number	2.5	5.0	10.0	50.0	90.0	95.0	97.5
1	0.505	1.021	2.085	12.945	36.904	45.072	52.182
2	5.274	7.644	11.223	31.381	58.389	65.741	71.642
3	14.663	18.926	24.644	50.000	75.336	81.074	85.337
4	28.358	34.259	41.611	68.619	88.777	92.356	94.726
5	47.818	54.928	63.096	87.055	97.915	98.979	99.495

Sample Size = 6

Order Number	2.5	5.0	10.0	50.0	90.0	95.0	97.5
1	0.421	0.851	1.741	19.910	31.871	39.304	45.926
2	4.327	6.285	9.260	26.445	51.032	58.180	64.123
3	11.812	15.316	20.091	42.141	66.681	72.866	77.722
4	22.278	27.134	33.319	57.859	79.909	84.684	88.188
5	35.877	41.820	48.968	73.555	90.740	93.715	95.673
6	54.074	60.696	68.129	89.090	98.259	99.149	99.579

Sample Size = 7

Order Number	2.5	5.0	10.0	50.0	90.0	95.0	97.5
1	0.361	0.730	1.494	9.428	28.031	34.816	40.962
2	3.669	5.338	7.882	22.489	45.256	52.070	57.872
3	9.899	12.876	16.964	36.412	59.618	65.874	70.958
4	18.405	22.532	27.860	50.000	72.140	77.468	81.595
5	29.042	34.126	40.382	63.588	83.036	87.124	90.101
6	42.128	47.930	54.744	77.151	92.118	94.662	96.331
7	59.038	65.184	71.969	90.752	98.506	99.270	99.639

Sample Size = 8

Order Number	2.5	5.0	10.0	50.0	90.0	95.0	97.5
1	0.316	0.639	1.308	8.300	25.011	31.234	36.942
2	3.185	4.639	6.863	20.113	40.625	47.068	52.651
3	8.523	11.111	14.685	32.052	53.822	59.969	65.086
4	15.701	19.290	23.966	44.016	65.538	71.076	75.514
5	24.486	28.924	43.462	55.984	76.034	80.710	84.299
6	34.914	40.031	46.178	67.948	85.315	88.889	91.477
7	47.349	52.932	59.375	79.887	93.137	95.361	96.815
8	63.058	68.766	74.989	91.700	98.692	99.361	99.684

Sample Size = 9

Order Number	2.5	5.0	10.0	50.0	90.0	95.0	97.5
1	0.281	0.568	1.164	7.413	22.574	28.313	33.627
2	2.814	4.102	6.077	17.962	36.836	42.914	48.250
3	7.485	9.775	12.950	28.624	49.008	54.964	60.009
4	13.700	16.875	21.040	39.308	59.942	65.506	70.070
5	21.201	25.137	30.097	50.000	69.903	74.863	78.799
6	29.930	34.494	40.058	60.692	78.960	83.125	86.300
7	39.991	45.036	50.992	71.376	87.050	90.225	92.515
8	51.750	57.086	63.164	82.038	93.923	95.898	97.186
9	66.373	71.687	77.426	92.587	98.836	99.432	99.719

Sample Size = 10

Order Number	2.5	5.0	10.0	50.0	90.0	95.0	97.5
1	0.253	0.512	1.048	6.697	20.567	25.887	30.850
2	2.521	3.677	5.453	16.226	33.685	39.416	44.502
3	6.674	8.726	11.583	25.857	44.960	50.690	55.610
4	12.155	15.003	18.756	35.510	55.173	60.662	65.245
5	18.709	22.244	26.732	45.169	64.578	69.646	73.762
6	26.238	30.354	35.422	54.831	73.268	77.756	81.291
7	34.755	39.338	44.827	64.490	81.244	84.997	87.845
8	44.390	49.310	55.040	74.143	88.417	91.274	93.326
9	55.498	60.584	66.315	83.774	94.547	96.323	97.479
10	69.150	74.113	79.433	93.303	98.952	99.488	99.747

Sample Size = 11

Order Number	2.5	5.0	10.0	50.0	90.0	95.0	97.5
1	0.230	0.465	0.953	6.107	18.887	23.840	28.491
2	2.283	3.332	4.945	14.796	31.024	36.436	41.278
3	6.022	7.882	10.477	23.579	41.516	47.009	41.776
4	10.926	13.508	16.923	32.380	51.076	56.437	60.974
5	16.749	19.958	24.053	41.189	59.947	65.019	69.210
6	23.379	27.125	31.772	50.000	68.228	72.875	76.621
7	30.790	34.981	40.053	58.811	75.947	80.042	83.251
8	39.026	43.563	48.924	67.620	83.077	86.492	89.074
9	48.224	52.991	58.484	76.421	89.523	92.118	93.978
10	58.722	63.564	68.976	85.204	95.055	96.668	97.717
11	71.509	76.160	81.113	93.893	99.047	99.535	99.770

Sample Size = 12

Order Number	2.5	5.0	10.0	50.0	90.0	95.0	97.5
1	0.211	0.427	0.874	5.613	17.460	22.092	26.465
2	2.086	3.046	4.524	13.598	28.750	33.868	38.480
3	5.486	7.187	9.565	21.669	38.552	43.811	48.414
4	9.925	12.285	15.419	29.758	47.527	52.733	57.186
5	15.165	18.102	21.868	37.583	55.900	60.914	65.112
6	21.094	24.530	28.817	45.951	63.772	68.476	72.333
7	27.667	31.524	36.228	54.049	71.183	75.470	78.906
8	34.888	39.086	44.100	62.147	78.132	81.898	84.835
9	42.814	47.267	52.473	70.242	84.581	87.715	90.075
10	51.586	56.189	61.448	78.331	90.435	92.813	94.514
11	61.520	66.132	71.250	86.402	95.476	96.954	97.914
12	73.535	77.908	82.540	94.387	99.126	99.573	99.789

Sample Size = 13

Order Number	2.5	5.0	10.0	50.0	90.0	95.0	97.5
1	0.195	0.394	0.807	5.192	16.232	20.582	24.705
2	1.921	2.805	4.169	12.579	26.784	31.634	36.030
3	5.038	6.605	8.800	20.045	35.978	41.010	45.447
4	9.092	11.267	14.161	27.528	44.426	49.465	53.813
5	13.858	16.566	20.050	35.016	52.343	57.262	61.426
6	19.223	22.396	26.373	52.508	59.824	64.520	68.422
7	25.135	28.705	33.086	50.000	66.914	71.295	74.865
8	31.578	35.480	40.176	57.492	73.627	77.604	80.777
9	38.574	42.738	47.657	64.984	79.950	83.434	86.142
10	46.187	50.535	55.574	72.472	85.839	88.733	90.908
11	54.553	58.990	64.022	79.955	91.200	93.395	94.962
12	63.970	68.366	73.216	87.421	95.831	97.195	98.079
13	75.295	79.418	83.768	94.808	99.193	99.606	99.805

Sample Size = 14

Order Number	2.5	5.0	10.0	50.0	90.0	95.0	97.5
1	0.181	0.366	0.750	4.830	15.166	19.264	23.164
2	1.779	2.600	3.866	11.702	25.067	29.673	33.868
3	4.658	6.110	8.148	18.647	33.721	38.539	42.813
4	8.389	10.405	13.094	25.608	41.698	46.566	50.798
5	12.760	15.272	18.513	32.575	49.197	54.001	58.104
6	17.661	20.607	24.316	39.544	56.311	60.959	64.862
7	23.036	26.358	30.455	46.515	63.087	67.497	71.139
8	28.861	32.503	36.913	53.485	69.545	73.642	76.964
9	35.138	39.041	43.689	60.456	75.684	79.393	82.339
10	41.896	45.999	50.803	67.425	81.487	84.728	87.240
11	49.202	53.434	58.302	74.392	86.906	89.595	91.611
12	57.187	61.461	66.279	81.353	91.852	93.890	95.342
13	66.132	70.327	74.933	88.298	96.134	97.400	98.221
14	76.836	80.736	84.834	95.170	99.250	99.634	99.819

Sample Size = 15

Order Number	2.5	5.0	10.0	50.0	90.0	95.0	97.5
1	0.169	0.341	0.700	4.516	14.230	18.104	21.802
2	1.658	2.423	3.604	10.940	23.557	27.940	31.948
3	4.331	5.685	7.586	17.432	31.279	36.344	40.460
4	7.787	9.666	12.177	23.939	39.279	43.978	48.089
5	11.824	14.166	17.197	30.452	46.397	51.075	55.100
6	16.336	19.086	22.559	36.967	53.171	57.744	61.620
7	21.627	24.373	28.218	43.483	59.647	64.043	67.713
8	26.586	29.999	34.152	50.000	65.848	70.001	73.414
9	32.287	35.957	40.353	56.517	71.782	75.627	78.733
10	38.380	42.256	46.829	63.033	77.441	80.914	83.664
11	44.900	48.925	53.603	69.548	82.803	85.834	88.176
12	51.911	56.022	60.721	76.061	87.823	90.334	92.213
13	59.540	63.656	68.271	82.568	92.414	94.315	95.669

| 14 | 68.052 | 72.060 | 76.443 | 89.060 | 96.396 | 97.577 | 98.342 |
| 15 | 78.198 | 81.896 | 85.770 | 95.484 | 99.300 | 99.659 | 99.831 |

Sample Size = 16

Order Number	2.5	5.0	10.0	50.0	90.0	95.0	97.5
1	0.158	0.320	0.656	4.240	13.404	17.075	20.591
2	1.551	2.268	3.375	10.270	22.217	26.396	30.232
3	4.047	5.315	7.097	16.365	29.956	34.383	38.348
4	7.266	9.025	11.380	22.474	37.122	41.657	45.646
5	11.017	13.211	16.056	28.589	43.892	48.440	52.377
6	15.198	17.777	21.041	34.705	50.351	54.835	58.662
7	19.753	22.669	26.292	40.823	56.544	60.899	64.565
8	24.651	27.860	31.783	46.941	62.496	66.663	70.122
9	29.878	33.337	37.504	53.059	68.217	72.140	75.349
10	35.435	39.101	43.456	59.177	73.708	77.331	80.247
11	41.338	45.165	49.649	65.295	78.959	82.223	84.802
12	47.623	51.560	56.108	71.411	83.944	86.789	88.983
13	54.354	58.343	62.878	77.526	88.620	90.975	92.734
14	61.652	65.617	70.044	83.635	92.903	94.685	95.953
15	69.768	73.604	77.783	89.730	96.625	97.732	98.449
16	79.409	82.925	86.596	95.760	99.344	99.680	99.842

Sample Size = 17

Order Number	2.5	5.0	10.0	50.0	90.0	95.0	97.5
1	0.149	0.301	0.618	3.995	12.667	16.157	19.506
2	1.458	2.132	3.173	9.678	21.021	25.012	28.689
3	3.779	4.990	6.667	15.422	28.370	32.619	36.441
4	6.811	8.465	10.682	21.178	35.187	39.564	43.432
5	10.314	12.377	15.058	26.940	41.639	46.055	49.899
6	14.210	16.636	19.716	32.704	47.807	52.192	55.958
7	18.444	21.191	24.614	38.469	53.735	58.029	61.672
8	22.983	26.011	29.726	44.234	59.449	63.599	67.075
9	27.812	31.083	35.039	50.000	64.961	68.917	72.188
10	32.925	36.401	40.551	55.766	70.274	73.989	77.017
11	38.328	41.971	46.265	61.531	75.386	78.809	81.556
12	44.042	47.808	52.193	67.296	80.284	83.364	85.790
13	50.101	53.945	58.361	73.060	84.942	87.623	89.686
14	56.568	60.436	64.813	78.821	89.318	91.535	93.189
15	63.559	67.381	71.630	84.578	93.333	95.010	96.201
16	71.311	74.988	78.979	90.322	96.827	97.868	98.542
17	80.494	83.843	87.333	96.005	99.382	99.699	99.851

Sample Size = 18

Order Number	2.5	5.0	10.0	50.0	90.0	95.0	97.5
1	0.141	0.285	0.584	3.778	12.008	15.332	18.530
2	1.375	2.011	2.995	9.151	19.947	23.766	27.294
3	3.579	4.702	6.286	14.58*	26.942	31.026	34.712

4	6.409	7.970	10.064	20.024	33.441	37.668	41.418
5	9.695	11.643	14.177	25.471	39.602	43.888	47.637
6	13.343	15.634	18.549	30.921	45.502	49.783	53.480
7	17.299	19.895	23.139	36.371	51.184	55.405	59.007
8	21.530	24.396	27.922	41.823	56.672	60.784	64.255
9	26.019	29.120	32.885	47.274	61.980	65.940	69.243
10	30.757	34.060	38.020	52.726	67.115	70.880	73.981
11	35.745	39.216	43.328	58.177	72.078	75.604	78.470
12	40.993	44.595	48.618	63.629	76.861	80.105	82.701
13	46.520	50.217	54.498	69.079	81.451	84.336	86.657
14	52.363	56.112	60.398	74.529	85.823	88.357	90.305
15	58.582	62.332	66.559	79.976	89.936	92.030	93.591
16	65.288	68.974	73.058	85.419	93.714	95.298	96.421
17	72.706	76.234	80.053	90.849	97.005	97.989	98.625
18	81.470	84.668	87.992	96.222	99.416	99.715	99.859

Sample Size = 19

Order Number	2.5	5.0	10.0	50.0	90.0	95.0	97.5
1	0.133	0.270	0.553	3.582	11.413	14.587	17.647
2	1.301	1.903	2.835	8.678	18.977	22.637	26.028
3	3.383	4.446	5.946	13.827	25.651	29.580	33.138
4	6.052	7.529	9.514	18.989	31.859	35.943	39.578
5	9.147	10.991	13.394	24.154	37.753	41.912	45.565
6	12.576	14.747	17.513	29.322	43.405	47.580	51.203
7	16.289	18.750	21.832	34.491	48.856	52.997	56.550
8	20.252	22.972	26.327	39.660	54.132	58.194	61.642
9	24.447	27.395	30.983	44.830	59.246	63.188	66.500
10	28.864	32.009	35.793	50.000	64.207	67.991	71.136
11	33.500	36.812	40.754	55.170	69.017	72.605	75.553
12	38.358	41.806	45.868	60.340	73.673	77.028	79.748
13	43.450	47.003	51.144	65.509	78.168	81.250	83.711
14	48.797	54.420	56.595	70.678	82.487	85.253	87.424
15	54.435	58.088	62.247	75.846	86.606	89.009	90.853
16	60.422	64.057	68.141	81.011	90.486	92.471	93.948
17	66.682	70.420	74.349	86.173	94.054	95.554	96.617
18	73.972	77.363	81.023	91.322	97.165	98.097	98.699
19	82.353	85.413	88.587	96.418	99.447	99.730	99.867

Sample Size = 20

Order Number	2.5	5.0	10.0	50.0	90.0	95.0	97.5
1	0.127	0.256	0.525	3.406	10.875	13.911	16.843
2	1.235	1.807	2.691	8.251	18.096	21.611	24.873
3	3.207	4.217	5.642	13.147	24.477	28.262	31.698
4	5.733	7.135	9.021	18.055	30.419	34.366	37.893
5	8.657	10.408	12.693	22.967	36.066	40.103	43.661
6	11.893	13.955	16.587	27.880	41.489	45.558	49.105
7	15.391	17.731	20.666	32.795	46.727	50.782	54.279
8	19.119	21.707	24.906	37.711	51.803	55.803	59.219
9	23.058	25.865	29.293	42.626	56.733	60.642	63.946
10	27.196	30.195	33.817	47.542	61.525	65.307	68.472
11	31.528	34.693	38.475	52.458	66.183	69.805	72.804

12	36.054	39.358	43.267	57.374	70.707	74.135	76.942
13	40.781	44.197	48.197	62.289	75.094	78.293	80.881
14	45.721	49.218	53.273	67.205	79.334	82.269	84.609
15	50.895	54.442	58.511	72.120	83.413	86.045	88.107
16	56.339	59.897	63.934	77.033	87.307	89.592	91.343
17	62.107	65.634	69.581	81.945	90.979	92.865	94.267
18	68.302	71.738	75.523	86.853	94.358	95.783	96.793
19	75.127	78.389	81.904	91.749	97.309	98.193	98.765
20	83.157	86.089	89.125	96.594	99.475	99.744	99.873

Sample Size = 21

Order Number	2.5	5.0	10.0	50.0	90.0	95.0	97.5
1	0.120	0.244	0.500	3.247	10.385	13.295	16.110
2	1.175	1.719	2.562	7.864	17.294	20.673	23.816
3	3.049	4.010	5.367	12.531	23.405	27.055	30.377
4	5.446	6.781	8.577	17.209	29.102	32.921	36.342
5	8.218	9.884	12.062	21.891	34.522	38.441	41.907
6	11.281	13.245	15.755	26.574	39.733	43.698	47.166
7	14.588	16.818	19.619	31.258	44.771	48.739	52.175
8	18.107	20.575	23.632	35.943	49.661	53.594	56.968
9	21.820	24.499	27.779	40.629	54.416	58.280	61.565
10	25.713	28.580	32.051	45.314	59.046	62.810	65.979
11	29.781	32.811	36.443	50.000	63.557	67.189	70.219
12	34.021	37.190	40.954	54.686	67.949	71.420	74.287
13	38.435	41.720	45.584	59.371	72.221	75.501	78.180
14	43.032	46.406	50.339	64.057	76.368	79.425	81.893
15	47.825	51.261	55.229	68.742	80.381	83.182	85.412
16	52.834	56.302	60.267	73.426	84.245	86.755	88.719
17	58.093	61.559	65.478	78.109	87.938	90.116	91.782
18	63.658	67.079	70.898	82.791	91.423	93.219	94.554
19	69.623	72.945	76.595	87.469	94.633	95.990	96.951
20	76.184	79.327	82.706	92.136	97.438	98.281	98.825
21	83.890	86.705	89.615	96.753	99.500	99.756	99.880

Sample Size = 22

Order Number	2.5	5.0	10.0	50.0	90.0	95.0	97.5
1	0.115	0.233	0.478	3.102	9.937	12.731	15.437
2	1.121	1.640	2.444	7.512	16.559	19.812	22.844
3	2.906	3.822	5.117	11.970	22.422	25.947	29.161
4	5.187	6.460	8.175	16.439	27.894	31.591	34.912
5	7.821	9.411	11.490	20.911	33.104	36.909	40.285
6	10.729	12.603	15.002	25.384	38.117	41.980	45.370
7	13.865	15.994	18.674	29.859	42.970	46.849	50.222
8	17.198	19.556	22.483	34.334	47.684	51.546	54.872
9	29.709	23.272	26.416	38.810	52.275	56.087	59.342
10	24.386	27.131	30.463	43.286	56.752	60.484	63.645
11	28.221	31.126	34.619	47.762	61.119	64.746	67.790
12	32.210	35.254	38.881	52.238	65.381	68.874	71.779
13	36.355	39.516	43.248	56.714	69.537	72.869	75.614
14	40.658	43.913	47.725	61.190	73.584	76.728	79.291
15	45.128	48.454	52.316	65.666	77.517	80.444	82.802

16	49.778	53.151	57.030	70.141	81.326	84.006	86.135
17	54.630	58.020	61.883	74.616	84.998	87.397	89.271
18	59.715	63.091	66.896	79.089	88.510	90.589	92.179
19	65.088	68.409	72.106	83.561	91.825	93.540	94.813
20	70.839	74.053	77.578	88.030	94.883	96.178	97.094
21	77.156	80.188	83.441	92.488	97.556	98.360	98.879
22	84.563	87.269	90.063	96.898	99.522	99.767	99.885

Sample Size = 23

Order Number	2.5	5.0	10.0	50.0	90.0	95.0	97.5
1	0.110	0.223	0.457	2.969	9.526	12.212	14.819
2	1.071	1.567	2.337	7.191	15.884	19.020	21.949
3	2.775	3.652	4.890	11.458	21.519	24.925	28.038
4	4.951	6.168	7.808	15.734	26.781	30.364	33.589
5	7.460	8.981	10.971	20.015	31.797	35.493	38.781
6	10.229	12.021	14.318	24.297	36.626	40.390	43.703
7	13.210	15.248	17.816	28.580	41.305	45.098	48.405
8	16.376	18.634	21.442	32.863	45.856	49.644	52.919
9	19.708	22.164	25.182	37.147	50.291	54.046	57.226
10	23.191	25.824	29.027	41.431	54.622	58.315	61.458
11	26.820	29.609	32.971	45.716	58.853	62.461	65.505
12	30.588	33.515	37.012	50.000	62.988	66.485	69.412
13	34.495	37.539	41.147	54.284	67.029	70.391	73.180
14	38.542	41.685	45.378	58.569	70.973	74.176	76.809
15	42.734	45.954	49.709	62.853	74.818	77.836	80.292
16	47.081	50.356	54.144	67.137	78.558	81.366	83.624
17	51.595	54.902	58.695	71.420	82.184	84.752	86.790
18	56.297	59.610	63.374	75.703	85.682	87.979	89.771
19	61.219	64.507	68.203	79.985	89.029	91.019	92.540
20	66.411	69.636	73.219	84.266	92.192	93.832	95.049
21	71.962	75.075	78.481	88.542	95.110	96.348	97.225
22	78.051	80.980	84.116	92.809	97.663	98.433	98.929
23	85.151	87.788	90.474	97.031	99.543	99.777	99.890

Sample Size = 24

Order Number	2.5	5.0	10.0	50.0	90.0	95.0	97.5
1	0.105	0.213	0.438	2.847	9.148	11.735	14.247
2	1.026	1.501	2.238	6.895	15.262	18.289	21.120
3	2.656	3.495	4.682	10.987	20.685	23.980	26.997
4	4.735	5.901	7.473	15.088	25.754	29.227	32.361
5	7.132	8.589	10.497	19.192	30.588	34.181	37.384
6	9.773	11.491	13.694	23.299	35.246	38.914	42.151
7	12.615	14.569	17.033	27.406	39.763	43.469	46.711
8	16.630	17.796	20.493	31.513	44.160	47.873	51.095
9	18.799	21.157	24.058	35.621	48.449	52.142	55.322
10	22.110	24.639	27.721	39.729	52.461	56.289	59.406
11	25.553	28.236	31.476	43.837	56.742	60.321	63.357
12	29.124	31.942	35.317	47.946	60.755	64.244	67.179
13	32.821	35.756	39.245	52.054	64.683	68.058	70.876
14	36.643	39.679	43.258	56.163	68.524	71.764	74.447
15	40.594	43.711	47.359	60.271	72.279	75.361	77.890

16	44.678	47.858	51.551	64.379	75.942	78.843	81.201
17	48.905	52.127	55.840	68.487	79.507	82.204	84.370
18	53.289	56.531	60.237	72.594	82.967	85.431	87.385
19	57.849	60.086	64.754	76.701	86.306	88.509	90.227
20	62.616	65.819	69.412	80.808	89.503	91.411	92.868
21	67.639	70.773	74.246	84.912	92.527	94.099	95.265
22	73.003	76.020	79.315	89.013	95.318	96.505	97.344
23	78.880	81.711	84.738	93.105	97.762	98.499	98.974
24	85.753	88.265	90.852	97.153	99.562	99.787	99.895

Sample Size = 25

Order Number	2.5	5.0	10.0	50.0	90.0	95.0	97.5
1	0.101	0.205	0.421	2.735	8.799	11.293	13.719
2	0.984	1.440	2.148	6.623	14.687	17.612	20.352
3	2.547	3.352	4.491	10.553	19.914	23.104	26.031
4	4.538	5.656	7.166	14.492	24.802	28.172	31.219
5	6.831	8.229	10.062	18.435	29.467	32.961	36.083
6	9.356	11.006	13.123	22.379	33.966	37.541	40.704
7	12.072	13.948	16.317	26.324	38.331	41.952	45.129
8	14.950	17.030	19.624	30.270	42.582	46.221	49.388
9	17.972	20.238	23.032	34.215	46.734	50.364	53.500
10	21.125	23.559	26.529	38.161	50.795	54.393	57.479
11	24.402	26.985	30.111	42.108	54.722	58.316	61.335
12	27.797	30.513	33.774	46.054	58.668	62.138	65.072
13	31.306	34.139	37.514	50.000	62.486	65.861	68.694
14	34.928	37.862	41.332	53.946	66.226	69.487	72.203
15	38.665	41.684	45.228	57.892	69.889	73.015	75.598
16	42.521	45.607	49.205	61.839	73.471	76.441	78.875
17	46.500	49.636	53.266	65.785	76.968	79.762	82.028
18	50.612	53.779	57.418	69.730	80.736	82.970	85.050
19	54.871	58.048	61.669	73.676	83.683	86.052	87.928
20	59.296	62.459	66.034	77.621	86.877	88.994	90.644
21	63.917	67.039	70.533	81.565	89.938	91.771	93.169
22	68.781	71.828	75.198	85.508	92.834	94.344	95.462
23	73.969	76.896	80.086	89.447	95.509	96.648	97.453
24	79.648	82.388	85.313	93.377	97.852	98.560	99.016
25	86.281	88.707	92.201	97.265	99.579	99.795	99.899

3 Common failure modes

RESISTOR TYPE COMPONENTS

Resistor, carbon composition

Open circuit	50%
Resistance value drift	50%

Potentiometer, carbon composition

Intermittent noise	60%
Open circuit	40%

Resistors, carbon film

Open circuit	50%
Resistance value drift	50%

Resistor, metal film

Resistance change	50%
Open circuit	50%

Resistor, metal oxide/cermet film

Open circuit	50%
Resistance value drift	50%

Resistor, power wirewound

Open circuit	90%
Short circuit	10%

Resistor, precision wirewound

Catastrophic failure open circuit	90%
Short circuit	10%

Potentiometers, wirewound

Open	53%
Noisy	21%
Shorted/contaminated or insulation breakdown	19%
Jammed/stuck	7%

Potentiometers, cermet

Noise	100%

Trimmers

Noise	100%

Metal thick-film networks

Open circuits	92%
Short circuits	8%

Potentiometers, conductive plastic

Noise	100%

CAPACITORS

Ceramic

Short circuits	99%
Open circuits	1%

Mica

Short circuits	99%
Open circuits	1%

Glass

Short circuits	99%
Open circuits	1%

Tantalum electrolytic

Short circuits	80%
Open circuits	20%

Aluminum electrolytic

Short circuits	80%
Open circuits	20%

INDUCTORS AND CHOKES

Inductors and chokes

Open circuits	43%
Parameter drift	19%
Shorted turns	19%
Insulation failure	11%
Lead damage	6%
Dielectric breakdown	1%
Unstable operation	1%

RF coils

Short circuits	39%
Insulation failures	23%
Wire failure due to overstress	20%
Open circuits	18%

Transformers

Open primary winding	50%
Shorted primary winding	30%
Open secondary winding	10%
Shorted secondary winding	10%

DELAY LINES

Delay lines

Degraded operation	52%
Solder joint failures	20%
Coil magnet wire failures	20%
Open circuits	4%
All output taps stuck high	4%

CONNECTORS

Connectors

High resistance	10%
Intermittent connections	20%

Open circuits   60%
Short circuits   10%

SWITCHES

Microswitches

High resistance   60%
No function   10%
Open circuit   30%

Rotary

Improper output   53%
Contact failure   47%

Push-button

Open   60%
Sticking   33%
Shorted   7%

Thermal

Parameter change   63%
Open   27%
No control   8%
Shorted   2%

Toggle

Open   65%
Sticking   19%
Shorted   16%

Magnetic

Mechanically damaged   60%
Intermittent/noisy   15%
Shorted-open circuit   13%
Parameter drift/high contact resistance   7%
Shorted   5%

Pressure

Loss of control, inoperative control,   30%
mechanically failed

Degraded operation (fluctuations)	25%
False operation	19%
Closed	13%
Open	13%

Keyboards

Mechanical failure	49%
Contact failure	23%
Connection/connector failure	22%
Locked up	6%

RELAYS

Relays

Coil failure	10%
Contact failure	90%

CABLES

Cables

Shorted	34%
Broken	26%
Opened	23%
Cracked/fractured	5%
Arcing or sparking	4%
Worn, frayed, chaffed, damaged	4%
Mechanical failure	4%

SEMICONDUCTOR DEVICES

Zener diode

Short circuit	50%
Open circuit	50%

Junction diode

High reverse	65%
Open circuit	23%
Short circuit	12%

SCR

Short circuit	98%

Open circuit   2%

Transistor

High leakage   20%
Low gain   20%
Open circuit   30%
Short circuit   30%

General purpose diode

Short circuit   49%
Open circuit   36%
Parameter change   15%

Diode rectifier

Short circuit   51%
Open circuit   29%
Parameter change   20%

Small signal diode

Short circuit   18%
Open circuit   24%
Parameter change   58%

Microwave diode

Open circuit   50%
Parameter change   23%
Short circuit   10%
Intermittent   17%

Zener diode reference

Parameter change   68%
Open circuit   17%
Short Circuit   13%
Intermittent   2%

Zener diode regulator

Parameter change   68%
Open circuit   17%
Short Circuit   13%
Intermittent   2%

Zener diode regulator

Open circuit	45%
Parameter change	35%
Short circuit	20%

Optoelectronic LED

Open circuit	70%
Short circuit	30%

Optoelectronic sensor

Short circuit	50%
Open circuit	50%

Thyristor

Failed off	45%
Short circuit	40%
Open circuit	10%
Failed on	5%

Triac

Failed off	90%
Failed on	10%

Bipolar transistor

Short circuit	73%
Open circuit	27%

Field effect transistor

Short circuit	51%
Low output	22%
Parameter change	17%
Open circuit	5%
Output high	5%

GaAs FET

Open circuit	61%
Short circuit	26%
Parameter change	13%

RF transistor

Parameter change	50%
Short circuit	40%
Open circuit	10%

INTEGRATED CIRCUITS

Digital bipolar

Output stuck high	28%
Output stuck low	28%
Output open	22%
Output open	22%

Digital MOS

Input open	36%
Output open	36%
Supply open	12%
Output stuck low	8%
Output stuck high	8%

Digital PAL

Failed truth table	80%
Short circuit	20%

Interface IC

Output stuck low	58%
Input open	16%
Output open	16%
Supply open	10%

Linear IC

Degraded/improper output	50%
No output	41%
Short circuit	3%
Open circuit	3%
Drift	3%

Linear operational amplifiers

Degraded	68%
Intermittent	13%

Short circuit	10%
Overstressed by transients	6%
No output	3%

Bipolar memory

Slow transfer of data	79%
Data bit loss	21%

MOS memory

Data bit loss	34%
Short circuit	26%
Open circuit	23%
Slow transfer of data	17%

Digital memory

Single bit error	30%
Column error	25%
Row error	25%
Row and column error	10%
Complete failure	10%

Digital memory RAM

No operation at cold temperature	26%
Parameter change	19%
Short circuit	18%
Open circuit	14%
Incorrect data	14%
Contaminated	9%

Memory UVEPROM

Open (unprogrammable) bit locations	94%
Would not erase	6%

Hybrid devices

Open circuit	51%
Degraded/improper output	26%
Short circuit	17%
No output	6%

4 Glossary

ACCELERATED TESTING

Testing at higher than normal stress levels to increase the failure rate and shorten the time to wearout.

ACCEPTABLE QUALITY LEVEL (AQL)

The maximum percent defective that, for the purpose of sampling inspection, can be considered satisfactory for a process average.

ACCEPTANCE

Sign-off by the purchaser.

ACTIVE REDUNDANCY

That redundancy wherein all redundant items are operating simultaneously.

AMBIENT

Used to denote surrounding, encompassing, or local conditions and is usually applied to environments.

ARCHIVING

The process of establishing and maintaining copies of controlled items such that previous items, baselines and configurations can be re-established should there be a loss or corruption.

ASSESSMENT

The review and auditing of an organization's quality management system to determine that it meets the requirements of the standards, that it is implemented, and that it is effective.

AUDITEE

An organization to be audited.

AUDITOR

A person who has the qualifications to perform quality audits.

BASELINE

A definition of configuration status declared at a point in the project life cycle.

BURN-IN

The operation of items prior to their end application to stabilize their characteristics and identify early failures.

CALIBRATION

The comparison of a measurement system or device of unverified accuracy to a measurement system or device of known and greater accuracy, to detect and correct any variation from required performance specifications of the measurement system or device.

CERTIFICATION

The process which seeks to confirm that the appropriate minimum best practice requirements are included and that the quality management system is put into effect.

CERTIFICATION BODY

An organization which sets itself up as a supplier of product or process certification against established specifications or standards.

CHANGE NOTICE

A document approved by the design activity that describes and authorizes the implementation of an engineering change to the product and its approved configuration documentation.

CHECKLIST

An aid for the auditor listing areas and topics to be covered by the auditors.

CHECKSUM

The sum of every byte contained in an input/output record used for assuring the integrity of the programmed entry.

CLIENT

A person or organization requesting an audit.

COMPLIANCE AUDIT

An audit where the auditor must investigate the quality system, as put into practice, and the organization's results.

CONDITIONING

The exposure of sample units or specimens to a specific environment for a specified period of time to prepare them for subsequent inspection.

CONFIDENCE

The probability that may be attached to conclusions reached as a result of application of statistical techniques.

CONFIDENCE INTERVAL

The numerical range within which an unknown is estimated to be.

CONFIDENCE LEVEL

The probability that a given statement is correct.

CONFIDENCE LIMITS

The extremes of a confidence interval within which the unknown has a designated probability of being included.

CONFIGURATION

A collection of items at specified versions for the fulfillment of a particular purpose.

CONTROLLED DOCUMENT

Documents with a defined distribution such that all registered holders of controlled documents systematically receive any updates to those documents.

CORRECTIVE ACTION

All action taken to improve the overall quality management system as a result of identifying deficiencies, inefficiencies, and non-compliances.

CREEP

Continuous increase in deformation under constant or decreasing stress.

CRITICAL ITEM

An item within a configuration item which, because of special engineering or logistic considerations, requires an approved specification to establish technical or inventory control.

CYCLE

An ON/OFF application of power.

DEBUGGING

A process to detect and remedy inadequacies.

DEFECT

Any non-conformance of a characteristic with specified requirements.

DEGRADATION

A gradual deterioration in performance.

DELIVERY

Transfer of a product from the supplier to the purchaser.

DERATING

The use of an item in such a way that applied stresses are below rated values.

DESIGN ENTITY

An element of a design that is structurally and functionally distinct from other elements and that is separately named and referenced.

DESIGN REVIEW

A formal, documented, comprehensive and systematic examination of a design to evaluate the design requirements and the capability of the design to meet these requirements and to identify problems and propose solutions.

DESIGN VIEW

A subset of design entity attribute information that is specifically suited to the needs of a software project activity.

DEVIATION

A specific written authorization, granted prior to manufacture of an item, to depart from a particular requirement(s) of an item's current approved configuration documentation for a specific number of units or a specified period of time.

DEVICE

Any functional system.

DISCRETE VARIABLE

A variable which can take only a finite number of values.

DOCUMENT

Contains information which is subject to change.

DOWN TIME

The total time during which the system is not in condition to perform its intended function.

EARLY FAILURE PERIOD

An interval immediately following final assembly, during which the failure rate of certain items is relatively high.

ENTITY ATTRIBUTE

A named characteristic or property of a design entity that provides a statement of fact about the entity.

ENVIRONMENT

The aggregate of all conditions which externally influence the performance of an item.

EXTERNAL AUDIT

An audit performed by a customer or his representative at the facility of the supplier to assess the degree of compliance of the quality system with documented requirements.

EXTRINSIC AUDIT

An audit carried out in a company by a third party organization or a regulatory authority, to assess its activities against specific requirements.

FAIL-SAFE

The stated condition that the equipment will contain self-checking features which will cause a function to cease in case of failure, malfunction, or drifting out of tolerance.

FAILURE

The state of inability of an item to perform its required function.

FAILURE ANALYSIS

Subsequent to a failure, the logical, systematic examination of any item, its construction, application, and documentation to identify the failure mode and determine the failure mechanism.

FAILURE MODE

The consequence of the mechanism through which the failure occurs.

FAILURE RATE

The probability of failure per unit of time of the items still operating.

FATIGUE

A weakening or deterioration of metal or other material, or of a member, occurring under load, specifically under repeated, cyclic, or continuous loading.

FAULT

The immediate cause of a failure.

FAULT ISOLATION

The process of determining the location of a fault to the extent necessary to effect repair.

FEASIBILITY STUDY

The study of a proposed item or technique to determine the degree to which it is practicable, advisable, and adaptable for the intended.

FIRMWARE

The combination of a hardware device and computer instructions or computer data that reside as read-only software on the hardware device.

FORM

The shape, size, dimensions, mass, weight, and other visual parameters which uniquely characterize an item.

GRADE

An indicator or category or rank relating to features or characteristics that cover different sets of needs for products or services intended for the same functional use.

INHERENT FAILURE

A failure basically caused by a physical condition or phenomenon internal to the failed item.

INHERENT RELIABILITY

Reliability potential present in the design.

INSPECTION

The examination and testing of supplies and services to determine whether they conform to specified requirements.

INSTALLATION

Introduction of the product to the purchaser's organization.

INTERNAL AUDIT

An audit carried out within an organization by its own personnel to assess compliance of the quality system to documented requirements.

ITEM

Any entity whose development is to be tracked.

MAINTAINABILITY

The measure of the ability of an item to be retained in or restored to a specified condition when maintenance is performed by personnel having specified skill levels, using prescribed procedures and resources, at each prescribed level of maintenance and repair.

MAINTENANCE

The servicing, repair, and care of material or equipment to sustain or restore acceptable operating conditions.

MAJOR NON-COMPLIANCE

Either the non-implementation, within the quality system of a requirement of ISO 9001, or a breakdown of a key aspect of the system.

MALFUNCTION

Any occurrence of unsatisfactory performance.

MANUFACTURABILITY

The measure of the design's ability to consistently satisfy product goals, while being profitable.

MEAN TIME BETWEEN FAILURE (MTBF)

A basic measure of reliability for repairable items.

MEAN TIME TO FAILURE (MTTF)

A basic measure of maintainability.

MEAN TIME TO REPAIR (MTTR)

The sum of repair times divided by the total number of failures, during a particular interval of time, under stated conditions.

METHOD

A prescribed way of doing things.

METRIC

A value obtained by theoretical or empirical means in order to determine the norm for a particular operation.

MINIMUM LIFE

The time of occurrence of the first failure of a device.

MINOR NON-COMPLIANCE

A single and occasional instance of a failure to comply with the quality system.

MODULE

A replaceable combination of assemblies, subassemblies, and parts common to one mounting.

NON-COMPLIANCE

The non-fulfillment of specified requirements.

OBJECTIVE EVIDENCE

Qualitative or quantitative information, records, or statements of fact pertaining to the quality of an item or service or to the existence and the implementation of a quality system element, which is based on observation, measurement, or test, and which can be verified.

OBSERVATION

A record of an observed fact which may or may not be regarded as a non-compliance.

PARAMETER

A quantity to which the operator may assign arbitrary values, as distinguished from a variable, which can assume only those values that the form of the function makes possible.

PARSING

The technique of marking system or subsystem requirements with specified attributes in order to sort the requirements according to one or more of the attributes.

PERFORMANCE STANDARDS

Published instructions and requirements setting forth the procedures, methods, and techniques for measuring the designed performance of equipments or systems in terms of the main number of essential technical measurements required for a specified operational capacity.

PHASE

A defined segment of work.

POPULATION

The total collection of units being considered.

PRECISION

The degree to which repeated observations of a class of measurements conform to themselves.

PREDICTED

That which is expected at some future time, postulated on analysis of past experience and tests.

PREVENTIVE MAINTENANCE

All actions performed in an attempt to retain an item in specified condition by providing systematic inspection, detection, and prevention of incipient failures.

PROBABILITY

A measure of the likelihood of any particular event occurring.

PROBABILITY DISTRIBUTION

A mathematical model which represents the probabilities for all of the possible values a given discrete random variable may take.

PROCEDURES

Documents that explain the responsibilities and authorities related to particular tasks, indicate the methods and tools to be used, and may include copies of, or reference to, software facilities or paper forms.

PRODUCT

Operating system or application software including associated documentation, specifications, user guides, etc.

PROGRAM

The program of events during an audit.

PROTOTYPE

A model suitable for use in complete evaluation of form, design, and performance.

PURCHASER

The recipient of products or services delivered by the supplier.

QUALIFICATION

The entire process by which products are obtained from manufacturers or distributors, examined and tested, and then identified on a qualified products list.

QUALITY

The totality of features or characteristics of a product or service that bear on its ability to satisfy stated or implied needs.

QUALITY ASSURANCE

All those planned and systematic actions necessary to provide adequate confidence that a product or service will satisfy given requirements for quality.

QUALITY AUDIT

A systematic and independent examination to determine whether quality activities and related results comply with planned arrangements and whether these arrangements are implemented effectively and are suitable to achieve objectives.

QUALITY CONTROL

The operational techniques and activities that are used to fulfill requirements for quality.

QUALITY MANAGEMENT

That aspect of the overall management function that determines and implements quality policy. A technique covering quality assurance and quality control aimed at ensuring defect-free products.

QUALITY POLICY

The overall intention and direction of an organization regarding quality as formally expressed by top management. Management's declared targets and approach to the achievement of quality.

QUALITY SYSTEM

The organizational structure, responsibilities, procedures, processes, and resources for implementing quality management.

RECORD

Provides objective evidence that the quality system has been effectively implemented. A piece of evidence that is *not* subject to change.

REDUNDANCY

Duplication, or the use of more than one means of performing a function in order to prevent an overall failure in the event that all but one of the means fails.

REGRESSION ANALYSIS

The fitting of a curve or equation to data in order to define the functional relationship between two or more correlated variables.

RELIABILITY

The probability that a device will perform a required function, under specified conditions, for a specified period of time.

RELIABILITY GOAL

The desired reliability for the device.

RELIABILITY GROWTH

The improvement of a reliability parameter caused by the successful correction of deficiencies in item design or manufacture.

REPAIR

All actions performed, as a result of failure, to restore an item to a specified condition.

REVIEW

An evaluation of software elements or project status to ascertain discrepancies from planned results and to recommend improvement.

REVIEW MEETING

A meeting at which a work product or a set of work products are presented to project personnel, managers, users, customers, or other interested parties for comment or approval.

REVISION

Any change to an original document which requires the revision level to be advanced.

RISK

The probability of making an incorrect decision.

SAFETY FACTOR

The margin of safety designed into the application of an item to ensure that it will function properly.

SCHEDULE

The dates on which the audit is planned to happen.

SCREENING

A process of inspecting items to remove those that are unsatisfactory or those likely to exhibit early failure.

SERVICE LEVEL AGREEMENT

Defines the service to be provided and the parameters within which the service provider is contracted to service.

SHELF LIFE

The length of time an item can be stored under specified conditions and still meet specified requirements.

SIMULATION

A set of test conditions designed to duplicate field operating and usage environments as closely as possible.

SINGLE-POINT FAILURE

The failure of an item which would result in failure of the system and is not compensated for by redundancy or alternative operational procedures.

SOFTWARE

A combination of associated computer instructions and computer data definitions required to enable the computer hardware to perform computational or control functions.

SOFTWARE DESIGN DESCRIPTION

A representation of a software system created to facilitate analysis, planning, implementation, and decision making. A blueprint or model of the software system.

SOURCE CODE

The code in which a software program is prepared.

SPECIFICATION

A document which describes the essential technical requirements for items, material, or services.

STANDARD DEVIATION

A statistical measure of dispersion in a distribution.

STANDARDS

Documents that state very specific requirements in terms of appearance, formal and exact methods to be followed in all relevant cases.

STANDBY REDUNDANCY

That redundancy wherein the alternative means of performing the function is not operating until it is activated upon failure of the primary means of performing the function.

SUB-CONTRACTOR

The organization which provides products or services to the supplier.

SUPPLIER

The organization responsible for replication and issue of product. The organization to which the requirements of the relevant parts of an ISO 9000 standard apply.

SYSTEM

A group of equipments, including any required operator functions, which are integrated to perform a related operation.

SYSTEM COMPATIBILITY

The ability of the equipments within a system to work together to perform the intended mission of the system.

TESTING

The process of executing hardware or software to find errors. A procedure or action taken to determine, under real or simulated conditions, the capabilities, limitations, characteristics, effectiveness, reliability, and suitability of a material, device, or method.

TOLERANCE

The total permissible deviation of a measurement from a designated value.

TOOL

The mechanization of the method or procedure.

TOTAL QUALITY

A business philosophy involving everyone for continuously improving an organization's performance.

TRACEABILITY

The ability to track requirements from the original specification to code and test.

TRADE-OFF

The lessening of some desirable factor(s) in exchange for an increase in one or more other factors to maximize a system's effectiveness.

USEFUL LIFE PERIOD

The period of equipment life following the infant mortality period, during which the equipment failure rate remains constant.

VALIDATION

The process of evaluating a product to ensure compliance with specified and implied requirements.

VARIABLE

A quantity that may assume a number of values.

VARIANCE

A statistical measure of the dispersion in a distribution.

VARIANT

An instance of an item created to satisfy a particular requirement.

VERIFICATION

The process of evaluating the products of a given phase to ensure correctness and consistency with respect to the products and standards provided as input to that phase.

VERSION

An instance of an item or variant created at a particular time.

WEAROUT

The process which results in an increase in the failure rate or probability of failure with increasing number of life units.

WEAROUT FAILURE PERIOD

The period of equipment life following the normal failure period, during which the equipment failure rate increases above the normal rate.

WORK INSTRUCTIONS

Documents that describe how to perform specific tasks and are generally only required for complex tasks which cannot be adequately described by a single sentence or paragraph with a procedure.

WORST CASE ANALYSIS

A type of circuit analysis that determines the worst possible effect on the output parameters by changes in the values of circuit elements. The circuit elements are set at the values within their anticipated ranges which produce the maximum detrimental output changes.

Index

A

AAMI. *See* Association for the Advancement of Medical Instrumentation
Abbreviated 510(k), 38–40
Accelerated testing, 356–358
Acceptable risk, 160
Acceptance program, 88–89
Acclaro (software), 227
Active failure testing, 347
Active Implantable Medical Devices Directive (AIMDD), 54, 56, 64, 68
Active redundancy, 233–234
Ada, 264
Advisory Group on the Reliability of Electronic Equipment (AGREE), 4
Advisory panel, 310
AIMDD. *See* Active Implantable Medical Devices Directive
Alarm circuit, fault tree analysis, 173–175
Alarms and signals, 320–322
ALARP. *See* As low as reasonably practical region
Allocated baseline, 411–412
American National Standards Institute (ANSI), 96, 109
American Society for Quality Control (ASQC), 96
American Society for Testing and Materials (ASTM), 96
Annexes. *See* Conformity assessment annexes
ANSI. *See* American National Standards Institute
Anthropometry, 303–306, 317
Architectural template, 258
As low as reasonably practical region (ALARP), 159–160
ASQC. *See* American Society for Quality Control

Assembler, 264
Association for the Advancement of Medical Instrumentation (AAMI), 45, 95–96, 399
ASTM. *See* American Society for Testing and Materials
Audible alarm, 322
Axiomatic design, 226–229

B

Basic, 264
Battery tests, 344
Benchmark usability testing, 310
Black box testing, 342
Block diagram, 232
Body mobility ranges, design and, 318
Bohm-Jacopini theorem, 276
Breach of warranty, 177, 179–180
British Standards Institute (BSI), 103
BSI. *See* British Standards Institute
Business proposal, 133–137

C

C (programming language), 264
Cables, failure modes, 441
Calibration, 86
Canada, standards, 104, 108
Canadian Standards Association (CSA), 104
Capacitors, failure modes, 438–439
CE mark, 54–55, 64, 73–74
CEN. *See* European Committee for Standardization
CENELAC. *See* European Committee for Electrotechnical Standardization
Certification, TickIT program, 106
CGMP. *See* Current Good Manufacturing Practice
Chance failure, 19

Chi square table, 425
Chokes, failure modes, 439
CISPR. *See* International Special
    Committee on Radio Interference
Class I devices, 28
    Medical Devices Directive (MDD),
        65, 67
    quality system regulation, 79, 81
Class I software, 47
Class II devices, 28–29
    Medical Devices Directive (MDD),
        65, 67–68
    quality system regulation, 78–79, 81
Class II software, 47–48
Class III devices
    Medical Devices Directive (MDD),
        65, 67–68
    Pre-Market Approval (PMA)
        application, 40–41
    quality system regulation,
        78–79, 81
    regulation, 29–30
Class III software, 48
Cleaning, documentation of, 87
Clinical studies, 30
Cobol, 264
Code generators, 270
Code reading, 268
Code review, 277
Codes of practice, 103
Coding (for software), 270, 275–282
    code reading, 268
    implementation checklist, 282
    implementation process, 279–282
    improving quality, 277–279
    lines of code (LOC), 290
    peer review, 277–278
    Program Design Language (PDL),
        279
    sign-offs, 278
    single-entry, single-exit constructs,
        276–277
    software metrics, 287–297
    sources of error, 20
    SQAP, 150
    structured coding, 275–276
    token count, 290–291
Comite Europeen de Normalisation. *See*
    European Committee for
    Standardization

Comite Europeen de Normalisation
    Electronique. *See* European
    Committee for Electrotechnical
    Standardization
Common test set (CTS), 374–375
Complaint procedures, 89
Complexity, 288, 292–293
Component data bank, 237
Component derating, 238–239
Component selection, 235–238
Components
    derating, 238–239
    failure rates, 237
    fitness for use, 236
    history, 237
    reliability, 236–237
    safety, 238
Computer-aided metrics, 295
Computer languages, 261–265
Computer products, regulation of, 47
Concurrent design, 311
Confidence level, 390
Confidence limits, 391–393
Configuration audits, 412–414
Configuration identification, 410–412
Configuration management, 409–415
    configuration audits, 412–414
    configuration identification, 410–412
    metrics, 414
    status accounting, 415
Configuration management
        metrics, 414
Conformity assessment annexes, 66–68
Connectors, failure modes, 439–440
Controls, interactive control, 327–328
Cooper Committee, 26–28
Copyright, 194–198, 205
Copyright Act of 1976, 195
Copyright infringement, 198
Copyright notice, 196–197
Copyright registration, 197
Coupled design, 229
Critical device requirements, Good
    Manufacturing Practices (GMP),
        401
CSA. *See* Canadian Standards
    Association
CTS. *See* Common test set
Current Good Manufacturing Practice
    (CGMP), 400

Customer complaints, 89–90
Customer survey, 123
Cycle testing, 350
Cyclomatic complexity, 292–293

D

Data abstraction, 262
Data analysis, field data, 418–422
Data encapsulation, 262
Data entry, 325
Data protection, error management, 329
DCCDI, 212
De facto standards, 102
De jure standards, 102
Declaration of Conformity, 35, 38, 40,
     55, 72–73
Decomposition description, in Software
     Design Description (SDD), 154
Decoupled design, 228–229
Default settings, 329
Defectiveness, test of, 181
Defects, 16, 180–182
Defects per million opportunities
     (DPMO), 210
Deficiency, 16
Delay lines, failure modes, 439
Department of Health (U.K.), 104
Dependency description, in Software
     Design Description (SDD), 154
Design
   alarms and signals, 320–322
   anthropometry, 303–306, 317
   changes, 249-250
   consistency and simplicity, 315
   defaults, 329
   design control, 45–46
   design specification, 147–148
   documentation, 316–317
   environmental/organizational
      considerations, 316
   error management/data protection,
      329
   feedback, 328
   functional dimensions, 317–319
   hardware design, 231–252
   human factors, 300–329
   human factors engineering, 44–45
   interactive control, 327–328
   labeling, 89–90, 323–324

   prompts, 328–329
   requirements vs., 142
   risk assessment, 160–161
   safety, 315
   Six Sigma, 209–229
   software design, 255–272
   Software Design Description (SDD),
      153–155
   software review, 266–269
   sources of error, 20
   user interface, 311–313
   verification and validation, 271–272
   workstation, 320
Design and Development Plan, 82
Design changes, 249–250
*Design Control Guidance for Medical
   Device Manufacturers*, 45
Design controls, 45–46, 81–83
   Good Manufacturing Practices
      (GMP), 400
   quality system regulation, 81
Design defects, 182
Design errors, 20
Design for Assembly (DFA), 403–404
Design for Manufacturability (DFM),
   402
Design for Six Sigma (DFSS). *See* Six
   Sigma
Design History File (DHF), 82, 83
Design patents, 189, 190–191
Design reviews, 250–252
Design simulation, 269
Design specification, 147–148
Detailed design description, in Software
   Design Description (SDD), 155
Deutsches Institut für Normung. *See*
   German Standardization Institute
Development Plan for an Improved
   Medical Devices Regulatory
   Program (Canada), 108
Developmental configuration, 411–412
Device failure. *See* Failure
Device History Record, 82, 92–93
Device Master Record, 82, 91–92
Device recalls, 46
Device registration number, 30
Device regulation. *See* Regulation
Device reliability, 10–11
   See also Reliability
DFA. *See* Design for Assembly

DFM. *See* Design for Manufacturability
DFSS. *See* Six Sigma
DHF. *See* Design History File
DIN. *See* German Standardization Institute
Display area, human, 304–305
Displays, human factors engineering, 325–327
DMADOV, 211
DMADV, 211
DMAIC, 210
DMEDI, 211–212
Do It By Design, 44–45
Document controls, quality system regulation, 83–84
Documentation
  of cleaning, 87
  device failure and, 21
  Device History Record, 82, 92–93
  Device Master Record, 82, 91–92
  quality system regulation, 92–93
  Software Quality Assurance Plan, 151
Dog-and-pony shows, 268–269
Domestic standards, 95–98
DPMO. *See* Defects per million opportunities
Drop testing, 353
Dynamic S/N ratio, robust design, 217

E

Early failures, 19
EC. *See* European Commission
Effort (metric), 294
Electrical stress usage rating, 239
Electromagnetic compatibility (EMC) testing, 355–356
Electronic reliability, 7–8
Electronic reliability curve, 7
Electrostatic discharge testing, 355
EMC testing. *See* Electromagnetic compatibility (EMC) testing
"End of life", 399
Environmental management system (EMS), 109
Environmental protection, 240
Environmental stress screening, 63
Environmental testing, 63, 338, 351–356

Ergonomics. *See* Human factors; Human factors engineering
Error management, 329
Essentials Requirements List, 55–58, 64
  Essential Requirement 1, 59–61
  Essential Requirement 2, 62
  Essential Requirement 3, 62
  Essential Requirement 4, 63–64
EU. *See* European Union
Europe, standards, 101
European Commission (EC), 101
European Committee for Electrotechnical Standardization (CENELAC), 58, 103
European Committee for Standardization (CEN), 58, 103
European Community (EC), medical device regulation, 54, 70
European Free Trade Association (EFTA), 54, 103
European Union (EU), 79
Event testing, 337
Exclusion of warranties, 180

F

Factor effects analysis, 218
Fail-safe tests, 346
Failure, 15–22
  causes, 16–17
  chance failure, 19
  customer's point of view, 21–22
  defined, 15–16, 339
  documentation, 21
  early failures, 19
  failure rate, 18
  hardware failure, 17, 18–20
  human error and, 21
  minimum life, 392
  Pareto analysis, 392, 420
  practical aspects, 17
  random failure, 17, 19
  safety testing, 346–347
  software failure, 10, 18, 20–21
  systematic failure, 16–17
  wearout failure, 19–20
Failure analysis, of field units, 421–422
Failure codes, 419

Failure mode and effects analysis
(FMEA), 169–171, 218
Failure mode and effects analysis form,
170–171
Failure modes
cables, 441
capacitors, 438–439
connectors, 439–440
delay lines, 439
inductors and chokes, 439
integrated circuits, 444–445
relays, 441
resistor type components, 437–438
semiconductor devices, 442–444
switches, 440–441
Failure rate, 18, 384–385
Failure related testing, 339
Failure-terminated confidence limits,
391–392
Failure-terminated, failed parts replaced
calculation, 387
Failure-terminated, no replacement
calculation, 387–388
Failures per million hours, 18
Fault, 16
Fault insertion tests, 346
Fault tree analysis, 172–175, 265
FDA. *See* Food and Drug
Administration
Federal Food, Drug and Cosmetic Act
(FFD&C), 26, 116
Federal regulation. *See* Regulation
FFD&C. *See* Federal Food, Drug and
Cosmetic Act
Field data, analysis, 418–422
Field service reports, 418–422
510(k) process, 28–40, 398–399
Abbreviated 510(k), 38–40
checklist, 35, 36–37
Declaration of Conformity, 35,
38, 40
format, 33–35
Special 510(k), 35, 37–38
FMEA. *See* Failure mode and effects
analysis
Focus groups, 309
Food and Drug Administration (FDA),
26–27
configuration management, 414–415
dealing with, 48–49

definition of medical device, 116
Good Laboratory Practices (GLP), 44
Good Manufacturing Practices
(GMP), 27, 44, 77–79, 397–407
history of medical device regulation,
398–399
Medical Device Reporting (MDR), 27
power to inspect, 48–49
Quality System Regulations, 27, 39
registration and listing, 30–31
Safe Medical Devices Act, 27
software and, 46–48
Formal design reviews, 251
Fortran, 264
France, standards, 101
Function count, 291–292
Functional baseline, 410–411
Functional configuration audit, 413
Functional modes, 344
Functional testing, 344

G

GB. *See* Ground benign environment
Generic mark, 200
German Standardization Institute
(DIN), 104
Germany, standards, 101, 104
GF. *See* Ground fixed environment
GIDEP, 237
GLP. *See* Good Laboratory Practices
GM. *See* Ground mobile environment
Good Laboratory Practices (GLP), 44
Good Manufacturing Practices (GMP),
27, 44, 77–79, 397–407
Design for Assembly (DFA),
403–404
Design for Manufacturability (DFM),
402
history, 398–399
recent changes to FDA regulation,
400–401
Graphic displays, 326
Graphical analysis, of test data,
392–394, 420
Ground benign environment (GB), 242
Ground fixed environment (GF), 242
Ground mobile environment
(GM), 242
Guidance document, 38, 39

H

Halstead measures, 293–295
Hand size, human, 306
Hardware
  design. *See* Hardware design
  medical devices composed of, 118
  testing, 343, 350–368
  verification and validation, 350–368
Hardware design, 231–252
  block diagram, 232
  component derating, 238–239
  component selection, 235–238
  design changes, 249–250
  design of experiments, 249
  design reviews, 250–252
  environmental protection, 240
  human factors engineering,
    302–304
  load protection, 240
  product misuse, 184, 240–241
  redundancy, 232–235
  reliability protection, 241–248
  safety margin, 239–240
  user interface design, 312, 315
  variation and, 248
Hardware failure, 17, 18–20
Hardware testing, 343, 350–368
  accelerated testing, 356–358
  cycle testing, 350
  drop testing, 353
  electromagnetic compatibility (EMC)
    testing, 355–356
  electrostatic discharge testing, 355
  environmental testing, 63, 338,
    351–356
  humidity testing, 353
  impact testing, 354–355
  mechanical shock testing, 353
  mechanical vibration testing, 354
  operating temperature
    testing, 352
  storage temperature testing, 352
  sudden death testing, 359–368
  10×10 testing, 350–351
  thermal shock testing, 352
  typical use testing, 350
  Weibull plotting, 359–364, 394
Hardware verification and validation,
  350–368

Harmonization, Good Manufacturing
    Practices (GMP), 401
Harmonized Standards, 55,
    58–64, 70
Hazard analysis, 60–61
  software hazard analysis, 264
Hazard analysis form, 60,
    167–168
Hazard/risk analysis, 166–169
Hazard severity, 168
High-priority alarm, 321–322
Horizontal standards, 58
Human error, failure and, 21
Human factors, 300–329
Human factors engineering, 44–45, 300,
    307
  alarms and signals, 320–322
  analysis, 307
  anthropometry, 303–306, 317
  consistency and simplicity, 315
  data entry, 325
  defaults, 329
  documentation, 316–317
  environmental/organizational
    considerations, 316
  error management/data protection,
    329
  feedback, 328
  functional dimensions, 317–319
  hardware element in, 302–304
  human element in, 301–302
  interactive control, 327–328
  labeling, 89–90, 323–324
  planning, 307
  prompts, 328–329
  psychological elements, 319
  risk assessment, 161–162
  safety, 315
  software design, 324
  software element in, 304–306
  usability goals, 310–311
  user studies, 308–310
  visual displays, 325–327
  workstation design, 320
*Human Factors Engineering Guidelines
    and Preferred Practices for the
    Design of Medical Devices*, 45
Human factors plan, 307
Human-machine interface, 302
Humidity testing, 353

I

IDE. *See* Investigational Device
    Exemption
IDEAS, 211
Identification, in quality system
    regulation, 85
IDOV, 211
IEC. *See* International Electrotechnical
    Committee
IEE. *See* Institution of Electrical
    Engineers
IEEE. *See* Institute of Electrical and
    Electronic Engineers
IES. *See* Institute of Environmental
    Sciences
Implied warranties, 179–180
In-process audit, 414
In Vitro Diagnostic Medical Devices
    Directive (IVDMDD), 56, 64, 68
Inductors and chokes, failure modes,
    439
Infant mortality, 7–8
Informal design reviews, 251–252
Infringement
    copyright, 198
    patents, 193–194
Input processing, 258
Inspection, 98
    by FDA, 48, 49
    software review, 266–267, 268
Institute for Interconnecting and
    Packaging Electronic Circuits
    (IPC), 97
Institute of Electrical and Electronic
    Engineers (IEEE), 96, 98
Institute of Environmental Sciences
    (IES), 96–97
Institution of Electrical Engineers (IEE),
    105
Institutional Review Board (IRB), 30,
    42–43
Instructional documentation, 316–317
Integrated circuits, failure modes,
    444–445
Intellectual property, 187–205
    copyrights, 194–198, 205
    patents, 188–194, 205
    trade secrets, 202–205
    trademarks, 198–202

Interface description, in Software
    Design Description
    (SDD), 155
International Electrotechnical
    Committee (IEC), 101–102, 105
International Organization for
    Standardization (ISO), 79, 105
International Special Committee on
    Radio Interference (CISPR), 104
International standards, 102–111
Interviews, by human factors engineers,
    308–309
Intolerable region, risk, 159
Inventions
    defined, 188
    patents, 188–194
Investigational Device Exemption
    (IDE), 28, 30, 41–43
    format, 43
IPC. *See* Institute for Interconnecting
    and Packaging Electronic Circuits
IRB. *See* Institutional Review Board
ISO. *See* International Organization for
    Standardization
ISO 9001 and 9002, 107–108
ISO 14000 standards, 108–110
Italy, standards, 101
IVDMDD. *See* In Vitro Diagnostic
    Medical Devices Directive

J

Japanese Standards Association (JSA),
    105

L

Labeling, 89–90, 323–324
Law, 177
    See also Intellectual property;
    Liability
Liability, 177–184
    breach of warranty, 177, 179–180
    defects, 16, 180–182
    failure to warn of danger, 182
    negligence, 177–179
    strict liability, 177, 179, 181
Line of sight, human, 303
Lines of code (LOC), 290
Listing, 30–31

Litigation
defendant's conduct, 183
failure to warn of danger, 182
plaintiff's conduct, 182–183
product liability, 177–184
Load protection, 240
LOC. *See* Lines of code
Log-on, 324
Long-term memory, 302
Low-priority alarm, 321

M

Malfunction, 16
Malpractice, 183
Manufacturer
defects and, 181–182
failure to warn of danger, 182
liability, 179, 183
Manufacturing
customer delivery, 407
Good Manufacturing Practices
(GMP), 27, 44, 77–79, 397–407
pilot run build, 406–407
pre-production activity, 405–406
production run, 407
Manufacturing defects, 181
Manufacturing planning chart, QFD,
130, 133
Mapping, of axiomatic design, 227–229
Materials, risk assessment, 161
Mathematical modeling, 269
MDD. *See* Medical Devices Directive
MDR. *See* Medical Device Reporting
Mean time between failure (MTBF),
146–147, 233, 241, 384, 385–388
Mechanical reliability, 8–9
Mechanical reliability curve, 9
Mechanical shock testing, 353
Mechanical vibration testing, 354
Media control, Software Quality
Assessment Plan, 150
Medical Device amendments (1976), 116
Medical Device Reporting (MDR), 27
Medical devices
classification, 28–30, 64–66
composition of, 118
computer products as, 47
defects, 16, 180–182
defined, 28, 54–55, 115–117

device recalls, 46
history, 117
intellectual property, 187–205
liability, 177–184
product development, 121–137
product misuse, 184, 240–241
See also Failure; Product
development; Regulation;
Reliability; Testing; Validation;
Verification
Medical Devices Amendments (1976),
26, 116
Medical Devices Directive (MDD),
53–69
Active Implantable Medical Devices
Directive (AIMDD), 54, 56, 64
CE marking, 54, 55, 64, 73–74
classification of the device, 64–66
conformity assessment annexes,
66–68
Declaration of Conformity, 35, 38, 40,
55, 72–73
definition of medical device, 116
Essentials Requirements List, 55,
56–58
Harmonized Standards, 55,
58–64, 70
In Vitro Diagnostic Medical Devices
Directive (IVDMDD), 56, 64
Notified Body, 68–72
process, 55–56
Medical Devices Regulatory Program
(Canada), 108
Medical informatics, 110–111
Medical malpractice, 183
Medical software, 47–48
See also Software
Medium-priority alarm, 321–322
Memory, human, 302
Meta-metrics, 289–290
Metrics
configuration management metrics,
414
software, 285–297
Military standards, 98
Minimum life, 392
Modula-2, 264
Module specifications (mspecs), 270
MTBF. *See* Mean time
between failure

N

National Electrical Manufacturers
    Association (NEMA), 97
National Fire Protection Association
    (NFPA), 97
Negligence, 177, 178–179
Non-conforming product, 89
Non-obviousness, patent criterion,
    189–190
Notified Body, 68, 69–72
Novelty, patent criterion, 189
Number of cycles to failure, 337
Numeric digital displays, 326

O

Object-oriented design, 260–261
Objective metrics, 287
Objective usability goals, 310
Observation, by human factors
    engineers, 308
Occupational Safety and Health
    Administration (OSHA), 97
"Off label" use, 184, 240–241
Office of Device Evaluation (ODE), 35
*Official Journal of the European
    Communities*, 58
Operating temperature testing, 352
Optimization, of reliability, 12
OSHA. *See* Occupational Safety and
    Health Administration
Output processing, 259

P

P-diagram, 215, 216, 218, 219–221
Packaging, 89–90
Parameter diagram. *See* P-diagram
Pareto analysis, 392, 420
Parsing, 144–145, 335–337
Part planning matrix, QFD, 129, 131
Parts count prediction, 242–248
Pascal (programming language), 264
Passive failure testing, 347
Patent claims, 192
Patent infringement, 193–194
Patents, 188–194
    claims, 192
    design patents, 189, 190–191

infringement, 193–194
    legal tests, 188–189
    patentable subject matter, 189
    process for application, 191–192
    protecting inventor's rights, 192–193
    trade secrets and, 205
PDL. *See* Program Design Language
Peer review, 62, 277–278
Percent rank tables, 427–435
Performance predictability, 269
Physical configuration audit, 413
Physicians, liability of, 183
Pilot run build, 406–407
Pilot run plan, 405
Plant patent, 189
Potential volume, 294
Pre-Market Approval Application
    (PMAA), 28, 29, 40–41
    contents, 41
Pre-Market Notification Process
    (510(k)), 28, 29, 30, 31–40
"Preproduction Quality Assurance
    Planning: Recommendations for
    Medical Device Manufacturers",
    398
Prescriptiveness, 289
Prior art, patents, 190
Probability, 264
Probability classification, hazard
    analysis, 60, 61
Probability of occurrence, 168
Problem reporting, 150
Process controls, 85–88
Process metrics, 289
Process planning matrix, QFD, 129, 132
Process validation, 87
Product baseline, 411, 412
Product definition, 121–124
Product design. *See* Design
Product development, 417
    business proposal, 133–137
    configuration management, 409–415
    defining the device, 121–137
    hardware verification and validation,
        350–368
    human factors, 300–329
    product specification, 144–145
    quality function deployment (QFD),
        124–133, 218
    requirements engineering, 139–155

Product development (*continued*)
  risk estimation, 166–175
  software design, 255–272
  Software Design Description (SDD),
    153–155
  Software Quality Assurance Plan
    (SQAP), 148–151
  Software Requirements Specification
    (SRS), 151–153, 255, 265
  software verification and validation,
    371–380
  See also Design
Product liability. *See* Liability
Product metrics, 289
Product misuse, 184, 240–241
Product recalls, 46
Product specification, 144–145, 147–148
Production control, 85–88
Production plan, 405
Production run, 407
Program Design Language (PDL), 279
Program level, 294
Program review, 251
Programming languages, 261–263, 264
Prompts, 328–329
Prospective standards, 103
Prototypes, 314
Purchasing controls
  Good Manufacturing Practices
    (GMP), 400
  quality system regulation, 84–85

Q

QFD. *See* Quality function deployment
QFD matrix, 125, 126
Quality, 5–6
Quality assurance, Software Quality
    Assurance Plan (SQAP), 148–151
Quality Assurance Unit, 44
Quality function deployment (QFD),
    124–133, 218
Quality measurement, robust design, 216
Quality system, 81
Quality System Record, 93
Quality system regulation, 27, 39, 77–94
  acceptance program, 88–89
  corrective and preventive action,
    89–90
  design controls, 81–83

Device History Record, 82, 92–93
Device Master Record, 82, 91–92
distribution, 91–92
document controls, 83–84
general provisions, 79–81
handling, 91
history, 78–79
identification and traceability, 85
installation, 91–92
labeling and packaging controls,
    90–91
non-conforming product, 89
production and process controls,
    85–88
purchasing controls, 84–85
Quality System Record, 93
recordkeeping, 92–93
servicing requirements, 93–94
storage, 91–92

R

Random failure, 17, 19
Rate Monotonic Analysis (RMA), 269
Real time logic, 265
Recordkeeping. *See* Documentation
Redundancy, 232–235
Reference models, 103
Registration, 30–31
Regression testing, 347–348
Regulation, 28
  CE mark, 54, 55, 64, 73–74
  Class I devices, 28
  Class II devices, 28–29
  Class III devices, 29–30
  clinical studies, 30
  of computer products, 47
  Cooper Committee, 26–28
  design control, 45–46
  device classification, 28–29
  domestic standards, 95–98
  Good Laboratory Practices
    (GLP), 44
  Good Manufacturing Practices
    (GMP), 27, 44, 77–79, 397–407
  history, 26–27
  human factors engineering, 44–45
  Institutional Review Board (IRB), 30,
    42–43
  international standards, 102–111

Investigational Device Exemption
(IDE), 28, 30, 41–43
Medical Device Directives (MDD),
53–69
Medical Device Reporting (MDR), 27
Pre-Market Approval Application
(PMAA), 28–29, 40–41
Pre-Market Notification Process
(510(k)), 28–40, 398–399
quality system regulation, 27, 39,
77–94
registration and listing, 30–31
Safe Medical Devices Act, 27
software, 46–48
substantial equivalence process, 31, 32
Reichelderfer, Brenda, 213
Relays, failure modes, 441
Reliability, 1–12, 383–384
calculation, 388–389
components, 236–237
defined, 3, 4–5, 9
device reliability, 10–11
electronic reliability, 7–8
history, 3–4
mechanical reliability, 8–9
optimization, 12
quality vs., 5–6
software reliability, 9–10
types, 7–11
unreliability vs., 6–7
See also Failure
Reliability assurance, 12
Reliability bathtub curve, 10–11
Reliability goal, requirements
engineering, 145–147
Reliability program, 12–13
Reliability protection, 241–248
Reliability tests, 356
Remote communications load
tests, 346
Remote communications protocol, 344
Requirements, design vs., 142
Requirements engineering, 139–155
assimilation of requirements, 141–142
design specification, 147–148
product specification, 144–145
refinement of requirements, 141
reliability goal, 145–147
Software Design Description (SDD),
153–155

Software Quality Assurance Plan
(SQAP), 148–151
Software Requirements Specification
(SRS), 151–153, 255, 265
specification review, 147
verification and validation, 140–141
Requirements traceability matrix
(RTM), 265–266
Resistor type components, failure
modes, 437–438
Resonant frequencies, 354
Retrospective standards, 103
Risk
acceptable risk, 160
defined, 158
probability of occurrence, 158–159
severity level, 158–159
See also Risk assessment; Risk
management
Risk analysis, 135–137
software design, 255–256
software risk analysis, 263–265
Risk assessment, 160–162
assessing risk probabilities, 164, 168
identifying risk factors, 164
Risk/benefit analysis, 179, 181
Risk-burden balancing, 181
Risk estimation, 166–175
failure mode and effects analysis
(FMEA), 169
fault tree analysis, 172–175
hazard/risk analysis, 166–169
Risk factors
identifying, 164
monitoring, 165
Risk levels, 171
Risk management, 162
action planning, 165
contingency plan, 166
failure mode and effects analysis
(FMEA), 169–171, 218
fault tree analysis, 172–175
monitoring risk factors, 165
process, 162–166
risk estimation, 166–175
Software Quality Assurance Plan, 151
Risk management plan, 162, 166
Risk probability, 164
Risk table, 171
RMA. *See* Rate Monotonic Analysis

Robust design, 213–218
Robust design failure mode and effects
    analysis (DFMEA), 218–226
Robustness, 289, 345
Robustness testing, 345
RTM. *See* Requirements traceability
    matrix

S

S/N ratio, robust design, 216–217
Safe Medical Devices Act (SMDA), 27,
    78, 398
Safety, 158
    human factors engineering, 315
    safety margin, 239–240
    testing, 346–347, 376
    tolerancing, 239
    See also Risk; Risk assessment; Risk
        management
Safety margin, 239–240
Safety review, 61–62
Safety testing, 346–347, 376
Screen hierarchy map, 314
Screen templates, 312
Screenplay, 312, 314
SDD. *See* Software Design Description
Second-level matrix, QFD,
    129, 130
Semi-horizontal standards, 58, 59
Semiconductor devices, failure modes,
    442–444
Service reports, 93–94
Servicing controls, Good Manufacturing
    Practices (GMP), 401
Severity classification, hazard analysis,
    60, 61
Short-term memory, 302
Signal to noise (S/N) ratio, robust
    design, 216–217
Signals, 321–322
Simulation, 269
Single-entry, single-exit constructs,
    276–277
Six Sigma, 209–229
    axiomatic design, 226–229
    methodologies, 210–212
    quality function deployment (QFD),
        124–133, 218
    robust design, 213–218

robust design failure mode and effects
    analysis (DFMEA), 218–226
structure, 212–213
tools, 213–229
Size metrics, 290–292
SMDA. *See* Safe Medical Devices Act
Software, 55
    classes, 47–48
    failure, 10, 18, 20–21
    hazard analysis, 264
    medical devices composed of, 118
    metrics, 285–297
    performance predictability, 269
    quality assurance, 148
    reliability, 9–10
    risk analysis, 263–265
    Software Design Description (SDD),
        153–155
    Software Quality Assurance Plan
        (SQAP), 148–151
    Software Requirements Specification
        (SRS), 151–153, 255, 265
    software review, 266–269
    standards, 98
    testing, 343–344, 371–380
    TickIT program, 106
    verification and validation, 371–380
    See also Coding; Software design
Software architecture, 257–259
Software coding. *See* Coding
Software complexity metrics, 288
Software design, 255–272
    alternatives and tradeoffs, 256–257
    choosing a methodology, 259–260
    coding, 270
    data entry, 325
    design simulation, 269
    detailed design, 256
    human factors engineering, 324
    metrics, 285–297
    module specifications, 270
    object-oriented design, 260–261
    programming languages, 261–264
    prompts, 328–329
    requirements traceability matrix
        (RTM), 265–266
    risk analysis, 255–256
    software architecture, 257–259
    Software Requirements Specification,
        151–153, 255, 265

software review, 266–269
software risk analysis, 263–265
structured analysis, 260
tools, 270–271
top-level design, 256
user interface design, 311–313
verification and validation, 271–272
visual displays, 325
Software Design Description (SDD),
    153–155
Software hazard analysis, 264
Software metrics, 285–297
    computer-aided metrics, 295
    function count, 291–292
    Halstead measures, 293–295
    lines of code (LOC), 290
    McCabe's complexity, 292–293
    meta-metrics, 289–290
    methodology, 295–296
    objective and algorithmic
        measurements, 288–289
    process and product metrics, 289
    quality requirements, 296–297
    size metrics, 290–292
    token count, 290–291
Software quality assurance, 148
Software Quality Assurance Plan
    (SQAP), 148–151
Software Quality System Registration
    (SQSR), 106–107
Software Quality System Registration
    Committee, 106
Software reliability, 9–10
Software reliability curve, 10–11
Software Requirements Specification
    (SRS), 151–153, 255, 265
Software review, 266–269
Software risk analysis, 263–265
Software standards, 98
Software testing, 343–344, 371–380
Software verification and validation,
    371–380
SOPs. *See* Standard Operating
    Procedures
Source code. *See* Coding
Special 510(k): Device Modification, 35,
    37–38
Specification errors, 20
Specification review, 147
Sphygmomanometers, 28

SQAP. *See* Software Quality Assurance
    Plan
SQSR. *See* Software Quality System
    Registration
SRS. *See* Software Requirements
    Specification
Standard Operating Procedures (SOPs),
    44
Standards
    defined, 102
    domestic standards, 95–98
    international standards, 102–111
    military standards, 98
    software design, 277
    Software Quality System Registration
        (SQSR), 106–107
    software standards, 98
    TickIT program, 106
Standby redundancy, 234–235
Static electricity, 355
Static S/N ratio, robust design, 217
Status accounting, 415
Stethoscopes, 28
Storage temperature testing, 352
Stress testing, 337–338, 345–346
Strict liability, 177, 179, 181
Structured analysis, 260
Structured coding, 275, 276
Style guide, for user interface, 314
Subjective usability goals, 310
Subjective metrics, 287
Substantial equivalence process, 31–32
Sudden death testing, 359–368
"Suggested Changes to the Medical
    Device Good Manufacturing
    Practices Regulation Information
    Document", 398
Supplier control, Software Quality
    Assessment Plan, 150
Supplier plan, 406
Switches, failure modes, 440–441
Symbols, in labeling, 324
Systematic failure, 16–17

T

Taguchi Method, 213, 249
    See also Robust design
Task analysis, 309
10×10 testing, 350–351

Test data
  analysis of results, 383–394
  confidence level, 390
  confidence limits, 391–393
  field service reports, 418–422
  graphical analysis, 392–394
  graphical plotting, 393–394
  Pareto analysis, 392, 420
  Weibull plotting, 359–364, 394
Test plan, 406
Testing, 333–348
  accelerated testing, 356–358
  analysis of test results, 383–394
  black box testing, 342
  confidence level, 390
  confidence limits, 391–392
  defined, 334–335
  environmental testing, 63, 338,
    351–356
  event testing, 337
  failure definition, 339
  failure related testing, 339
  functional testing, 344
  hardware testing, 343, 350–368
  parsing test requirements, 335–337
  purpose of the test, 339
  regression testing, 347–348
  robustness testing, 345
  safety testing, 346–347, 376
  sample size and test length,
    339–342
  software testing, 343–344, 371–380
  stress testing, 337–338, 345–346
  sudden death testing, 359–368
  test methodology, 337–339
  test protocol, 337
  test severity, 356–357
  time-related testing, 338–339
  time testing, 337
  types of, 342–348
  user interface, 313–315
  validation, 342
  verification, 342
  white box testing, 342
  See also Usability testing
Theories of recovery, 177
Thermal derating, 239
Thermal shock testing, 352
TickIT program, 106
Time-related testing, 338–339

Time-terminated confidence limits,
    390–391
Time-terminated, failed parts replaced
    calculation, 385–386
Time-terminated, no replacement
    calculation, 386
Time testing, 337
Timing tests, 344
Token count, 290–291
Tolerancing, 239
Tongue depressors, 28
Top-level design, 256
Traceability, 85
Trade secrets, 202–205
Trademarks, 198–202
Type testing, 68–69
Typical use testing, 350
Typographical errors, in coding, 20

U

UL. *See* Underwriters Laboratory
Uncoupled design, 228
Underwriters Laboratory (UL),
    97–98
Uniform Trade Secrecy Act, 203
United Kingdom
  standards, 101, 103, 104, 105
  TickIT program, 106
"Unreasonable danger", 181
Usability goals, 310–311
Usability testing, 310
  user interface, 313–315
Use/misuse evaluation, 64
Useful life period, 8
Usefulness, patent criterion, 189
User interface, 302
  design process, 311–313
  modeling, 313
  specifying, 314–315
  testing, 313–315
User interface processing, 258
User profiles, 310
Users
  field service reports, 418–422
  liability, 184
  risk assessment, 161
  See also Human factors; Human
    factors engineering
Utility patent, 189

V

Validation
  hardware, 350–368
  software, 371–380
  software design, 271–272
  testing, 342
Validation testing, 62, 371–380
Variation reduction, 214–215
Verification
  hardware, 350–368
  software, 371–380
  software design, 271–272
  testing, 342
Vertical standards, 58, 59
Vibration testing, 354
Visual displays, software design, 325
Vocabulary of the software,
  293–294
Voice alarms, 321–322

Voice of the Customer, 210
Volume (of the software), 294

W

Walkthrough, software review, 267–268
Warranty
  exclusion of warranties, 180
  implied warranties, 179–180
Warranty action, 179
Warranty analysis, 422
Warranty cost, 146
Wearout failure, 19–20
Wearout period, 8
Weibull plotting, 359–364, 394
White box testing, 342
Workstation design, 320
World Health Organization (WHO), 102
Worst-case scenario tests, 346